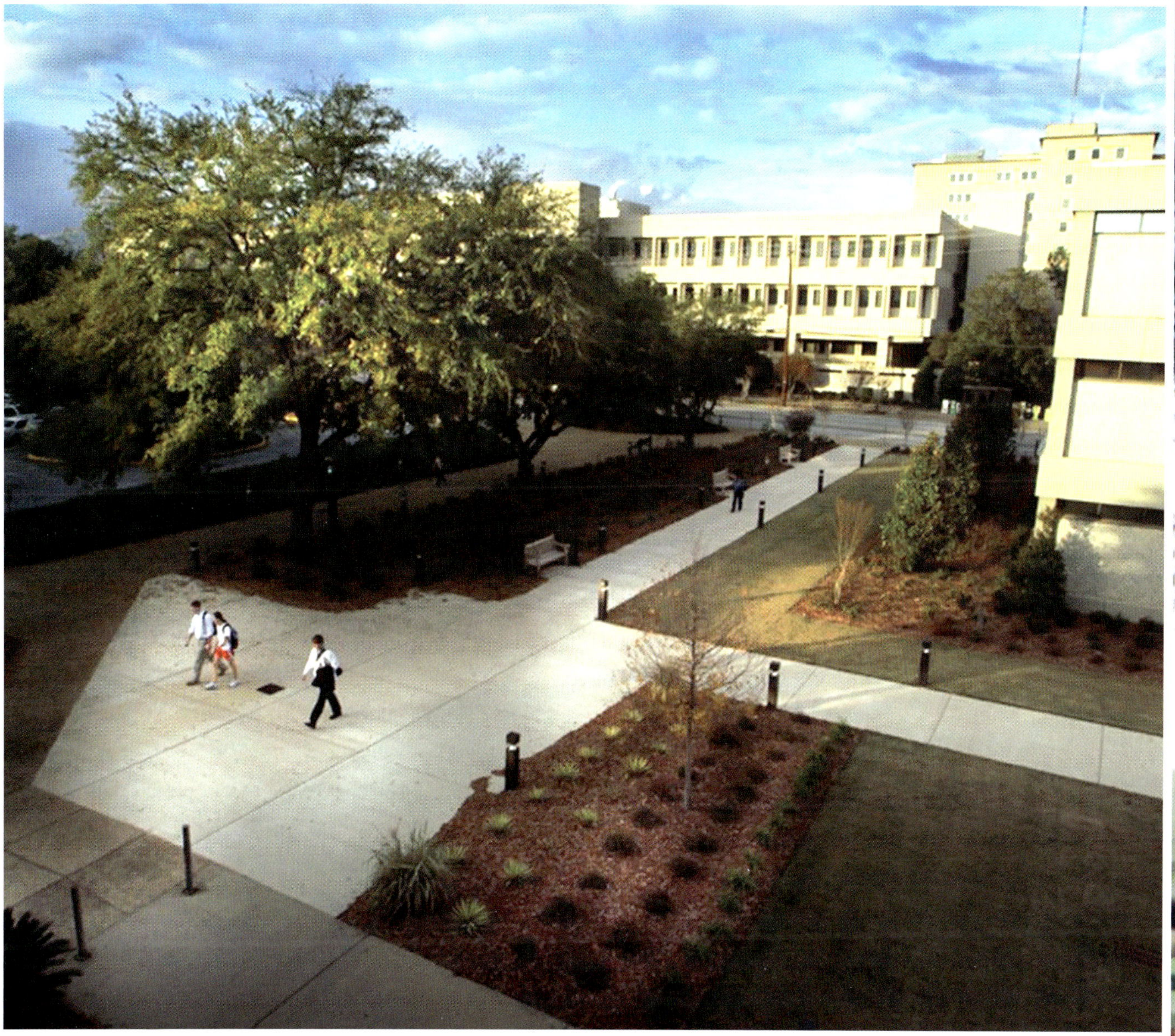

GRU GEORGIA REGENTS UNIVERSITY
AUGUSTA

# *Dedication*

*This volume is dedicated to the thousands of faculty, staff, students, alumni, and friends who have participated in the growth and success of Georgia Regents University and its legacy institutions. You have made this university great.*

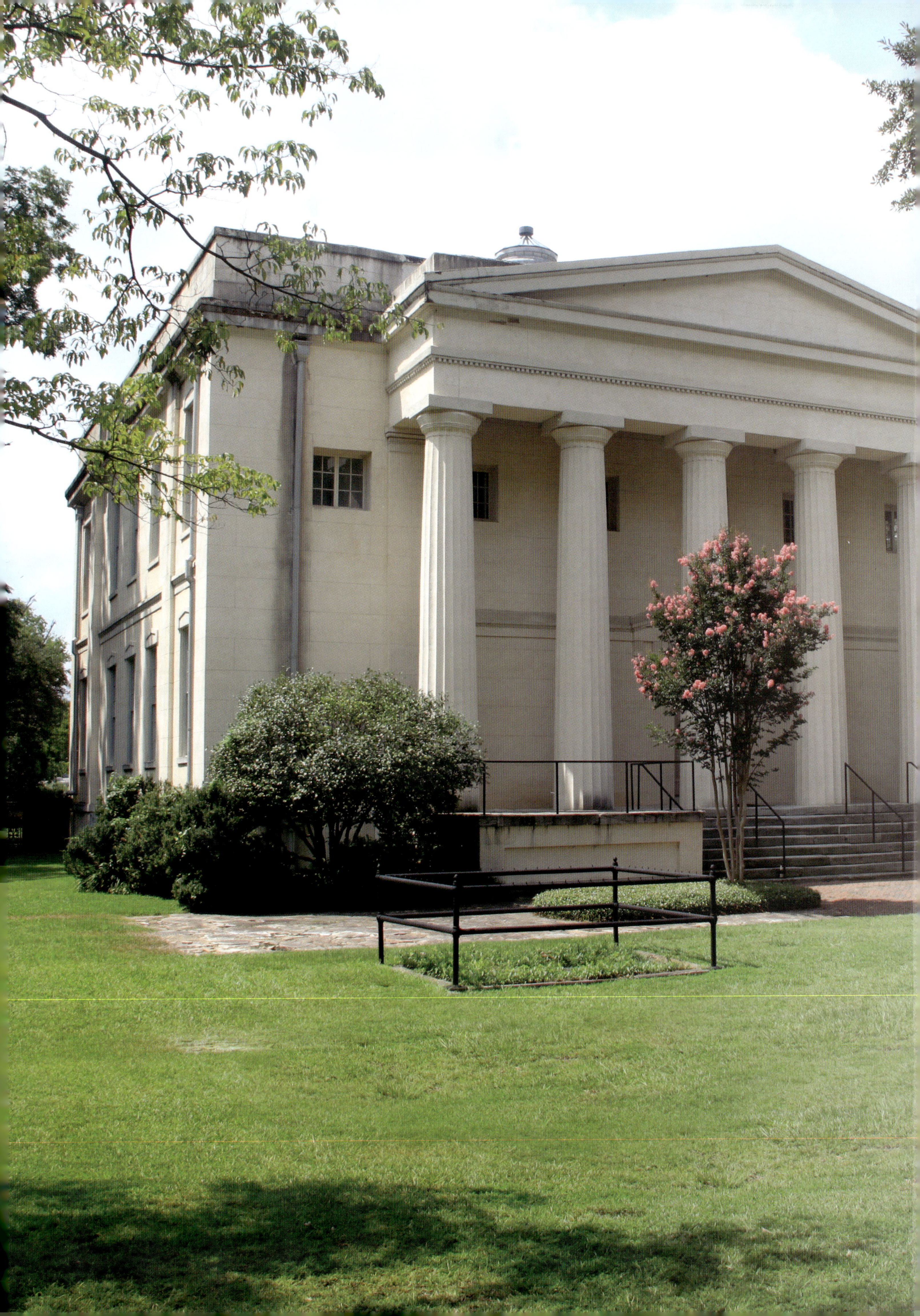

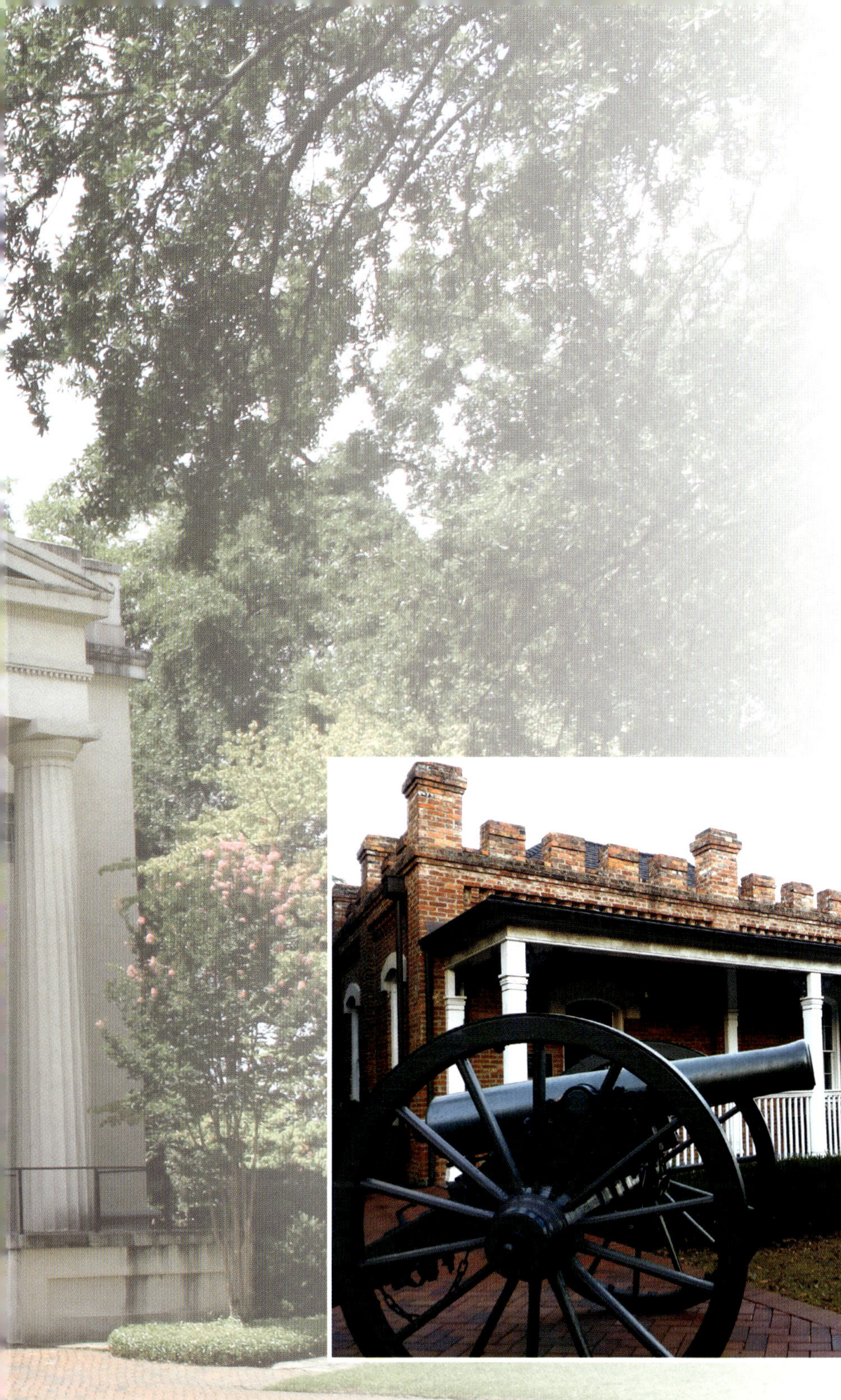

# SHARED LEGACIES

## *A Pictorial History of Georgia Regents University*

For information, please write:

The Donning Company Publishers
184 Business Park Drive, Suite 206
Virginia Beach, VA 23462

Steve Mull, General Manager
Barbara Buchanan, Office Manager
Anne Burns, Editor
Rick Boley, Graphic Designer
Kathy Adams, Imaging Artist
Jennifer Elam, Project Research Coordinator
Nathan Stufflebean, Research and Marketing Supervisor
Katie Gardner, Marketing Advisor

Lynn Walton, Project Director

THE DONNING COMPANY PUBLISHERS

Library of Congress Cataloging-in-Publication Data

Shared legacies : a pictorial history of Georgia Regents University.
pages cm
Includes index.
ISBN 978-1-57864-950-1
1. Georgia Regents University--History--Pictorial works. 2. Augusta State University (Augusta, Ga.)--History--Pictorial works. 3. Medical College of Georgia (1950-)--History--Pictorial works.
LD1961.G66233S53 2014
379.758'64--dc23
2014043483

Printed in the United States of America at Walsworth Publishing Company

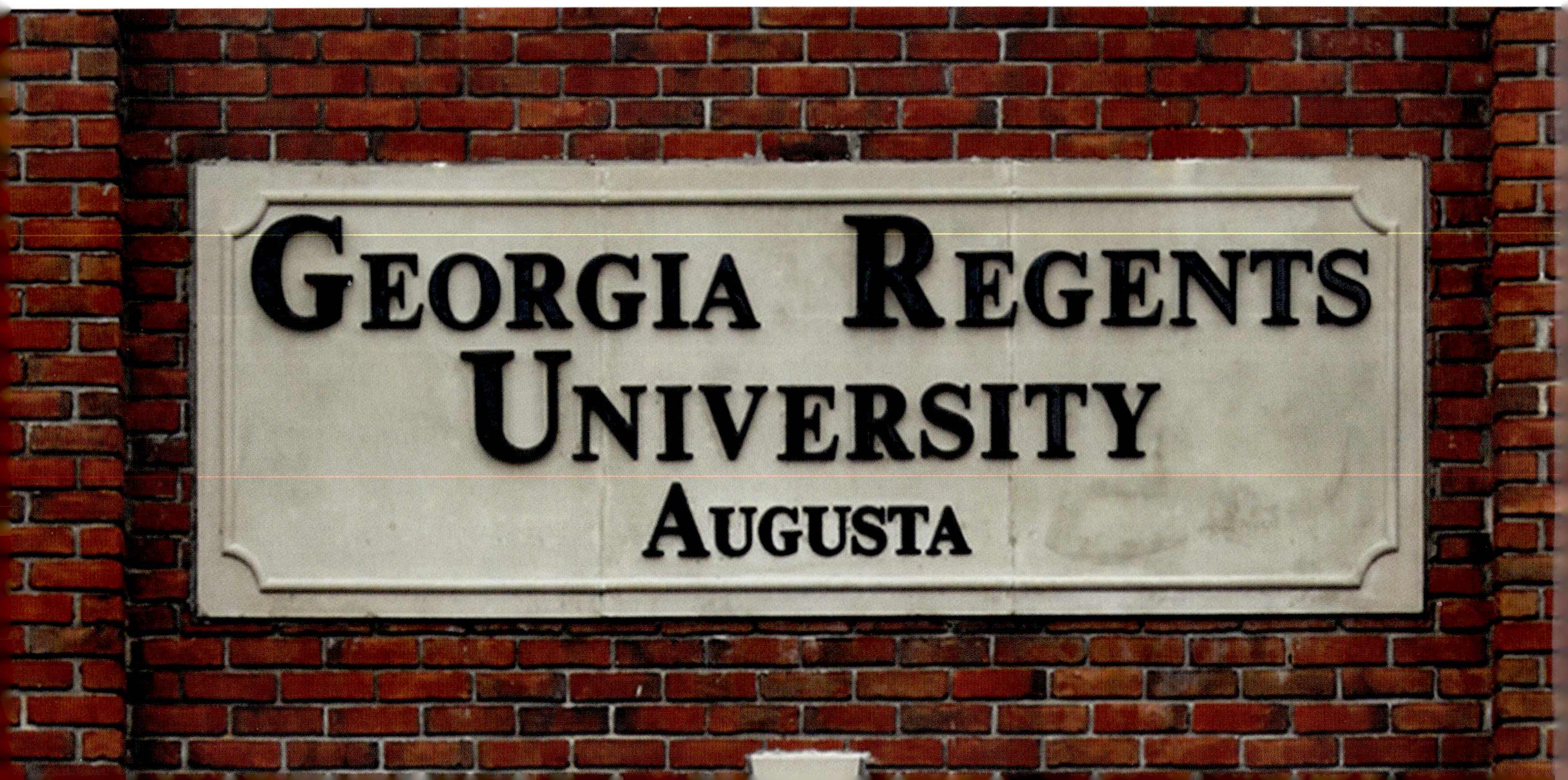

# CONTENTS

# Foreword

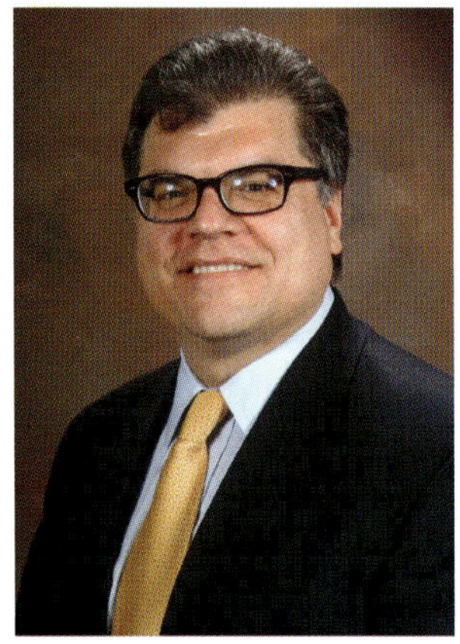

In 1783, the Georgia state legislature passed the charter that established the Academy of Richmond County to offer college-level classes for boys.

In 1826, Dr. Milton Antony began informally teaching a handful of apprentices at Augusta's City Hospital. Joined the following year by Dr. Joseph Eve, they petitioned and received a state charter in 1828 to provide medical education.

These proverbial first steps in a thousand-mile journey were the genesis of Augusta State University and Georgia Health Sciences University, respectively, combined in 2013 to create Georgia Regents University (GRU).

It is doubtful that even at their most grandiose and hopeful, these original leaders ever conjured today's GRU—one of only four public research institutions in the state, comprising over 110 programs in eight colleges and one school, complete with an aligned and integrated health system, employing more than 12,000 faculty and staff, enrolling more than 9,500 students, and with a direct economic impact across the enterprise that exceeds $2.2 billion.

In these pages, we preserve and recount GRU's long and fascinating history in hundreds of photographs from every era. From the founding of each legacy institution to the end of the 2012–2013 academic year; encompassing academics, research, campus development, athletics, and student life; this pictorial history is an exploration of a university's proud heritage and celebration of its unique spirit, honored traditions, and proud accomplishments.

GRU's history has witnessed many changes, not the least in its name. At various times the legacy institutions were called the Junior College of Augusta (1925), Augusta College (1958), and Augusta State University (1996); the Medical Academy of Georgia (1828), Medical Institute of Georgia (1829), Medical College of Georgia (1833), Medical Department of the University of Georgia (1873), University of Georgia School of Medicine (1933), Medical College of Georgia (1950), and Georgia Health Sciences University (2011).

Today we honor that evolving past, are invigorated by a transforming present, and steward an ascendant future. Throughout it all, GRU maintains an abiding commitment to academic excellence, personal integrity, clinical and translational discovery, a collaborative learning and working environment, and a tradition of service to our community, state, and world.

Enjoy this journey into GRU's storied past, and may it inspire an even greater future—a future that has truly only just begun.

Ricardo Azziz, MD, MPH, MBA
Professor, Obstetrics & Gynecology, Medicine, and Medical Humanities
President, Georgia Regents University
CEO, Georgia Regents Health System

# Preface

Created by the Board of Regents of the University System of Georgia's consolidation of Augusta State University and Georgia Health Sciences University, Georgia Regents University brought together the strong academic traditions of each institution, as well as the rich histories of both. The beginning of this new era provides a unique opportunity for a retrospective glance at the important paths, sometimes intersecting, these institutions have taken on their way to this significant point.

Over two hundred photographs and the accompanying text reveal some of the people, places, and events that have been part of the development of Augusta State University and Georgia Health Sciences University. These images are only a tiny portion of the thousands that preserve their pasts. In limited space, only a representative portion could be used and difficult choices had to be made. With so many significant faculty, students, and staff, unfortunately many other faces not pictured here are also part of this legacy.

Beginning with a brief general history, this book examines physical growth and expansion, academic programs, faculty research and creative activity, campus life beyond the classroom, and sports activities—formal and informal. All have helped create the legacy that now becomes part of the ongoing story of Georgia Regents University.

From these two parent institutions, thousands have received the education and training they needed for productive careers, continued learning, and fulfilling personal lives that have contributed to our community, state, nation, and world. Faculty have made discoveries that alleviated suffering and brought healing, contributed to increased knowledge and better practices in many fields of endeavor, and created works of beauty and meaning. It is on this legacy that Georgia Regents University will build as the institution strives to become the next great research university, offering continued excellence in teaching, innovative and creative research, and a strong ethic of service and commitment to the betterment of our society.

Lee Ann Caldwell, PhD
Director, Center for the Study of Georgia History
GRU Historian-in-Residence
Professor of History

GRU

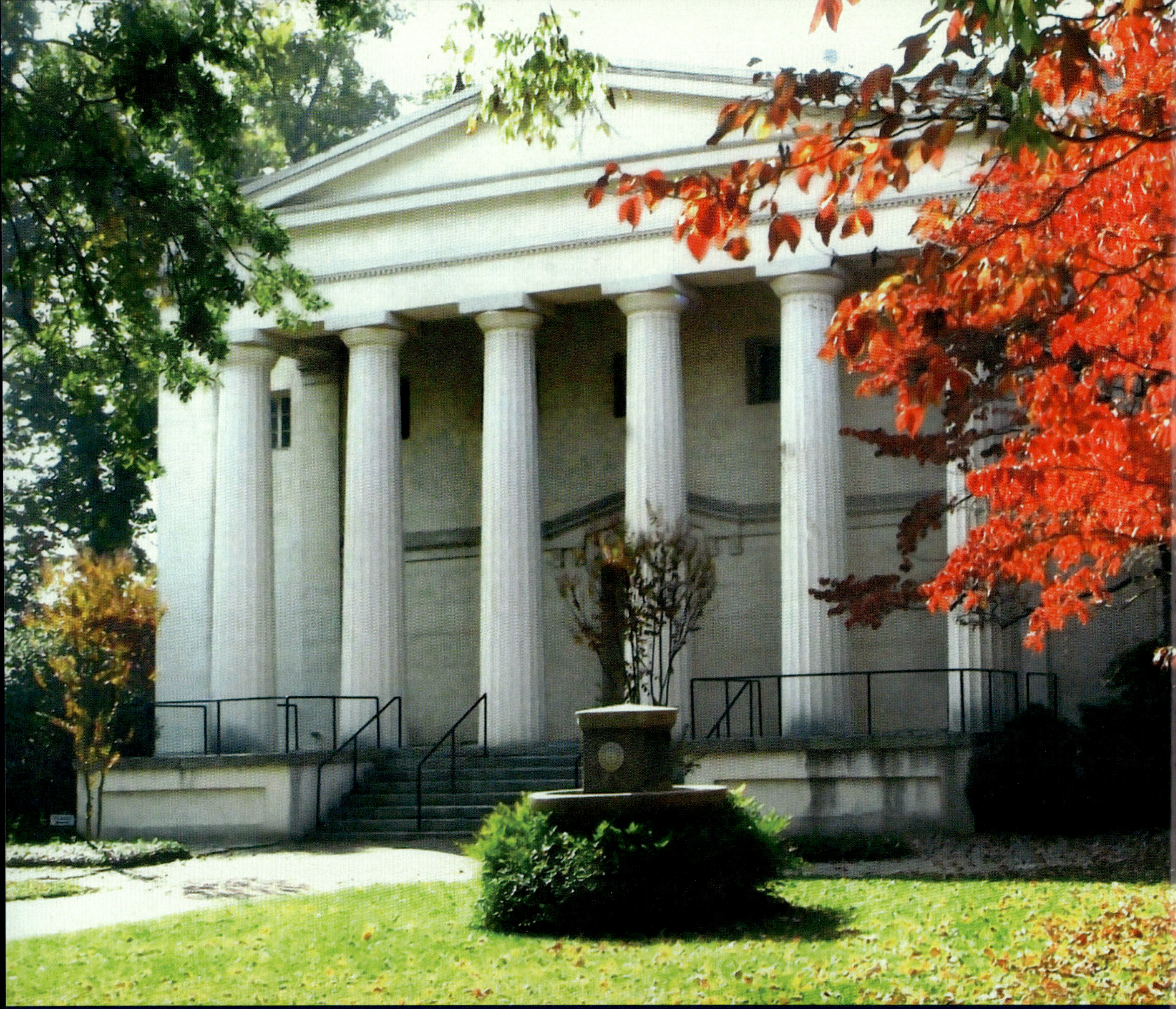

# HISTORY:
## *The Past is Prologue*

Following the American Revolution, a zeal for education spread through the new United States. Augustans, too, caught this fire and chartered the state's first academy in 1783, the Academy of Richmond County (ARC). In 1791, President George Washington attended the examinations at the academy where he heard an address by student Edmund Bacon, who had graduated two years before. Bacon was still a student because the academy offered post-secondary studies in Latin, French, Greek, algebra, and trigonometry to prepare students for transfer to universities as sophomores. This year of college work at the academy was the beginning of higher education in Augusta.

In the early nineteenth century the seeds of medical education were also germinating. In 1817, the city established a board to oversee the health problems of the town. The next year, on property purchased from the ARC Trustees, a ten-bed City Hospital was constructed. In 1822, Dr. Milton Antony and seven physicians organized the Medical Society of Augusta to improve healthcare and physician education. Four years later, Antony began instructing students in the City Hospital, and the following year, he was joined by Dr. Joseph Adams Eve. In 1828, the two physicians secured a state charter to establish the Medical Academy of Georgia, which could award bachelor of medicine degrees. The following year, in order to grant the MD degree, the Georgia General Assembly was asked to revise the 1828 charter; in doing so, they changed the medical academy's name to the Medical Institute of Georgia and in 1833 to the Medical College of Georgia (MCG) to more accurately reflect its true mission and status. MCG moved into a new building on Telfair Street in 1835, on property adjoining ARC.

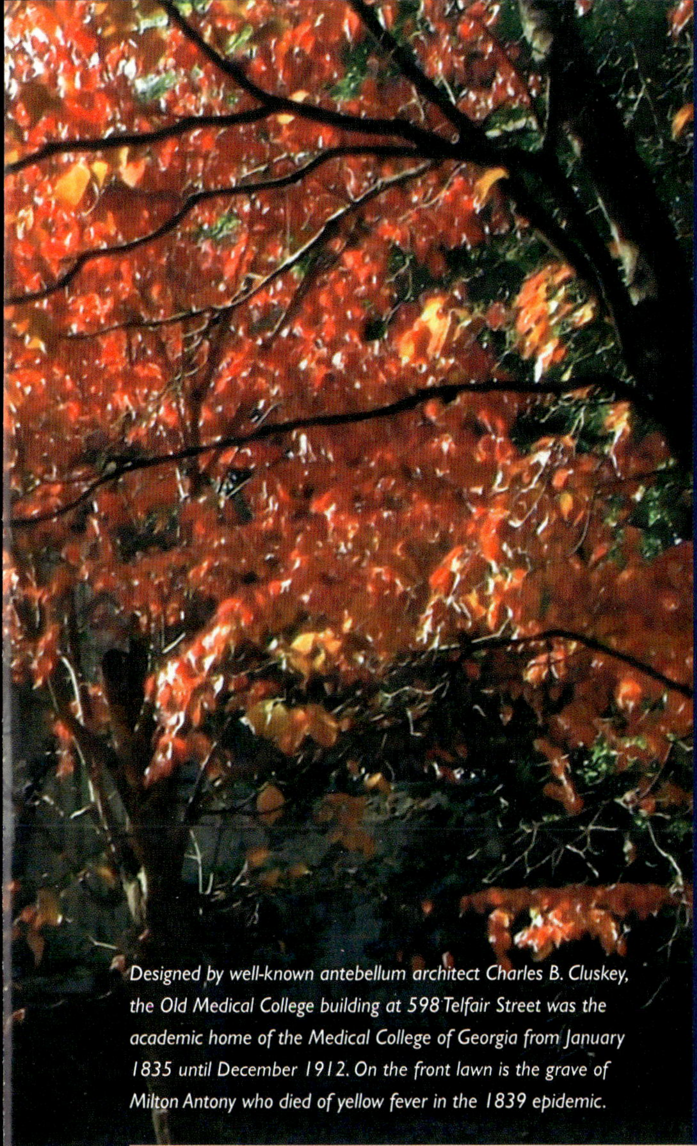

*Designed by well-known antebellum architect Charles B. Cluskey, the Old Medical College building at 598 Telfair Street was the academic home of the Medical College of Georgia from January 1835 until December 1912. On the front lawn is the grave of Milton Antony who died of yellow fever in the 1839 epidemic.*

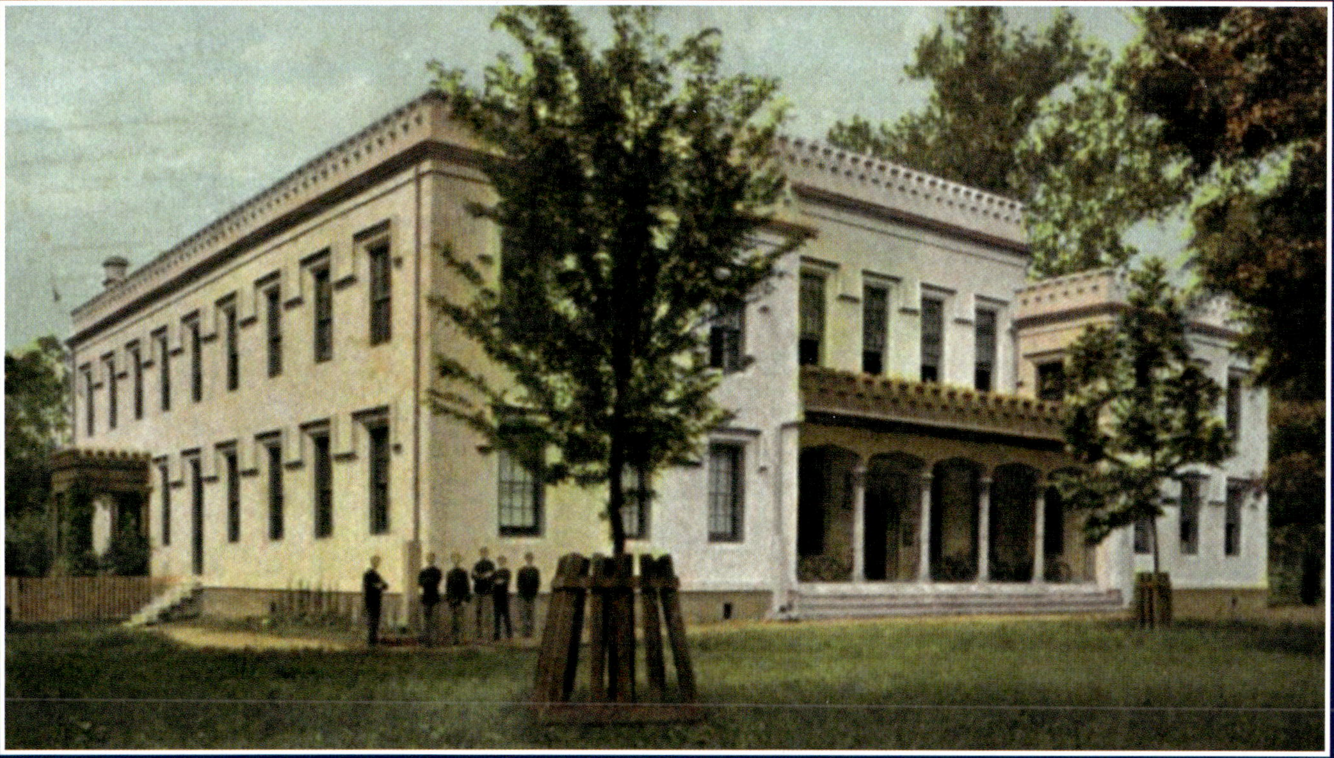

*Operated by trustees, the Academy of Richmond County prepared young men for leadership roles and for admission with advanced standing to colleges and universities (a trend that continued into the twentieth century). In 1802, ARC moved from its site on Bay Street to a new building on Telfair Street. This postcard, courtesy of the Augusta Museum of History, shows the building after an 1840s addition.*

Throughout the remaining years of the antebellum era, the two institutions operated side by side, with ARC students even being allowed to attend certain lectures at MCG. When the Civil War began in 1861, both institutions suspended classes as faculty and students took roles in the war efforts. ARC's building became a hospital, and the MCG building became surgeons' quarters, with its amphitheater serving as an operating room. When the war ended in 1865, MCG resumed classes the same year while ARC served as headquarters for federal troops for two more years before resuming operation.

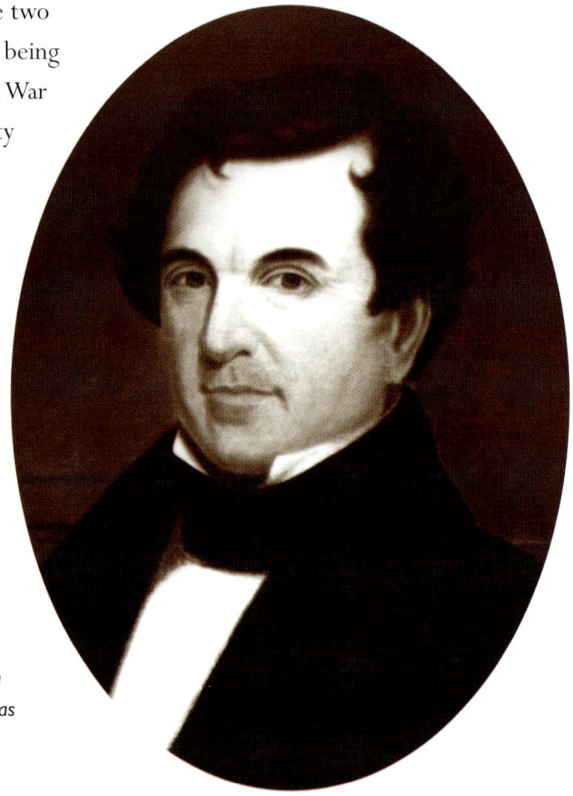

*Right: In 1826, Milton Antony began teaching medicine in two rooms of the wooden frame structure, Augusta's City Hospital, located at 124 Greene Street. Dr. Joseph Adams Eve joined him a year later.*

*Below: When physicians Milton Antony and Joseph A. Eve received the charter for the Medical Institute of Georgia, City Hospital underwent $457 in renovations to accommodate the new school, which in 1833 became known as the Medical College of Georgia.*

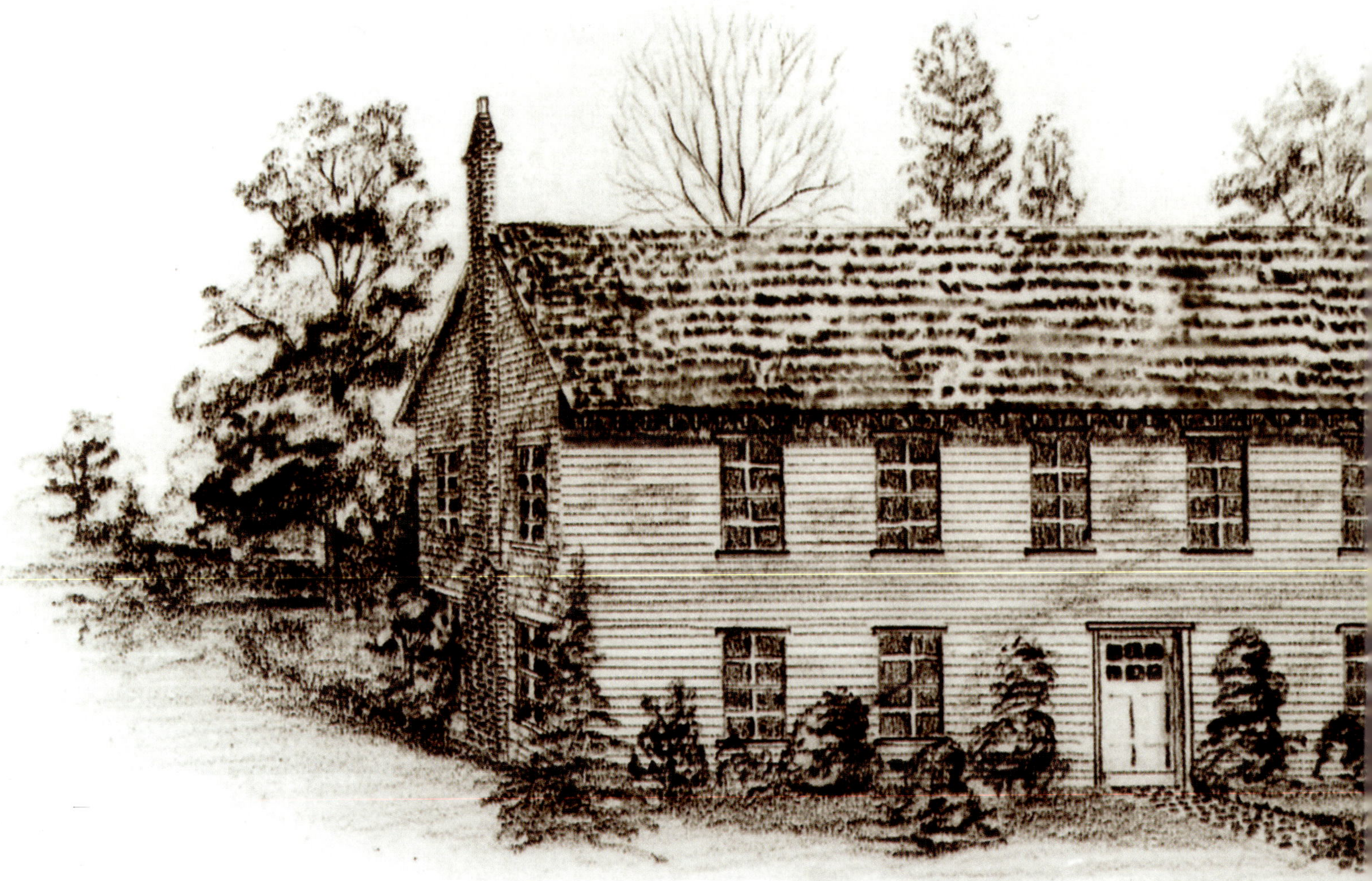

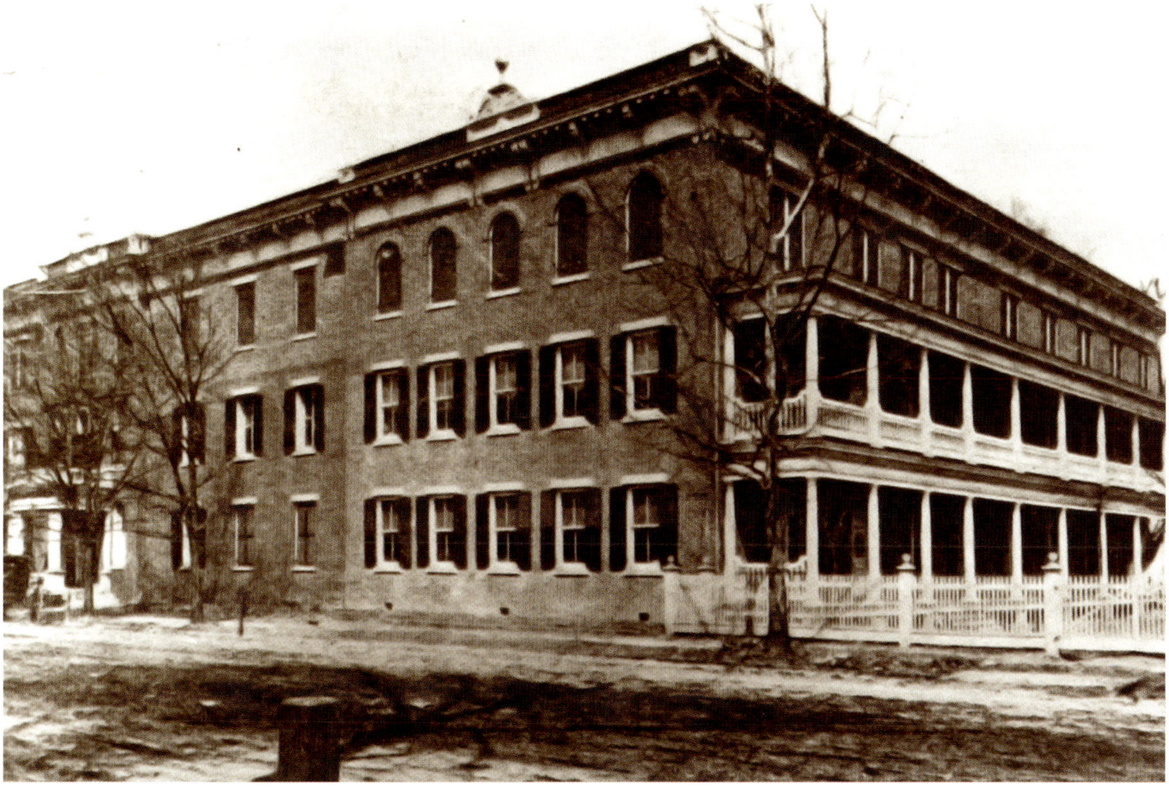

*The "new" City Hospital opened in 1869 on the corner of Washington (Sixth) and Walker Streets behind the old MCG building. Accommodating between eighty to one hundred patients, the hospital served as a community hospital and teaching facility for MCG faculty until 1915.*

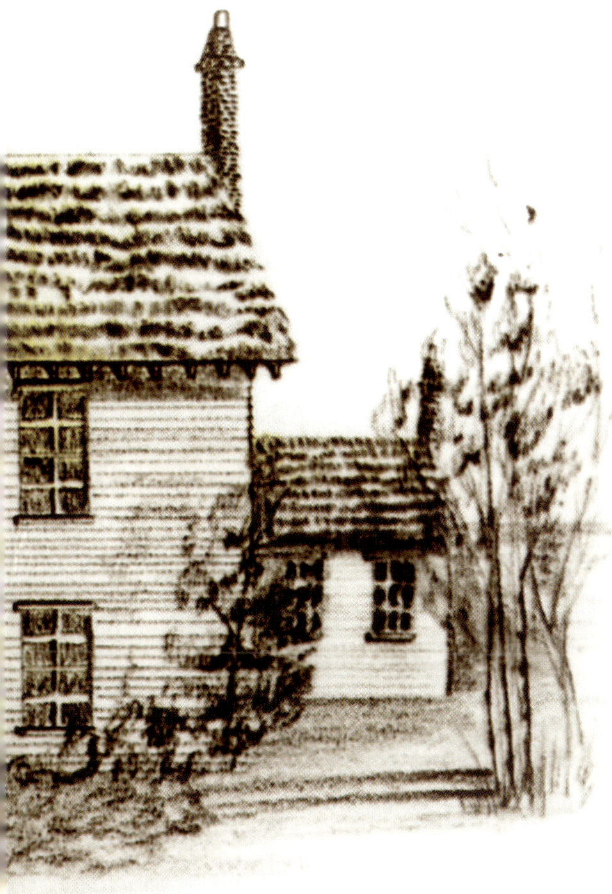

At that time, Colonel George Washington Rains, the Confederate commandant of the Augusta Arsenal and the Augusta Powder Works, was asked to reopen ARC. He became regent (headmaster) and established the new Scientific Department. Rains also taught chemistry at MCG next door and later became its dean. In 1873, MCG became the Medical Department of the University of Georgia (UGA). This union was strengthened by a legislative act of 1911 transferring all assets and properties to the UGA Board of Trustees, which was accomplished the following year. The early twentieth century saw major reforms in the medical school. In January 1913, the institution moved into a renovated Tuttle Newton Building, formerly the Augusta Orphan Asylum.

By then, ARC had come under control of the Richmond County Board of Education. In 1910, the board added a formal fifth year of study as preparation for college, and Augustans boasted that it was the only high school in the state offering college credit.

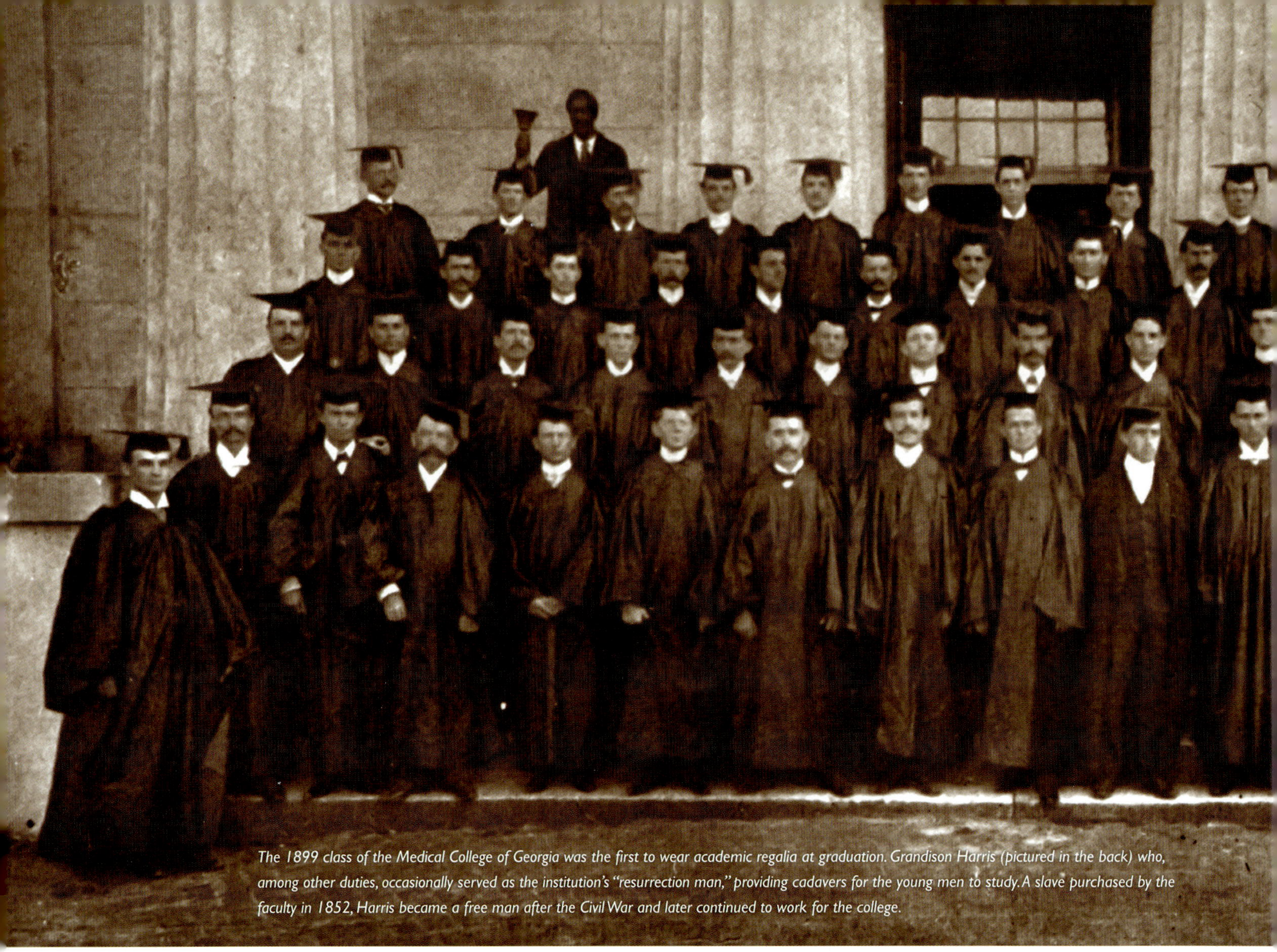

*The 1899 class of the Medical College of Georgia was the first to wear academic regalia at graduation. Grandison Harris (pictured in the back) who, among other duties, occasionally served as the institution's "resurrection man," providing cadavers for the young men to study. A slave purchased by the faculty in 1852, Harris became a free man after the Civil War and later continued to work for the college.*

As a national junior college movement gained momentum, ARC's fifth year evolved in 1925 into the first chartered junior college in the state—the Junior College of Augusta (JCA). The following year, 1926, ARC and the JCA moved to a new location on Baker Avenue, where they would share space for the next thirty-one years.

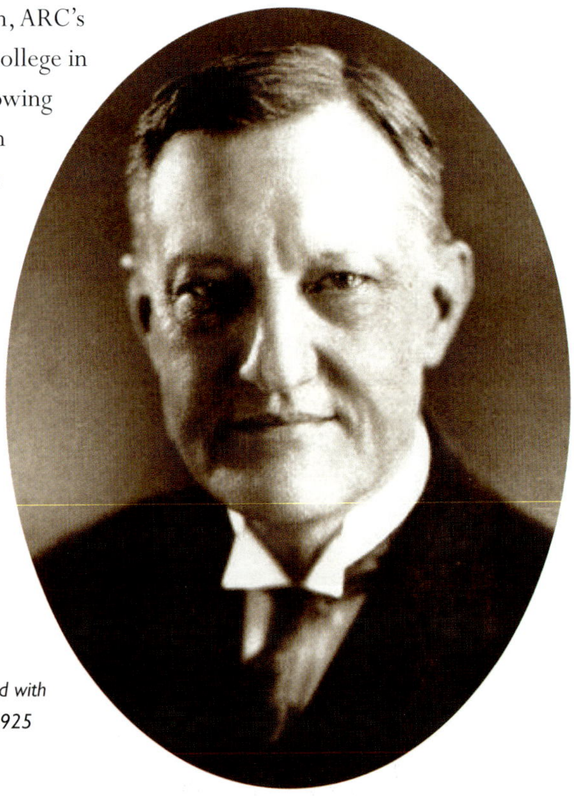

The medical college was also evolving. New facilities advanced its academic, research, and clinical care mission. Following its admission into the newly created University System of Georgia in 1932, the medical department was renamed the University of Georgia School of Medicine the following year.

Both institutions made contributions in World War II and in the post-war years began periods of expansion

*Lawton B. Evans (right), superintendent of Richmond County Schools, worked with ARC Principal George P. Butler to add a fifth year of study in 1910 and in 1925 chartered the Junior College of Augusta.*

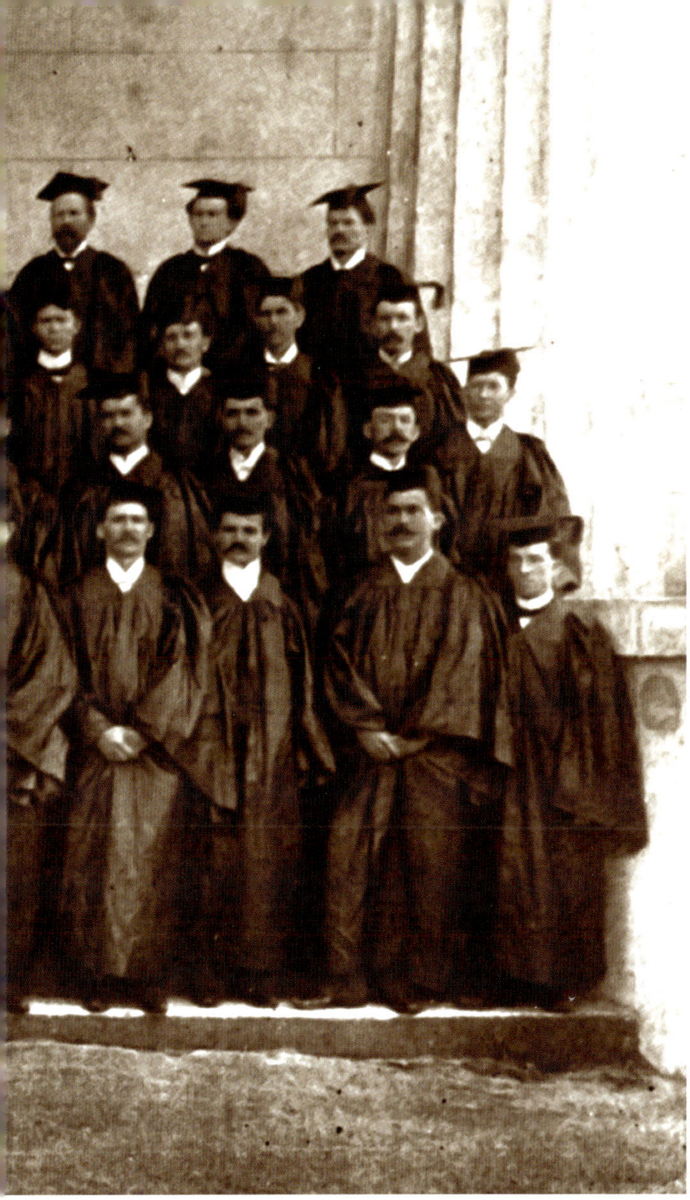

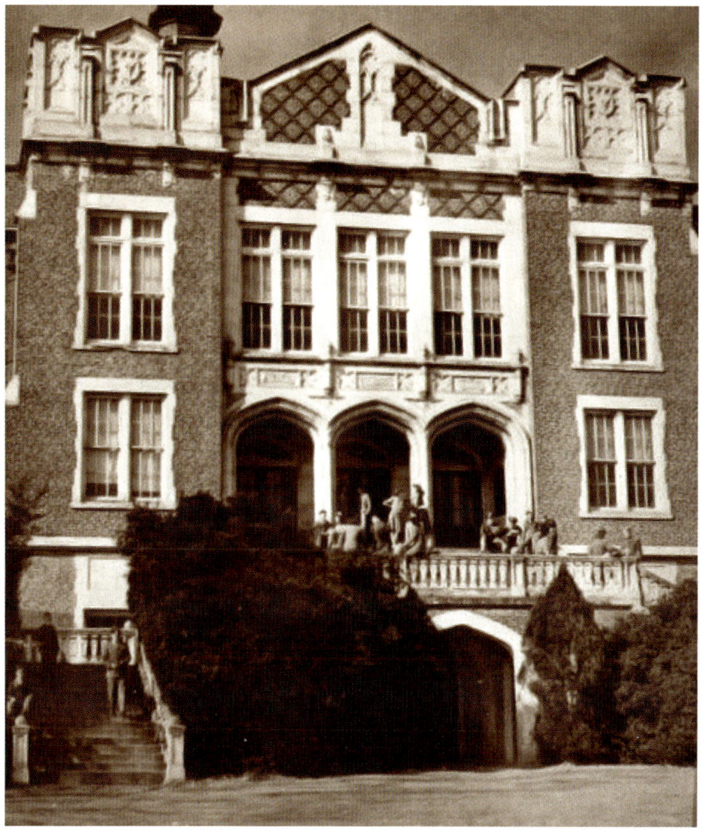

*Above and below: The JCA and ARC moved into their new building on Baker Street in 1926 and shared the facility for thirty-one years.*

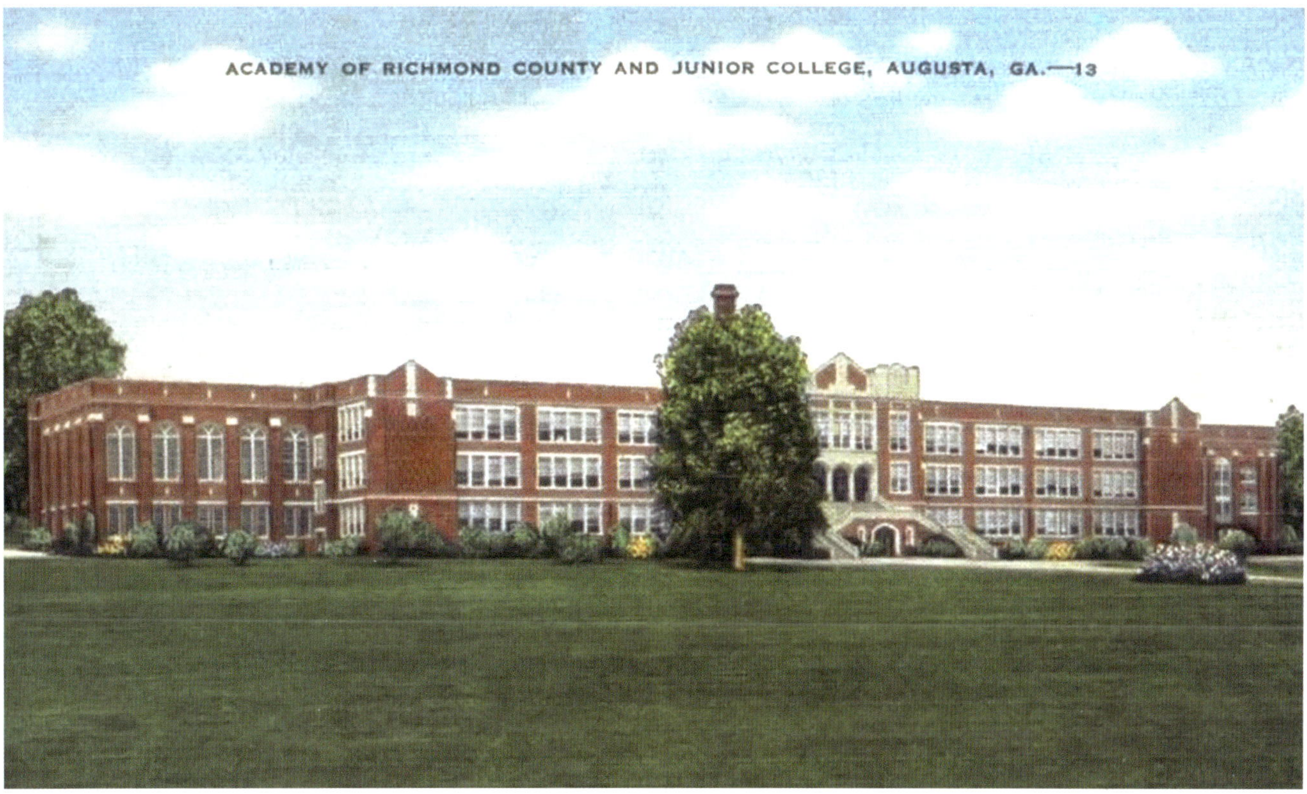
ACADEMY OF RICHMOND COUNTY AND JUNIOR COLLEGE, AUGUSTA, GA.—13

and growth. In 1950, MCG regained its autonomy and was known once again as the Medical College of Georgia, a name it retained for over sixty years. In 1956, the institution gained its own teaching hospital and by the late 1960s had added the state's only public dental school.

Meanwhile in the 1950s, overcrowding reached a critical point at the building shared by ARC and JCA. A remedy was found when the U.S. government abandoned the Augusta Arsenal in 1955. Following a move to the Walton Way property

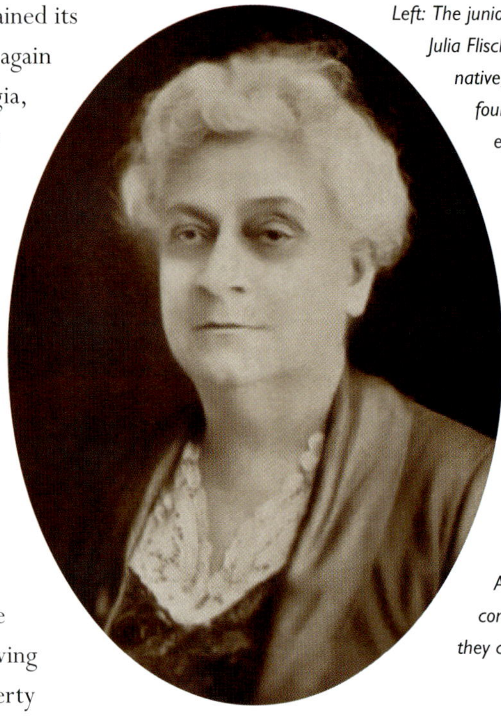

*Left: The junior college was co-ed from its beginning. Ms. Julia Flisch served as dean of women. An Augusta native, she had been one of the forces behind the founding of the first public institution of higher education for women—Georgia Normal & Industrial Institute, later Georgia State College for Women, in Milledgeville. She was a trained historian who also wrote fiction.*

*Below: The U.S. Army Specialized Training Program and the U.S. Navy's V-12 program accounted for 80 percent of MCG's enrollment during World War II. With government funding, qualified privates and seamen, in uniform and under military regulations, took an accelerated three-year course. After receiving their MDs, they were commissioned and put on inactive status until they completed their internships.*

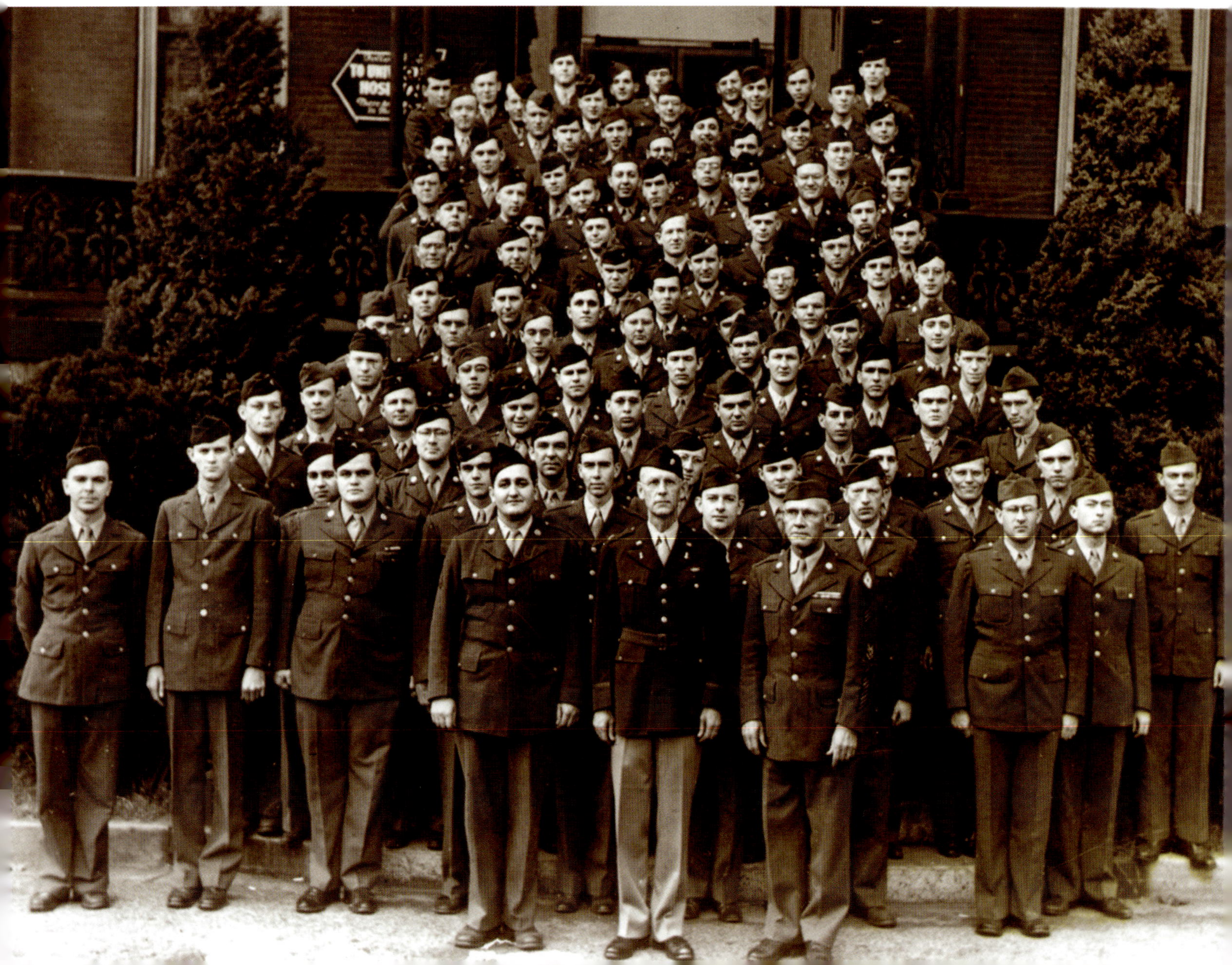

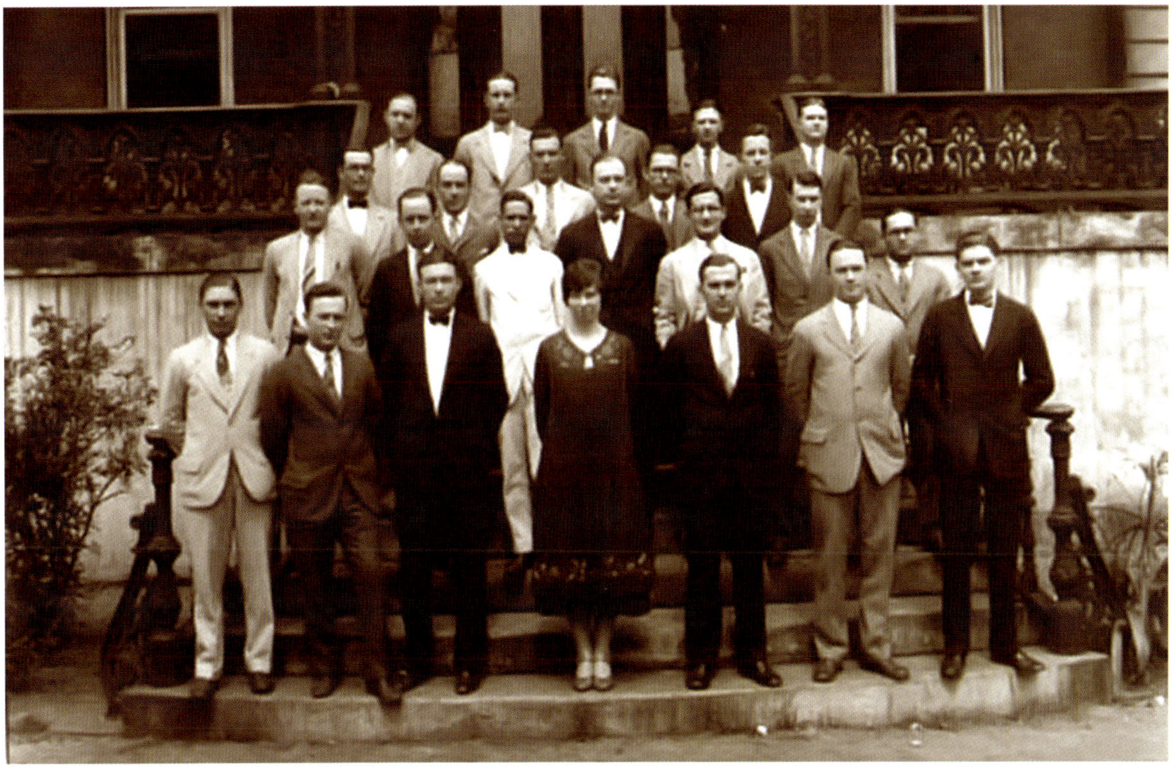

*Above: A new era for medical training in Georgia began when Loree Florence (front row, center) matriculated at the medical school in 1922 and graduated in 1926, ending almost one hundred years of single sex education. Ellen Marsh graduated the same year with a BS in public health.*

*Right: Henry Kitchens broke the gender barrier in MCG's nursing school in 1960, becoming the first male nursing graduate.*

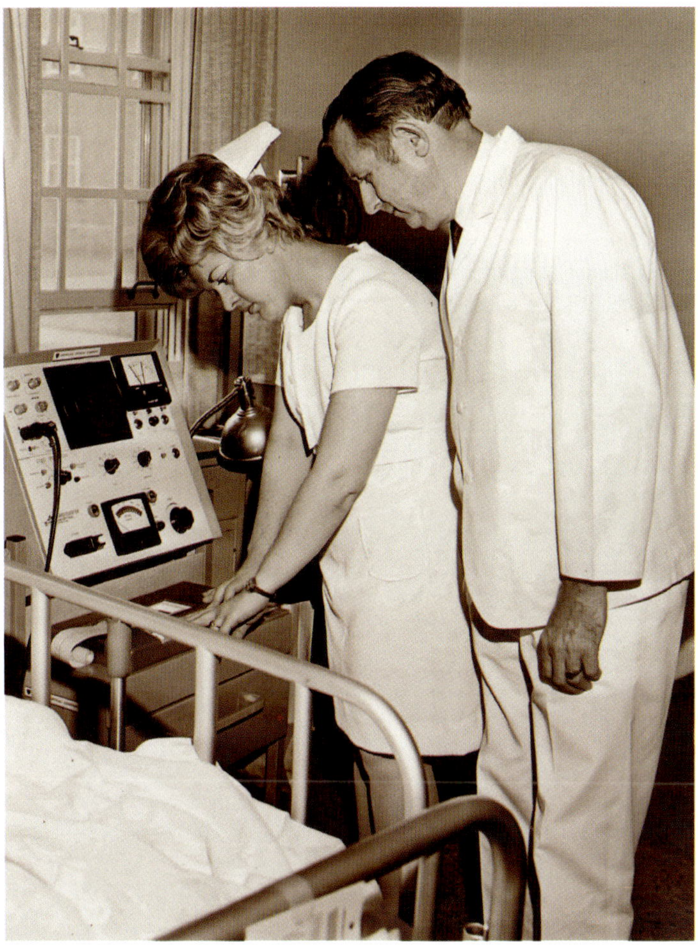

in 1957, the JCA joined the university system the following year and was renamed Augusta College (AC). In 1963, the college became a four-year institution, and the first graduate degrees were added in the 1970s.

Throughout the post-war years both institutions continued to modernize and made significant and, in some cases, long overdue changes. One major change sought to overcome the mistakes of the past. While the junior college was co-ed from the beginning and the medical college began admitting women in 1922, both institutions had remained racially segregated under the Jim Crow laws. In the 1960s this historical discrimination ended when the first African Americans matriculated at both schools.

Both campuses continued to expand physically, acquiring additional properties and building badly needed new structures to house ever-growing enrollments. AC acquired the last arsenal tract on Walton Way in the 1970s as well as the 240-plus acres of the former Oliver General Hospital site that would become the Forest Hills campus.

Both schools grew programmatically to meet the educational and professional needs of society of the late twentieth and twenty-first centuries. In 1996, AC acquired university status, becoming Augusta State University (ASU). In 2011, MCG's name was changed

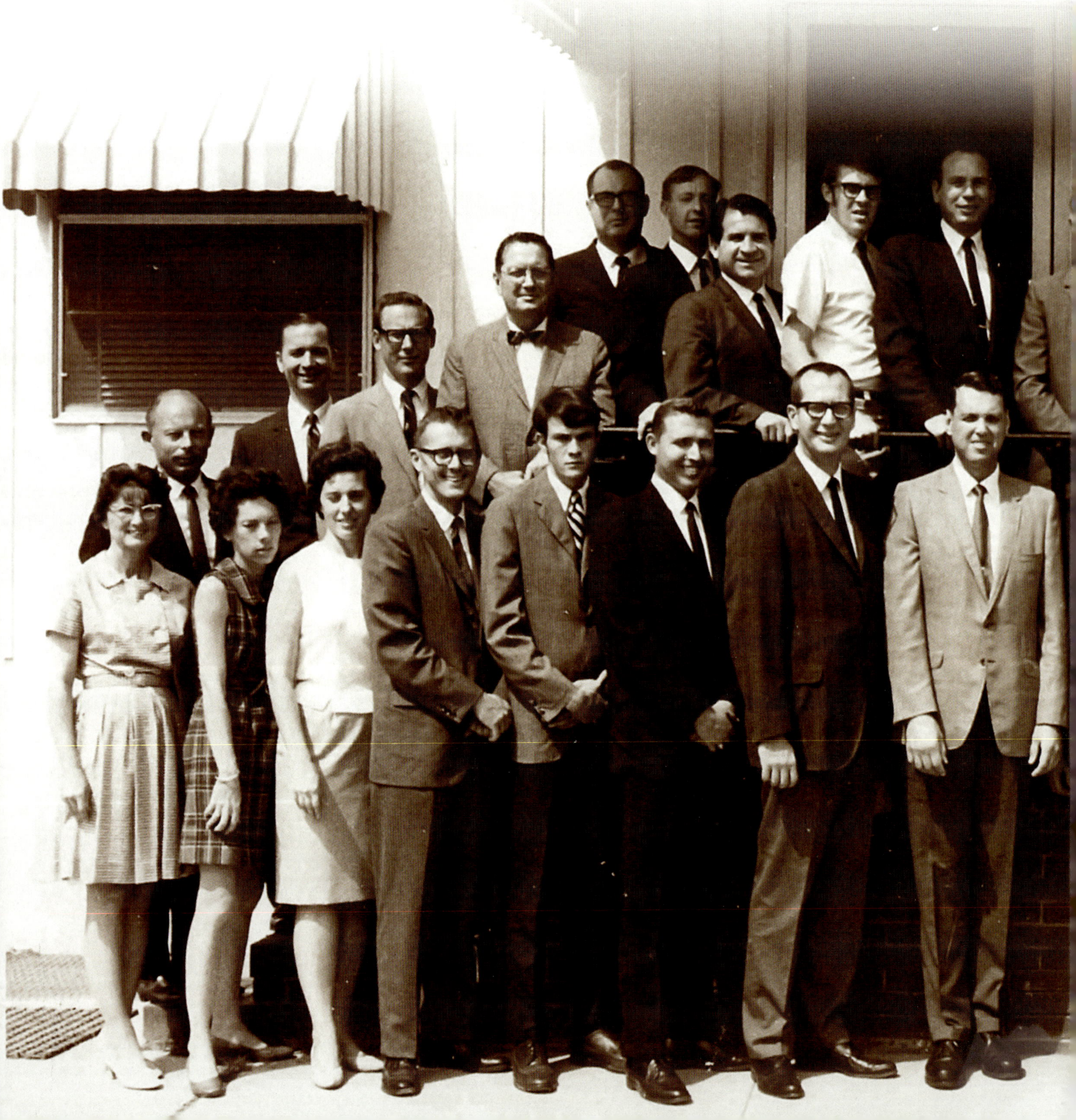

*Right: In the 1960s MCG ended its history of racial discrimination when African Americans joined the student body. In 1971, the Black Student Medical Alliance was formed. (Pictured left to right: Vice President Tommy Leonard Jr., Treasurer Ronald Spearman, President Joseph Hobbs, and Secretary Benjamin Rucker.)*

*Below: MCG's School of Dentistry was only two years old when this 1969 photo of its faculty and staff was taken.*

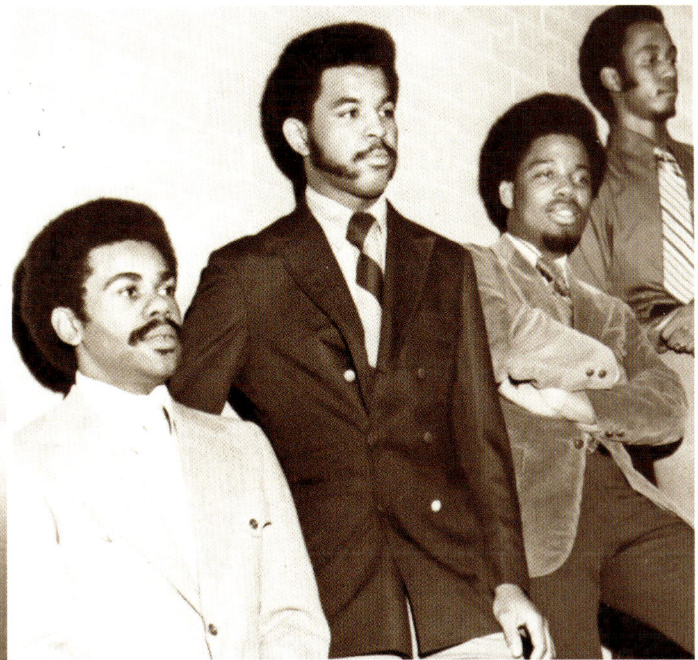

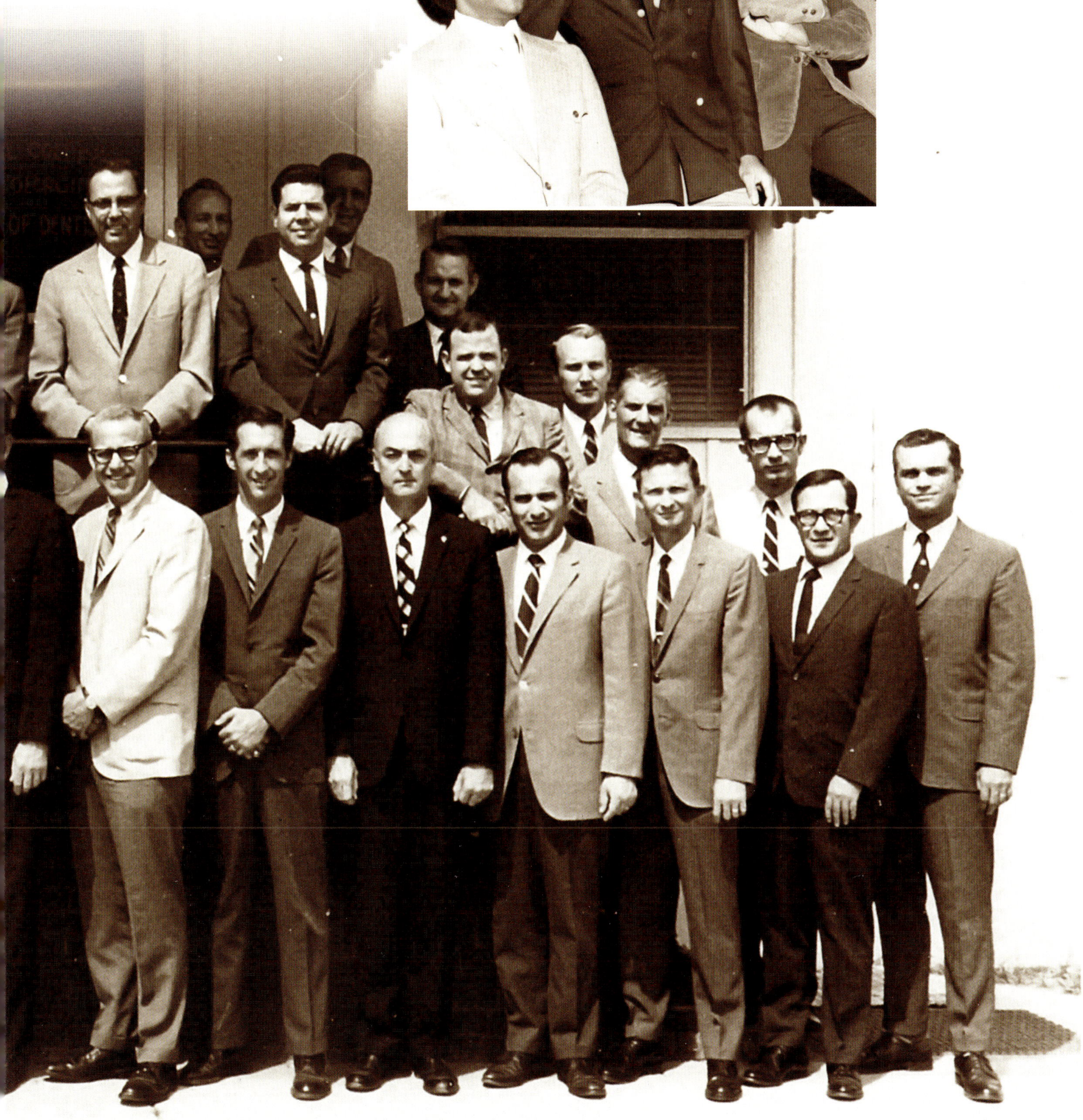

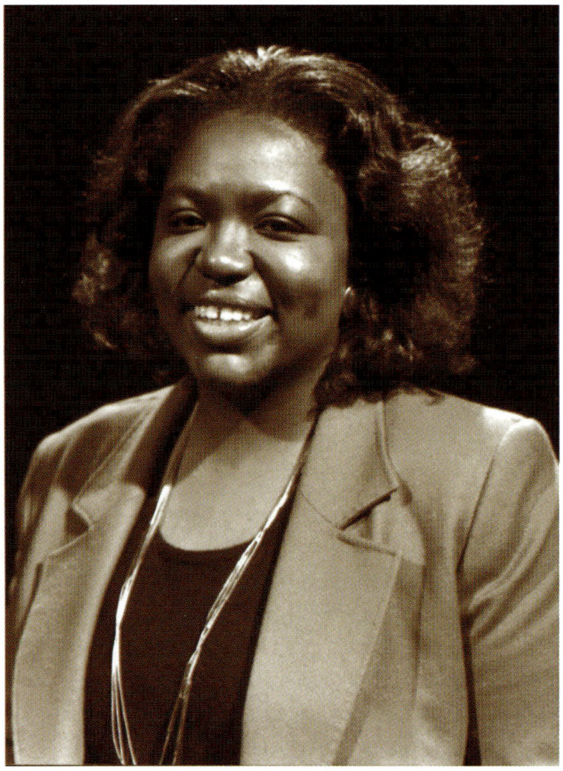

to Georgia Health Sciences University (GHSU). The Board of Regents of the University System of Georgia created Georgia Regents University on January 8, 2013, when it approved the consolidation of ASU and GHSU.

As William Shakespeare said, "What's past is prologue." The tribulations and triumphs in these institutional pasts have set the stage for the opportunities now before this newly created institution as it begins to write its own story.

*Left: In 1971, Lillie Butler became the first African American valedictorian at AC. With a PhD in English, Dr. (Butler) Johnson returned to her alma mater and became a faculty member and later chair of the Department of English and Foreign Languages until her retirement in 2013.*

*Below: In 1997, Augusta State University hosted President Bill Clinton when he announced a national educational initiative similar to Georgia's HOPE scholarship.*

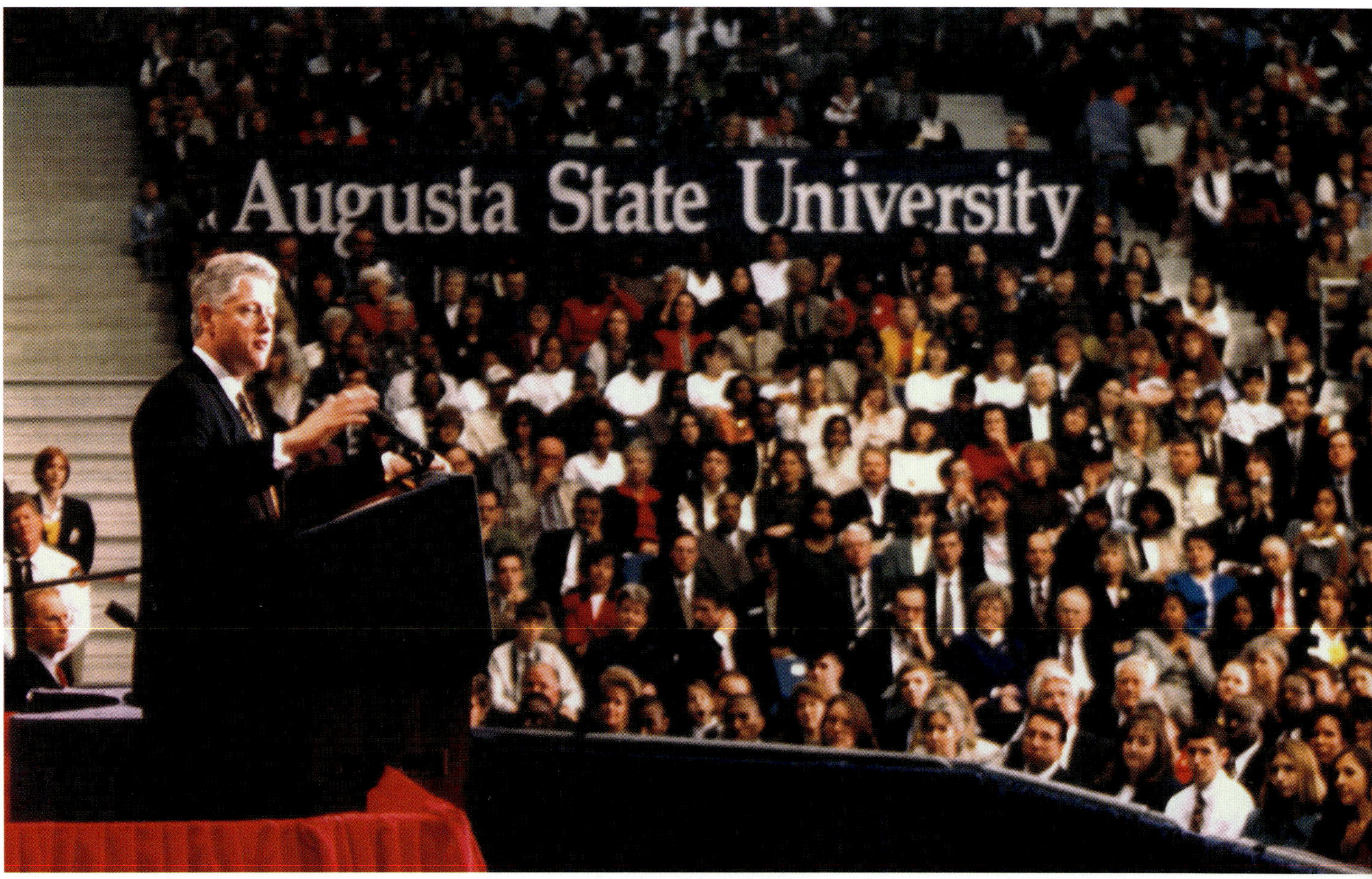

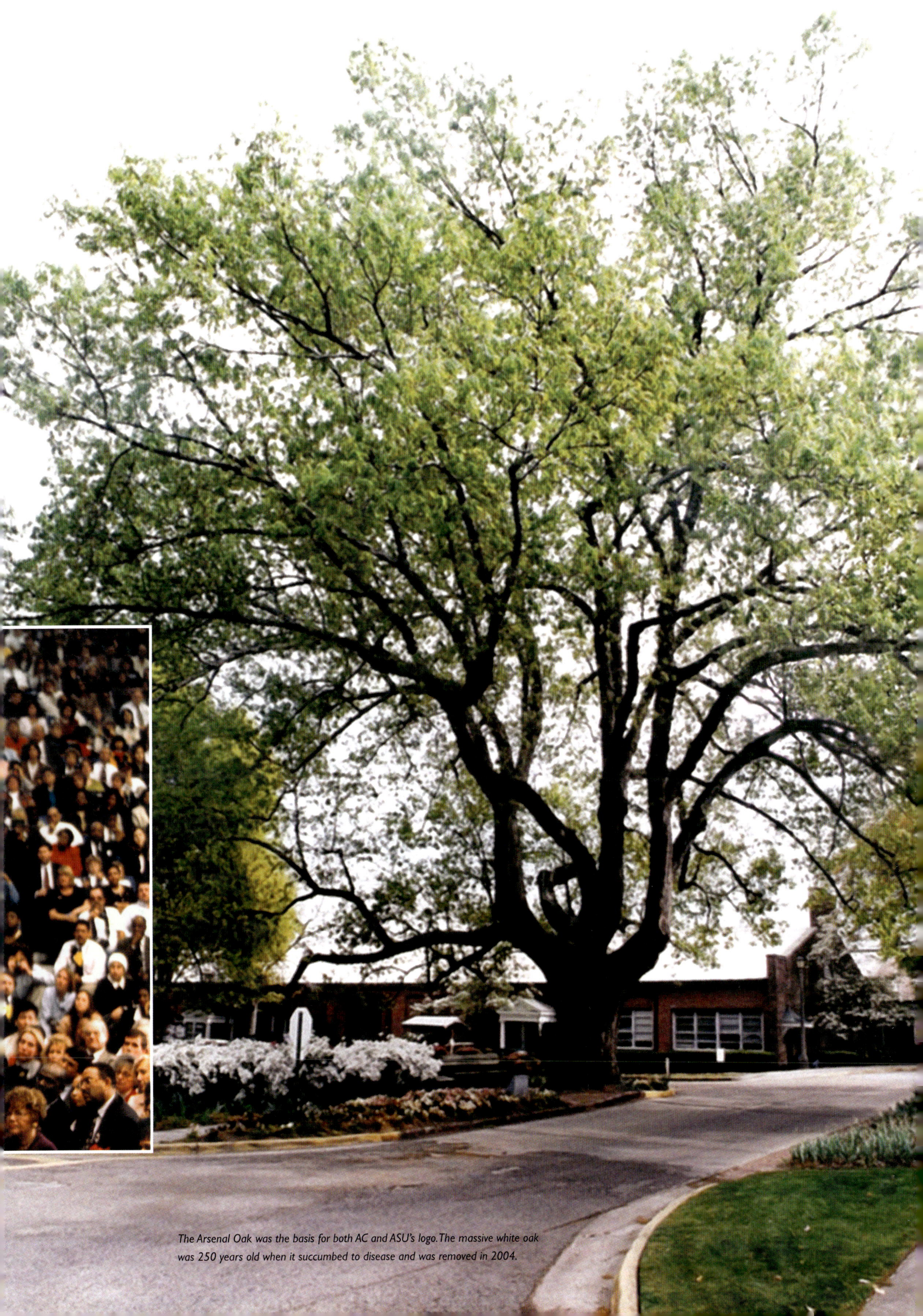

*The Arsenal Oak was the basis for both AC and ASU's logo. The massive white oak was 250 years old when it succumbed to disease and was removed in 2004.*

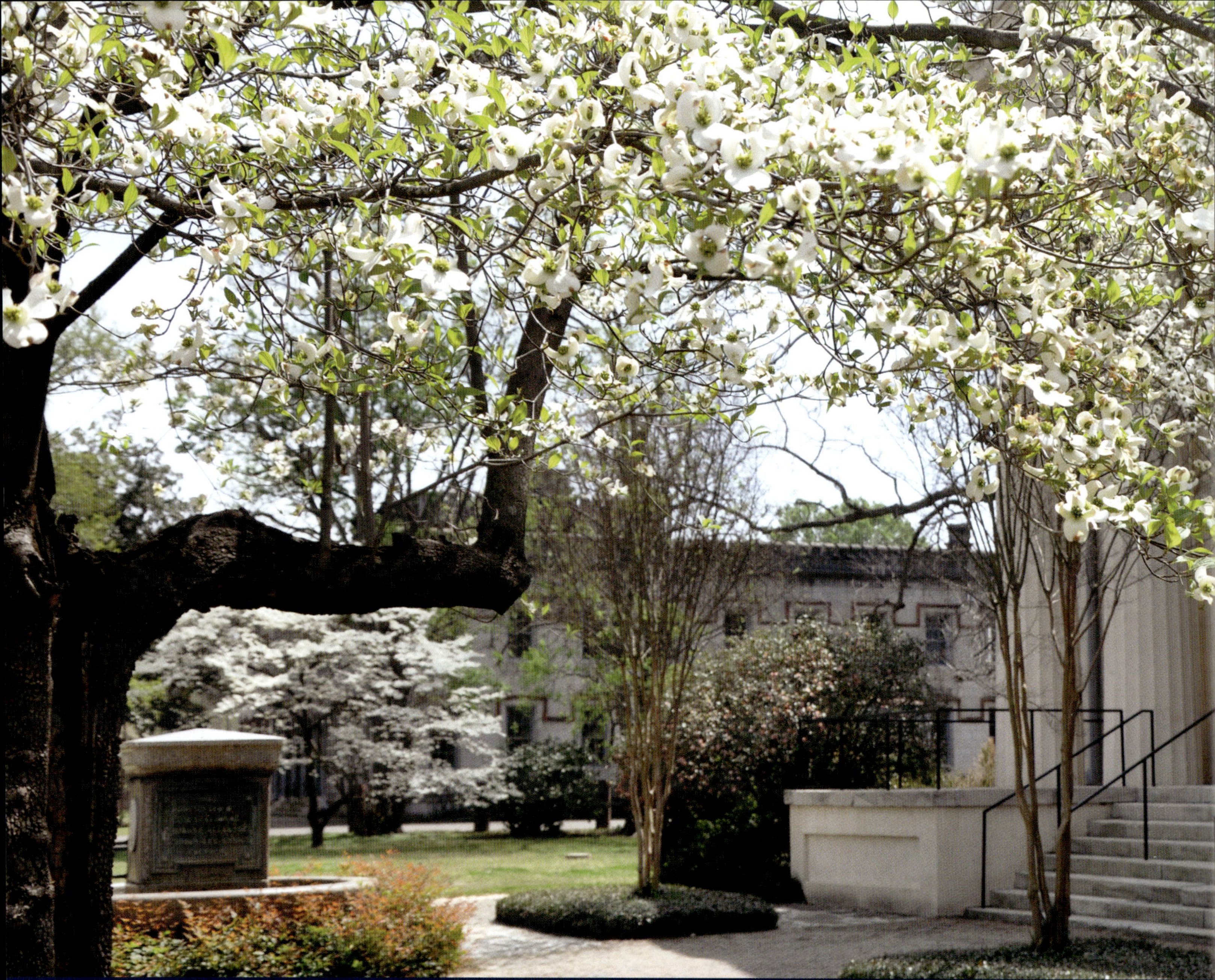

# LEADERSHIP:

## *On the Shoulders of Giants*

Georgia Regents University has a strong legacy of leadership, a nearly two-hundred-year history that includes educational trailblazers, research pioneers, medical innovators, and visionary advocates for academic excellence and better health. This chapter pays homage to the founders and the individuals who served as chief administrative officers of the legacy institutions from establishment through the consolidation of Augusta State University and Georgia Health Sciences University. While these men served as the de facto leaders of the legacy institutions, leadership is not limited to circumstances of appointed power or influence. That is why leadership—a shared commitment to courage, honor, professionalism, transparency, and vision—was embraced as one of GRU's core values.

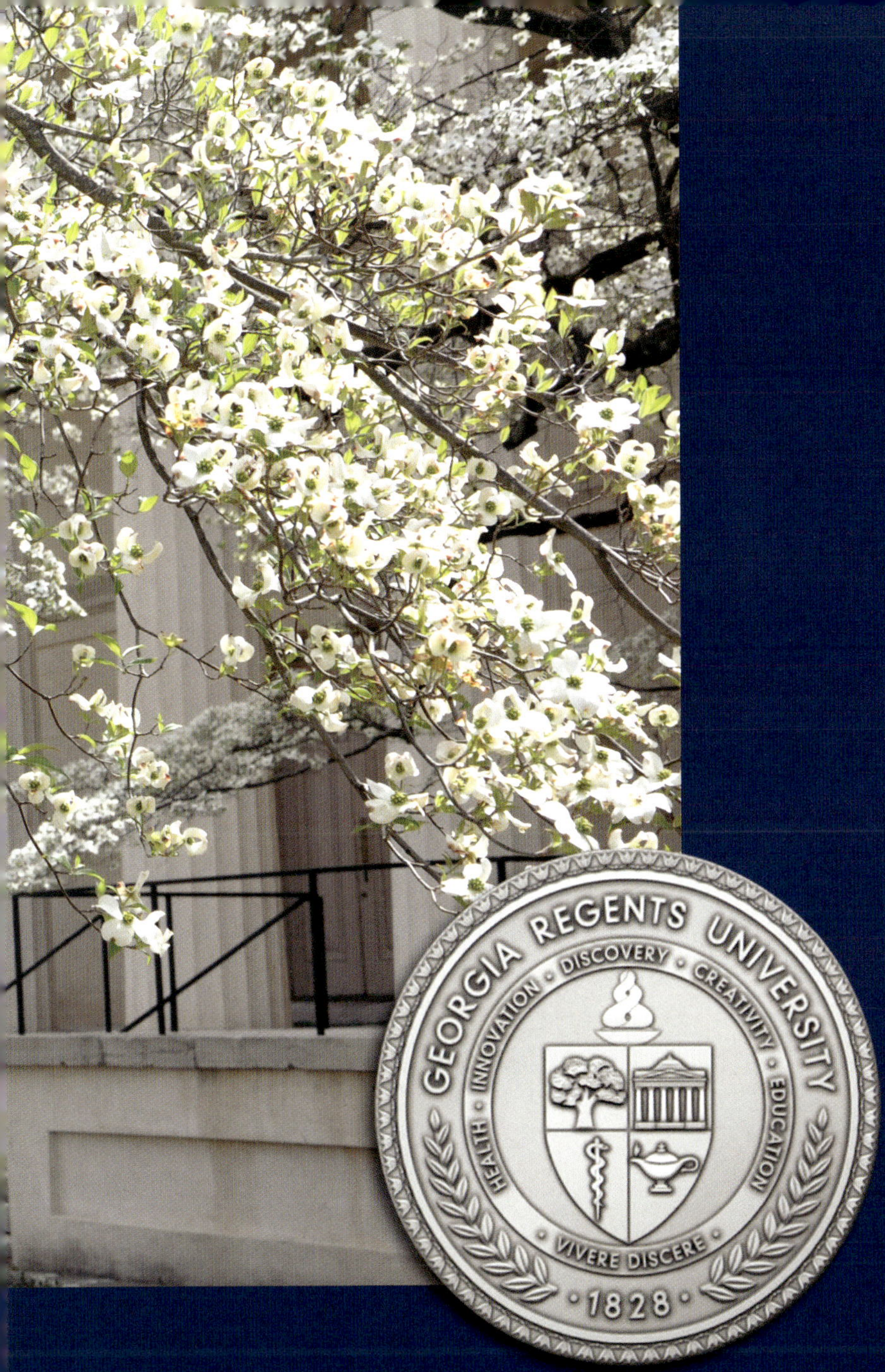


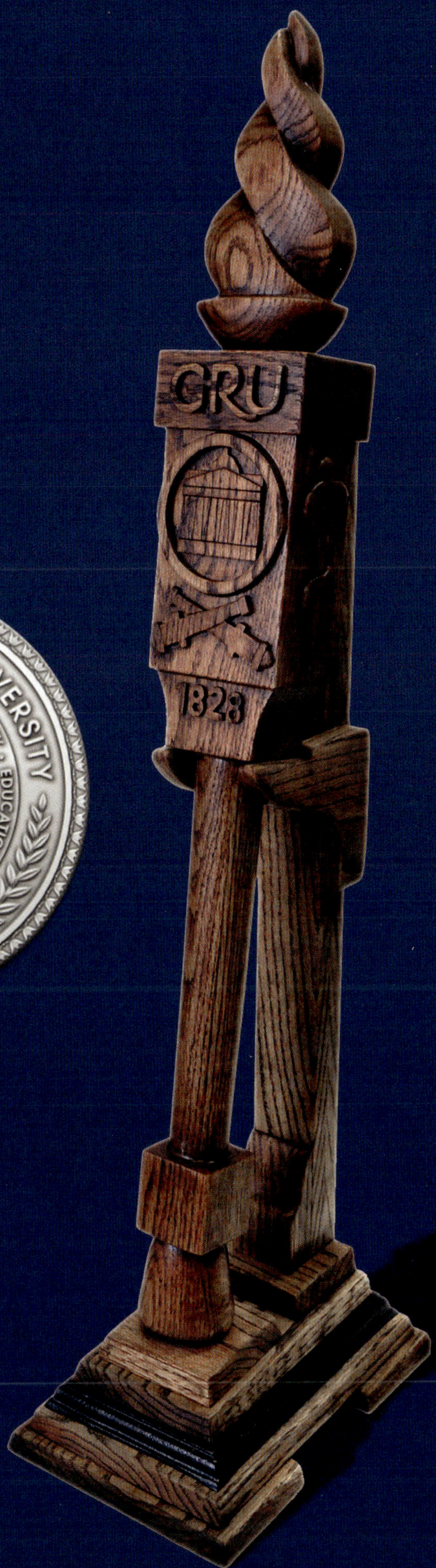


NOTES

- *The title of MCG's chief administrative officer changed from dean to president in 1950 when the institution became an independent unit in the University System of Georgia.*
- *The legacy institution Georgia Health Sciences University was known by multiple names over the course of its history; the name in use the longest being Medical College of Georgia. Therefore, the acronym MCG is used as the default identifier in the following biosketches for ease of reference.*
- *While the following collection of biosketches does not include interim deans/presidents of the legacy institutions, their commitment to "filling the gap" during times of transition is much appreciated.*

# Georgia Health Sciences University

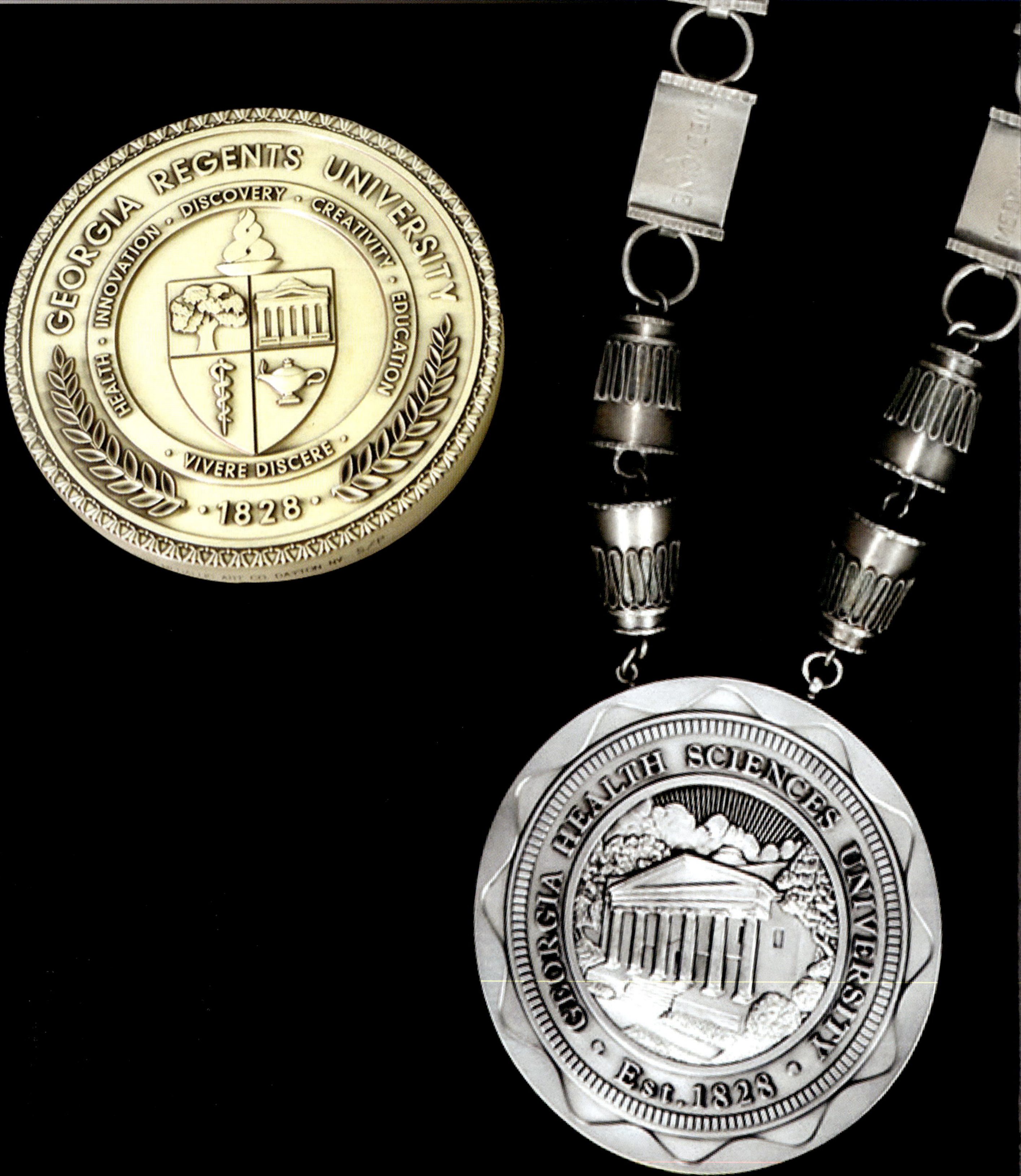

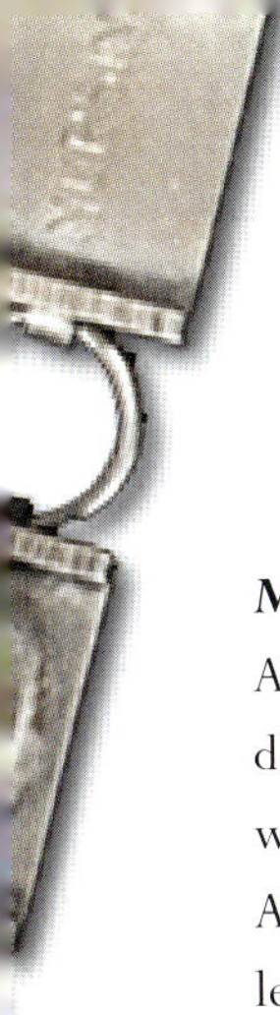

**MILTON ANTONY, FOUNDER**

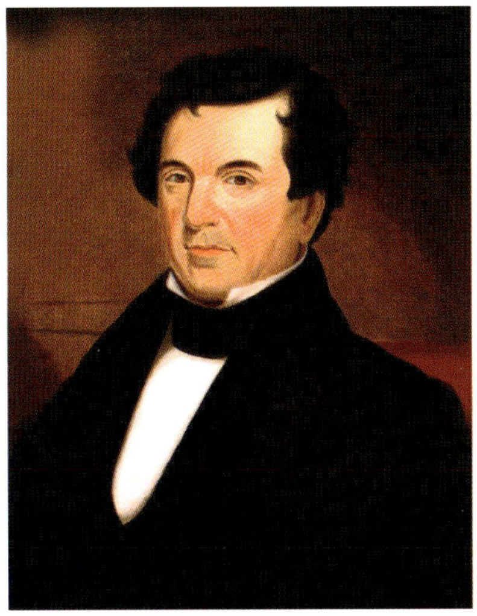

Antony was one of Georgia's most important medical pioneers. Suspicious of herb doctors and quacks, Antony felt formal education and the licensing of practitioners would stamp out the medical superstitions that were so prominent during his day. After serving as a physician's apprentice, Antony attended a year's course of medical lectures at the University of Pennsylvania but, as a result of financial challenges, was unable to complete the second year. Antony's greatest strengths were his organizational ability and the ease with which he cut through political bureaucracy. He took advantage of a promising situation in Augusta and created the state's first medical college and one the South's most respected medical journals, the *Southern Medical and Surgical Journal*. When a yellow fever epidemic raged in Augusta in 1839, Antony made the ultimate sacrifice—treating those with the disease until he himself contracted and eventually succumbed to it in September 1839. He is buried on the grounds of the Old Medical College on Telfair Street.

**LEWIS DESAUSSURE FORD (1829–1836)**

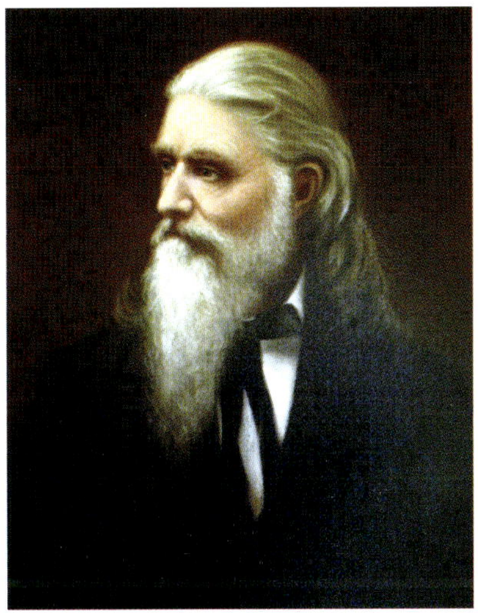

Ford was educated in New York and moved south to practice medicine in 1822. He was one of MCG's founding fathers and the school's first dean. Ford was well known for his benevolence and encouraged this attitude in his students as a duty of the profession. He was an expert on epidemic diseases and advocated better sanitary conditions to improve the health of the citizens. He served as president of the Board of Health of Augusta for several years and was chosen as the first president of the Georgia Medical Association when it was organized in 1849. He served on the Augusta City Council and was elected mayor in 1846. He served the Confederacy in the Civil War despite being sixty years old at the time. A resolution from the faculty of the Medical College of Georgia upon his death stated, ". . . he will long be remembered as one of the founders of medical science in our State . . . an early cultivator of correct methods of medical reasoning."

**PAUL FITZSIMMONS EVE (1836–1844)**

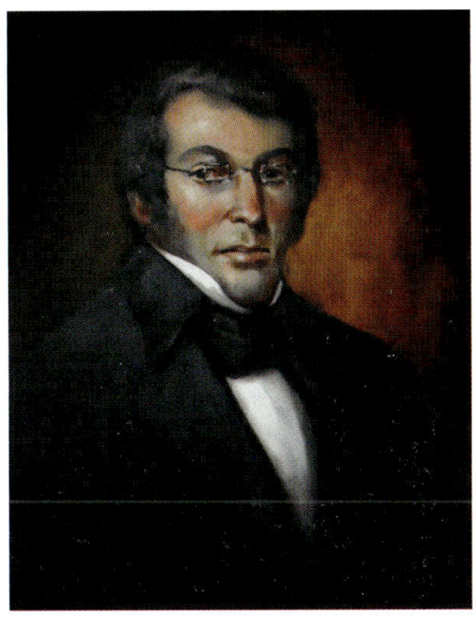

After receiving his MD degree from the University of Pennsylvania in 1828, Eve traveled to Europe to study under some of the finest physicians and in the best clinics of the time. An adventurer, he participated in the Paris Revolution of 1830 and in the Polish bid for independence as a soldier and surgeon. After his appointment to the MCG faculty in 1832, he became a well-known teacher and surgeon and contributed to the growth and reputation of the new school. He served as the second dean of the school and was editor of the prestigious *Southern Medical and Surgical Journal* for five years. Eve left Augusta in 1850 to continue his teaching and surgical practice, primarily in Nashville, Tennessee. He served as president of the American Medical Association in 1857 and as Centennial Representative to the Medical Congress of Nations in 1876. The Polish government, one hundred years after Eve's contributions during the Polish war, honored him by erecting a monument in Augusta.

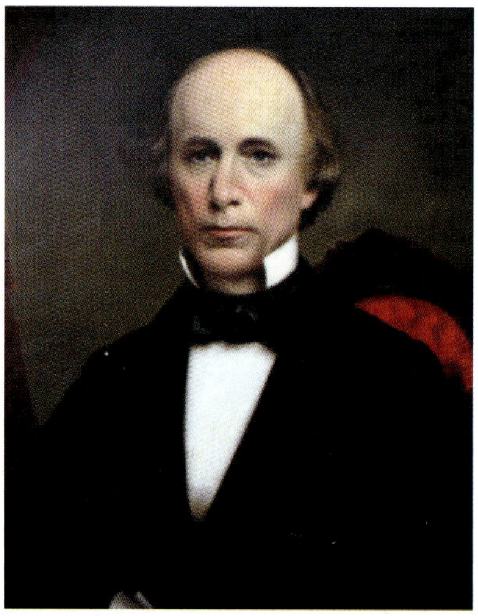

**GEORGE MADISON NEWTON (1844–1857)**

Newton was raised in Augusta and obtained his MD degree from the University of Pennsylvania School of Medicine. Newton was appointed to the faculty of MCG in 1833 and served as chair of anatomy. He was appointed the school's third dean in 1844 and served in that position for thirteen years. Because of his family's solid financial position, Newton was the first faculty member to devote his time fully to teaching, administration, and civic duties without having a private practice of medicine. He joined his stepfather, Isaac Tuttle, in providing philanthropic care to the orphans of the city. Their estates provided for the construction of the Augusta Orphanage Asylum, later known as the Newton Building. The building bearing Newton's name was occupied by the medical school from 1913 to 1956 and was demolished in 1960. Tuttle-Newton is still in existence serving families and at-risk children.

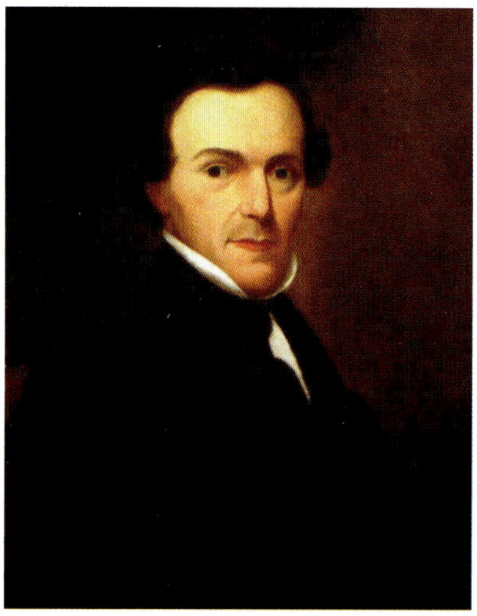

**IGNATIUS POULTNEY GARVIN (1857–1861)**

Garvin graduated with the first class of the Medical College of South Carolina in 1825. He was a founding member of the board of trustees and a member of the original faculty of MCG. He held the professor of anatomy and surgery chair for one year, leaving the school for private practice. He returned to the school and served as dean from 1857 to 1861. After Augusta's devastating yellow fever epidemic of 1839, Garvin and his colleagues were appointed to study its causes. The subsequent report was hailed as a valuable contribution to medical literature. Garvin was elected to represent the school at the national medical convention in 1847 where he proposed implementing educational standards for all medical schools, a theme common to the founding fathers. Besides his active professional life, he also participated in the civic affairs of Augusta. He was elected mayor of Augusta in 1848 and also served as treasurer of Augusta for more than fifteen years. He retired from MCG in 1867 at the age of sixty-three.

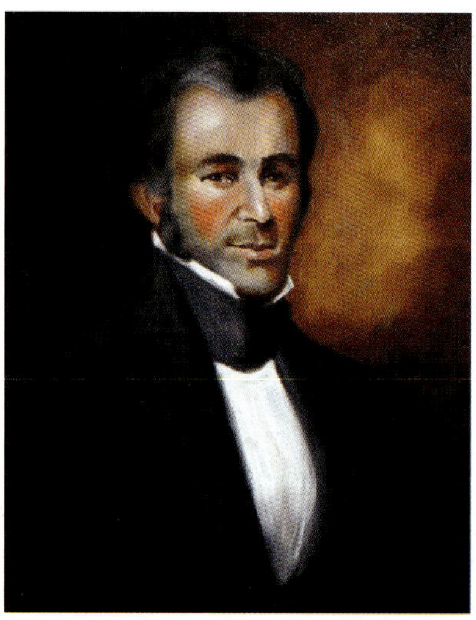

**LOUIS ALEXANDER DUGAS (1861–1876)**

Dugas came from an accomplished French West Indies family. He studied under renowned professors and physicians in Philadelphia, Maryland, and France. Three years after he joined MCG, each faculty member contributed $1,000 for Dugas to travel to Europe to purchase materials for an anatomical museum and a library. He returned with a valuable collection, most of which is housed in the archives of the Greenblatt Library. His service as dean came during the trying times of the Civil War and its aftermath. He served as editor of the *Southern Medical and Surgical Journal* for seven years and made voluminous contributions to medical literature. His insights into the origins of yellow fever foreshadowed the discovery of its transmission by mosquito, and he used animal sutures years before it became commonplace. The Dugas Test, a clinical examination performed to determine whether an injured shoulder is due to dislocation or a fracture, is still used today. Dugas also was involved with civic affairs, helping erect the Signers Monument in Augusta that recognizes the three Georgia signers of the Declaration of Independence.

**WILLIAM HENRY DESAUSSURE FORD (1876–1880, 1893–1894, 1903–1906)**

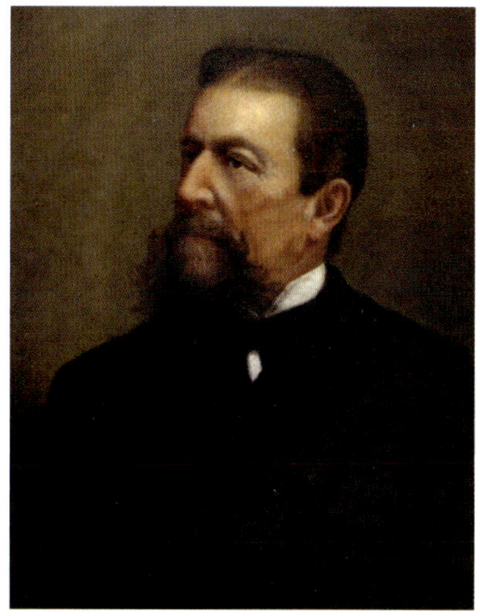

Son of the first dean of MCG, the younger Ford received his education at Richmond Academy, University of Georgia, and MCG. After his medical training, he accepted a position in Philadelphia, but left at the outbreak of the Civil War. After serving the Confederacy as a surgeon, he returned to MCG as professor of anatomy. He helped found the "New" City Hospital and chaired its governing board. He was involved in other civic activities as a city council member, president of Richmond Academy, physician to the Augusta Orphanage Asylum and Tubman Home, and surgeon to the Georgia Railroad and other railroads in the South. He had the unusual distinction of serving as dean of MCG three times in four decades—a testimony to his ability and character as a leader.

**GEORGE WASHINGTON RAINS (1880–1884)**

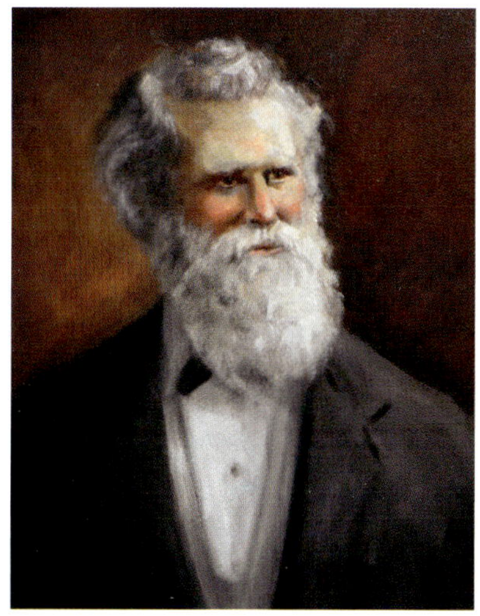

Rains served as dean of MCG after spending more than two decades as an army officer, chemist, and engineer. In 1842 he graduated from West Point Military (third in a class of fifty-six) and rose through the ranks of the army to major during the Mexican War. In the late 1850s he resigned from the army and secured patents on inventions related to steam engines. When the Civil War began, Rains enlisted in the Confederate army. Assigned the task of producing gunpowder, Rains established the powder mill in Augusta that manufactured gunpowder for the Confederacy. He and his brother Gabriel, also a munitions/ordnance expert, were known as "The Bomb Brothers." A former commandant of the Augusta Arsenal, Rains joined MCG after the war as professor of chemistry and received an honorary MD degree. He served as dean from 1880 to 1884 and continued on faculty until his retirement in 1893. Rains Hall on the Summerville Campus is named in his honor.

**EDWARD WYATT GEDDINGS (1884–1893)**

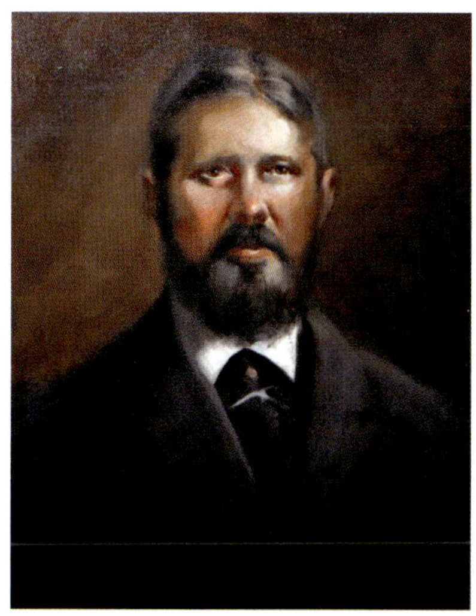

Geddings graduated from the University of Berlin with high honors in 1854. He also received his MD degree in Berlin, after which he returned to Charleston, South Carolina, to practice medicine before and after the Civil War. During the war, he served as a surgeon with the rank of major. In 1866, he joined the MCG faculty and remained affiliated with the school for the next twenty-five years. Shortly after assuming the deanship, Geddings encouraged the faculty to abandon the old didactic form of lecturing for the newer, fresher, question-and-answer technique. There is no evidence the faculty followed his request. During Geddings's tenure as dean, the faculty started the first formal residency training at City Hospital in 1888. In 1891, the Sisters of Mercy ended their twenty years of service to City Hospital, leaving the facility without nurses, maintenance workers, and administrators. The school entered into an agreement with the city council to control the hospital. Geddings resigned from the deanship in 1893, after nine years as the school's leader.

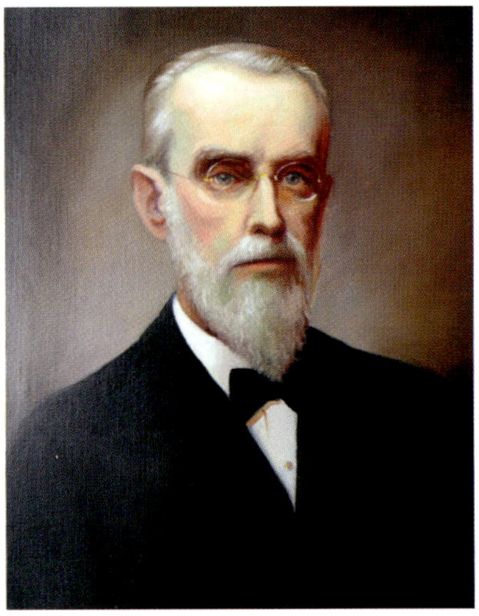

**THOMAS RUSSELL WRIGHT (1894–1896)**

Wright received his MD degree from MCG in 1876. He taught at the school for forty-seven years, first as professor of anatomy and later as professor of surgery. Wright became dean in 1894 during a national depression, just in time, as it happened, to preside over a drastic decline in attendance. Wright apparently did not care for his administrative duties. This consideration, coupled with the enrollment problems, led the trustees to conclude that another dean should be sought. Despite his short tenure as dean, Wright remained intricately involved in the workings of the school and is credited, along with William Henry Doughty Jr., of being responsible for the school's survival and rejuvenation following the 1910 publication of Abraham Flexner's landmark critique of American medical education, in which Flexner recommended the University of Georgia sever its ties with the medical program in Augusta. Wright died in 1923. Doughty, his colleague and fellow dean, passed away less than a month later.

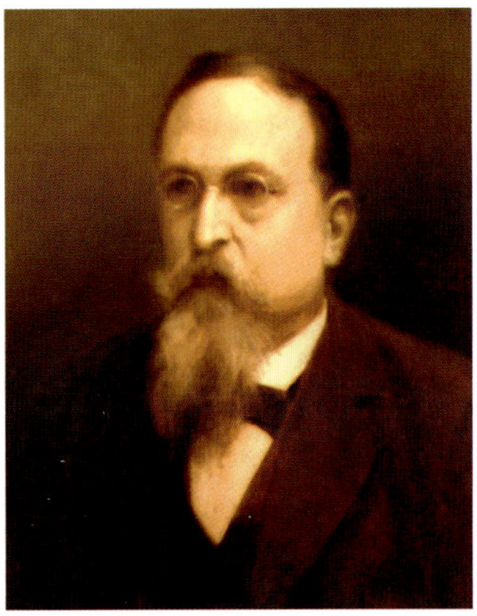

**EUGENE FOSTER (1896–1903)**

Foster was born in Augusta and received his MD degree from MCG in 1872. He did postgraduate work at University Medical College in New York and returned to Augusta to oversee the smallpox hospital. He was an advocate for public health programs throughout his life, serving on the Augusta Board of Health, backing Augusta's implementation of its sewerage system, and serving as an active member of the American Public Health Association. In 1892, Foster gave the address at the first annual alumni association meeting in conjunction with commencement. He urged more cooperation among doctors and lashed out against quacks. During his tenure as dean, Foster lobbied to require four years for the medical degree in order to expand the curriculum to include emerging knowledge, such as bacteriology. As a proponent of using sound business principles to run the institution, his term as dean saw prosperous times. He improved the physical plant with new equipment and expanded facilities. Foster died in January 1903.

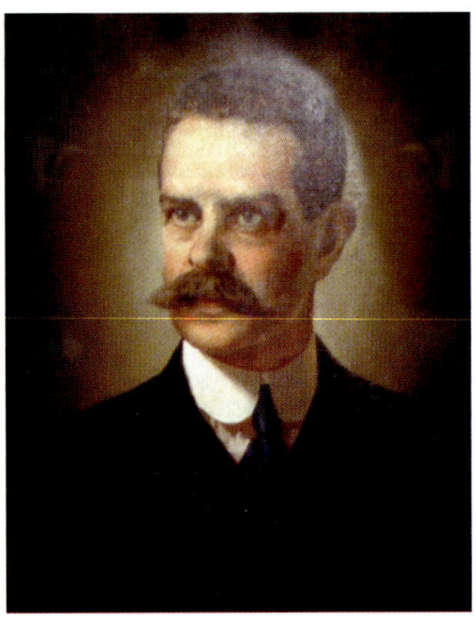

**JOSEPH EVE ALLEN (1906–1910)**

Allen, the grandson and namesake of MCG co-founder Joseph Eve, was educated in Augusta and received his MD degree from MCG in 1877. When he was named dean in 1906, the students hoisted him on their shoulders and carried him into the assembly. That same year, the institution fielded its first football team, the Medicos. As dean, Allen made needed changes to the curriculum and improved clinical instruction and laboratory facilities. The teaching staff also was strengthened by the addition of more faculty members. Despite this progress, in 1910 the Flexner Report gave the school a less than favorable review, recommending the University of Georgia no longer be affiliated with the medical program. The school, the report detailed, should close its doors or move to Athens due to inadequate financial support and the tenuous affiliation with the university. Allen's term as dean ended in 1910 with much work yet to be done to redeem the school's reputation on the national medical scene.

**WILLIAM HENRY DOUGHTY JR. (1910–1923)**

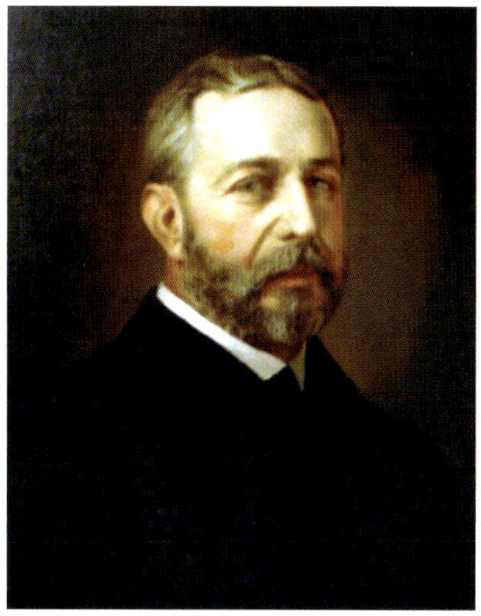

Doughty, a native Augustan, received an undergraduate degree from the University of Georgia in 1875 and a degree of doctor of medicine in 1878. After completing postgraduate studies in New York City, he began his practice in Augusta, and in 1881, began his career at MCG as assistant demonstrator of anatomy and clinical assistant. In 1910, after many years as professor of surgery, he assumed the deanship. He continued in this position until 1923 when he died from a gas bacillus that developed following a tooth extraction. Doughty guided MCG through a stormy period following the publication of the Flexner Report. During his tenure, a new committee on curriculum was formed, a new set of bylaws and rules governing the faculty was put into place, and a board of directors was created. Doughty's time in office changed the old face of the college. He brought in grants and community backing to fund more full-time faculty members and faculty chairs which enabled the school to produce "an all-round physician." Doughty facilitated the institution's relocation from Telfair Street to its present campus. Within a short time of this relocation, he helped to establish the University Hospital.

**WILLIAM HENRY GOODRICH (1923–1931)**

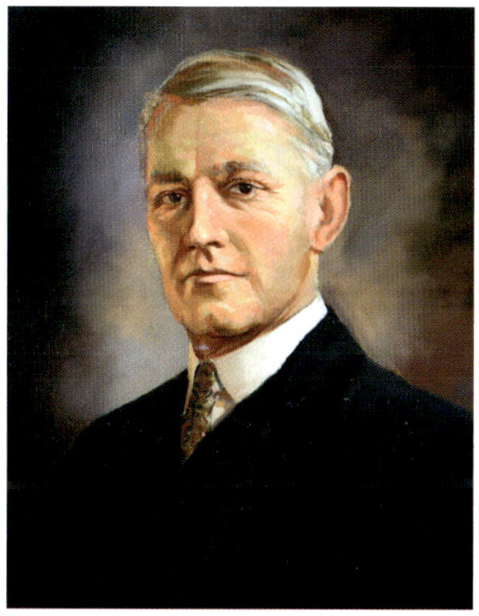

Goodrich graduated from MCG with honors in 1897 and began his teaching career with the institution shortly thereafter. After the sudden death of Doughty in 1923, Goodrich was elected dean and served until 1931. During his tenure, two women achieved major milestones: Loree Florence became the first woman to graduate with an MD degree and Ellen Marsh was the first female at the college to earn a degree in public health. In 1927, fire destroyed the south wing of the Newton Building and caused smoke damage to the north wing. The insurance money helped the school construct new animal surgery quarters. In 1928, Goodrich authored the first history of the college to honor its centennial. In 1939, he was appointed superintendent of University Hospital, a post he held until 1945. At the time of his death, he was chief surgeon for the Georgia & Florida Railroad and local surgeon for the Central of Georgia Railroad. Goodrich died in a boating accident in 1947.

**WILLIAM LORENZO MOSS (1931–1934)**

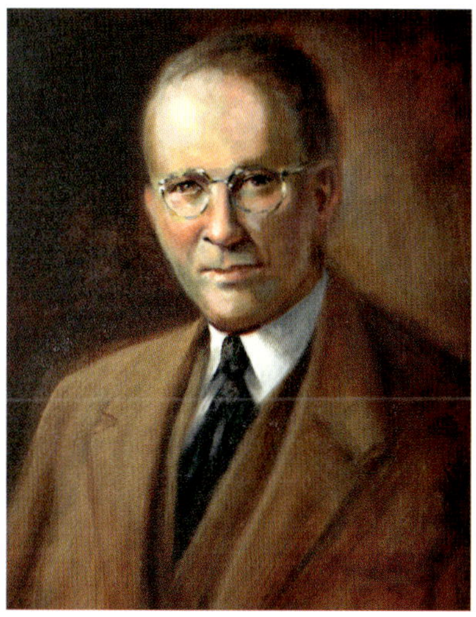

Moss, a native of Athens, Georgia, earned his medical degree at Johns Hopkins Medical School in 1905. Moss spent many years as a teacher and researcher at Johns Hopkins, Yale, and Harvard, heading numerous international medical research expeditions in the Caribbean, South America, and the South Pacific. In 1931, he was named dean of MCG, the same year the Georgia legislature united all state institutions into the University System of Georgia and established the Board of Regents. Within two years, the board assumed complete control of the universities, and in one of its first meetings, it closed eight schools including MCG. Local and gubernatorial support prompted the regents to overturn the decision, but problems continued. The Great Depression and lack of finances kept Moss from fully implementing the regents-recommended improvements, leading to two negative reviews from independent councils. The regents asked Moss to resign in 1934, leaving his successor—George Lombard Kelly—to address the school's lack of funds, insufficient number of full-time teachers, and inadequate equipment, classrooms, and clinical areas.

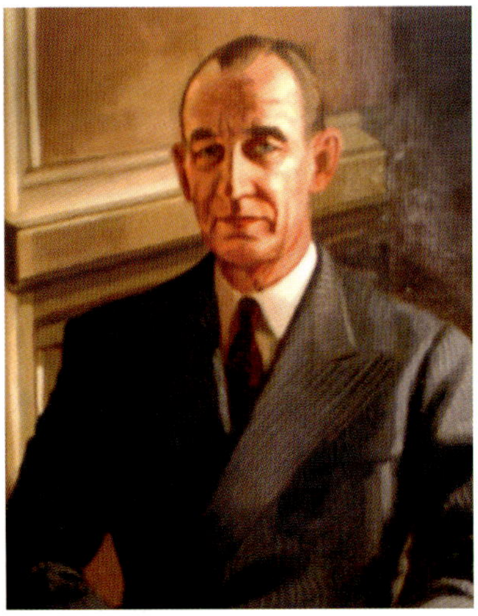

**GEORGE LOMBARD KELLY (1935–1953)**

Kelly, a native Augustan, withdrew twice from medical schools because of illness before he received his MD degree from MCG in 1924. Before he graduated, he began teaching at the school as assistant professor of anatomy. The school promoted him to professor of anatomy five years later. In 1935, Kelly was appointed dean and embarked on a twenty-year mission to build a strong foundation that would assure the school's continued existence and growth. He developed a master plan that included establishing a state owned and controlled teaching hospital in Augusta to replace the city owned and controlled University Hospital. In 1950, Kelly became the first president of the school after the regents separated the institution from the University of Georgia and renamed it the Medical College of Georgia. He retired in 1953 to practice reproductive physiology full time. One month after his retirement, construction started on the state hospital. The bold vision of developing a comprehensive health sciences university in Augusta was Kelly's; his successors executed the ambitious plan.

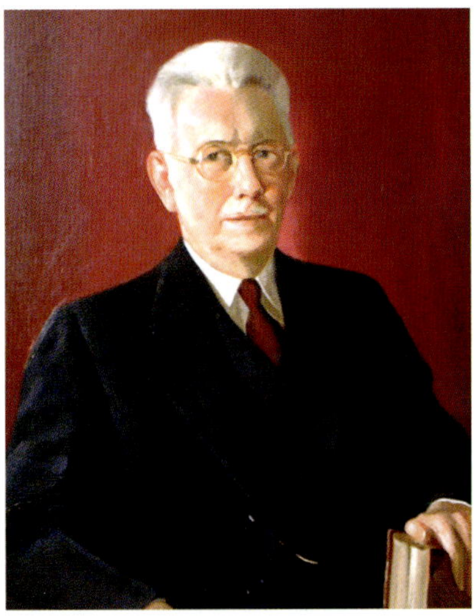

**EDGAR RUDOLPH PUND (1953–1958)**

Pund, a native of Augusta, was the long-serving chair of the Department of Pathology until his appointment as MCG's second president in 1953. One year after his appointment, he met with four MCG alumni to determine how to best solidify the institution's well being and optimize its impact. Within an hour, the men had reached into their pockets and donated the $450 they collectively had on hand to form the Medical College of Georgia Foundation—the first of GRU's three partner foundations. Another highlight of Pund's presidency was the opening of Eugene Talmadge Memorial Hospital in 1956, a teaching hospital to support the college's medical program. Strong but modest, it was a matter of understandable pride to Pund that the college's instruction budget had more than doubled during his presidency and funds to support patient care had been secured through a direct appropriation to the hospital. Pund stepped down from the presidency in 1958. He remained an advocate of the college until his death in 1975.

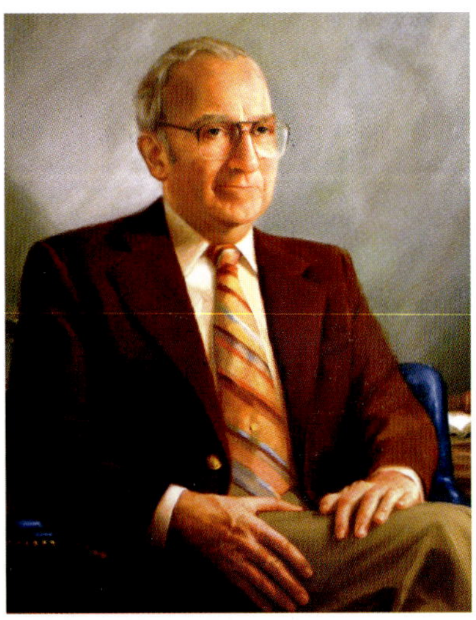

**HARRY BARRON O'REAR (1960–1972)**

O'Rear joined MCG in 1950, the year the college became an independent unit in the University System of Georgia, and rose through the faculty ranks to become professor of pediatrics, dean of the School of Medicine, and eventually the third president. During his presidency, the university acquired twenty-six acres of land for future growth and built several new facilities, including the college's library, the Student Center, and the original home of the dental college on Laney-Walker Boulevard. When he assumed the presidency, MCG had two schools (Medicine and Nursing). He left it with five. Even though the presidency occupied most of his time, O'Rear found time to pursue his favorite hobby, photographing flowers in their natural settings. He resigned as president in 1972 to accept the full-time position of vice chancellor for health affairs at the University System of Georgia, a position he held until his retirement in 1985. O'Rear passed away in 2008 in the mountains of North Carolina where he and his wife had built their retirement home.

**WILLIAM HENRY MORETZ (1972–1983)**

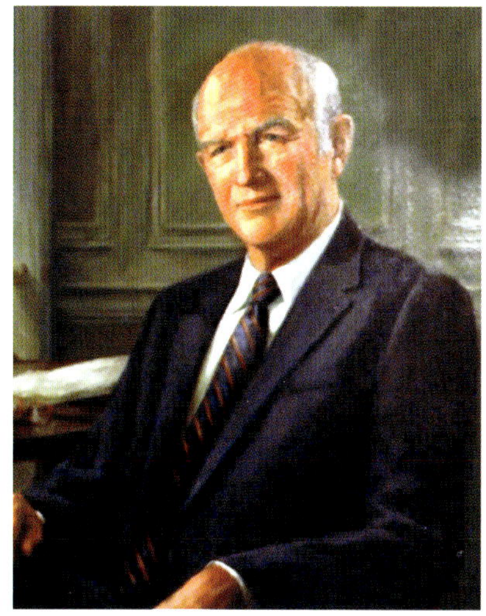

Moretz, a 1939 graduate of Harvard Medical School, joined MCG in 1955 as professor and chair of the Department of Surgery. The board of regents appointed Moretz MCG's fourth president in 1972, and he began expanding MCG's student body and physical plant. During his tenure, the number of MCG graduates almost doubled and more than $25 million in renovations and new construction were completed. Moretz oversaw the opening of the hospital's Sydenstricker Wing in 1976, adding 240 beds and doubling the hospital's research potential. Other additions to the campus included the radiation therapy center, the Research and Education Building, and that building's Hamilton Wing. The Greenblatt Library also was expanded under his leadership, increasing the facility to more than 60,000 square feet. The Moretz Surgical Society, established in 1972, was named in his honor to promote the exchange of scientific research and observation by surgeons affiliated with MCG who worked under Moretz when he chaired the department. Moretz retired from the presidency in 1983 and died in 1989.

**JESSE LEONARD STEINFELD (1983–1987)**

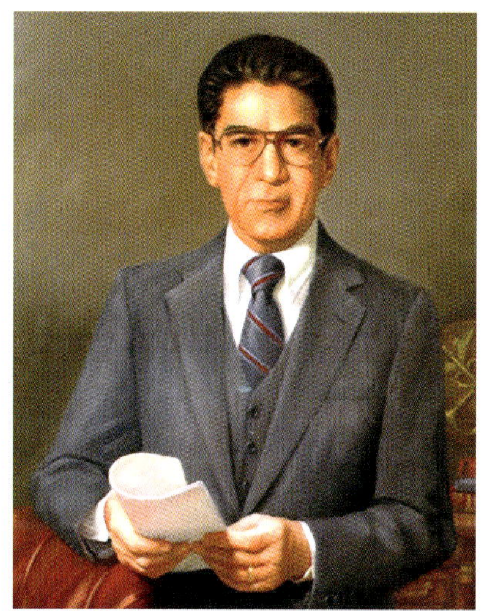

Steinfeld served as United States surgeon general from 1969 to 1973 under President Nixon. An ardent advocate of building public awareness of the dangers of tobacco and smoking, Steinfeld developed a contentious relationship with the tobacco industry, which lobbied for his eventual dismissal. He became president of MCG in 1983 after serving in various posts in academic medicine, including director of the Mayo Clinic Comprehensive Cancer Center and dean of the medical school at the Medical College of Virginia. Administrative streamlining and a new emphasis on planning marked his years at MCG's helm. He also oversaw construction of two parking decks and computerization of the Greenblatt Library. Early in his presidency, Steinfeld instituted a no smoking policy, a mandate that failed to take hold until a more inclusive Tobacco Free Campus campaign was waged during the Rahn presidency more than twenty years later. Steinfeld retired in 1987 after developing debilitating osteoarthritis. He passed away in California in 2014.

**FRANCIS JOSEPH TEDESCO (1988–2001)**

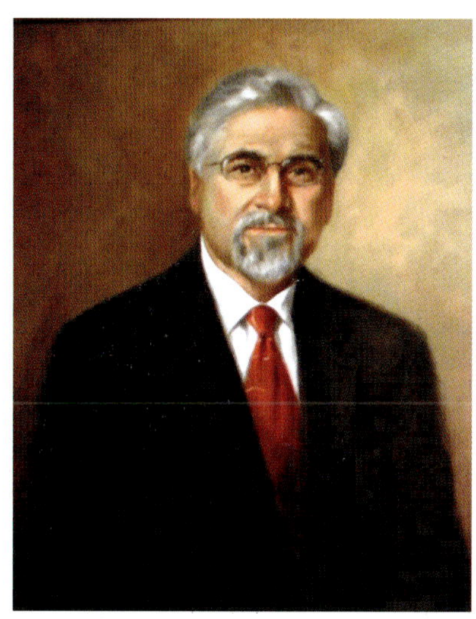

Tedesco joined the MCG faculty in 1978 as section chief for gastroenterology. He quickly ascended the academic ranks—named full professor in 1981, acting vice president for clinical activities in 1984, and interim dean for the medical school in 1986. He was appointed president in 1988. During his tenure, Tedesco focused on developing a rigorous and state-of-the-art research program before that was popular at universities. He oversaw the construction of the institution's first interdisciplinary research facility, an Ambulatory Care Center/Specialty Care Center, the nationally recognized Children's Hospital of Georgia, and the Center for Sports Medicine. The quality of education at MCG increased during Tedesco's presidency with competitive admission and most students passing their board exams. Tedesco remained in Augusta following his retirement in 2001, serving on the boards of several nonprofits within the health care and education sectors and spending time with his grandsons.

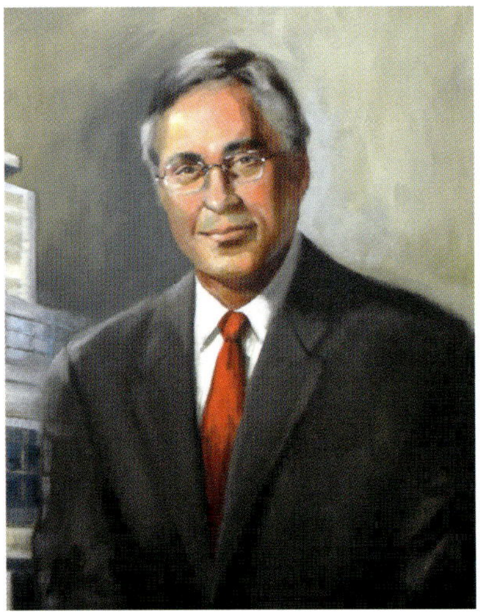

**DANIEL WALLACE RAHN (2001–2009)**

A nationally recognized expert in Lyme disease, Rahn joined the faculty of MCG in 1991 and was named the university's seventh president in 2001. He served as senior vice chancellor for health and medical programs for the University System of Georgia concurrent with his presidency. The campus saw great physical growth under Rahn's leadership, including construction of the Cancer Research Center, Health Sciences Building, phase II of the Interdisciplinary Research Center (which doubled research space), and a Wellness Center. Rahn also laid the groundwork for construction of a modern facility to house the university's College of Dental Medicine and shaped an enhanced statewide presence for the university's medical college. Rahn led the institution during a particularly challenging period marked by the separation of the clinical system from the operations of the university. An accomplished pianist, Rahn frequently participated in the university's Noon Arts Conference, a concert series highlighting the performing arts talent of MCG faculty, staff, and students. Rahn left MCG in 2009 to become the chancellor of the University of Arkansas for Medical Sciences.

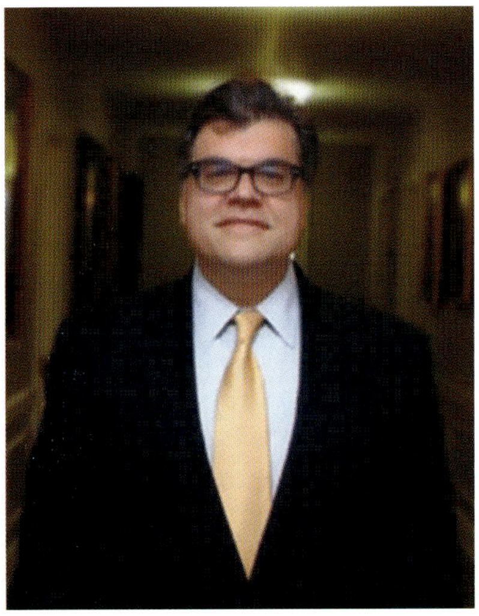

**RICARDO AZZIZ (2010–2013)**

An educator, clinician, researcher, academic leader, and accomplished visual artist, Azziz was named president of the Medical College of Georgia in 2010. Early in his term, he championed a name change to more clearly reflect the scope of the health sciences university. He also led the reunification of the clinical system and the university, serving as CEO of the health system concurrent with his presidency. Azziz led the consolidation of Augusta State University and Georgia Health Sciences University to create Georgia Regents University, serving as the new university's first president. Bold by some accounts and brash by others, Azziz articulated a big vision for GRU and encouraged the university community to "make noise" about it. Azziz revitalized philanthropy, nearly tripling yearly contributions and achieving the largest donation to a capital project in the university's history and, separately, the largest philanthropic gift ever given to a public institution in Georgia. Citing the end of his work as a change agent, Azziz stepped down from the presidency of GRU in 2015 to re-engage with his research and academic writing.

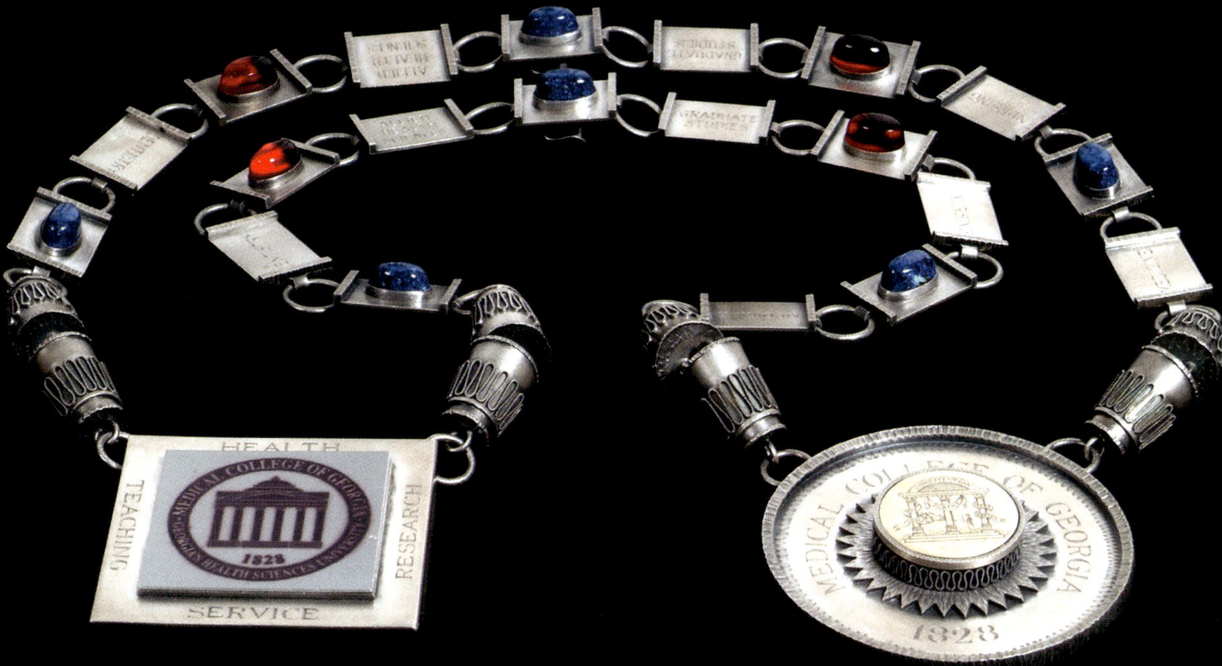
HEALTH
TEACHING
RESEARCH
SERVICE
MEDICAL COLLEGE OF GEORGIA
1828
MEDICAL COLLEGE OF GEORGIA
1828

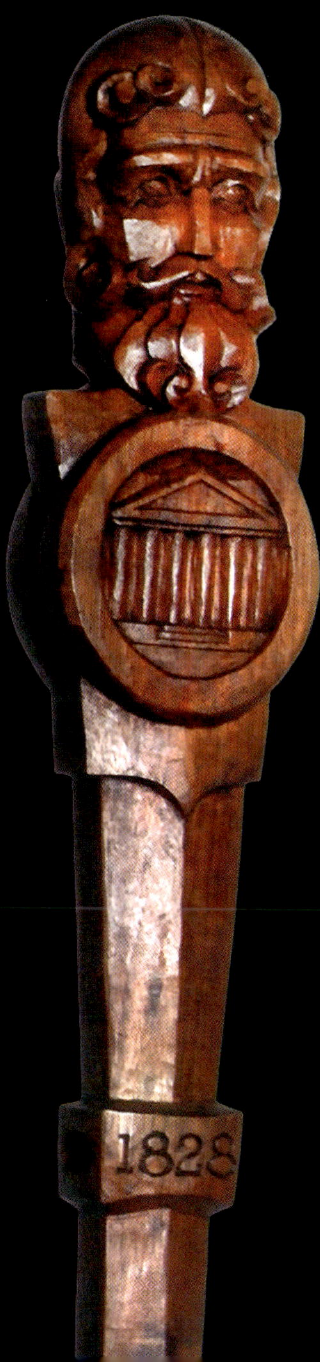
1828

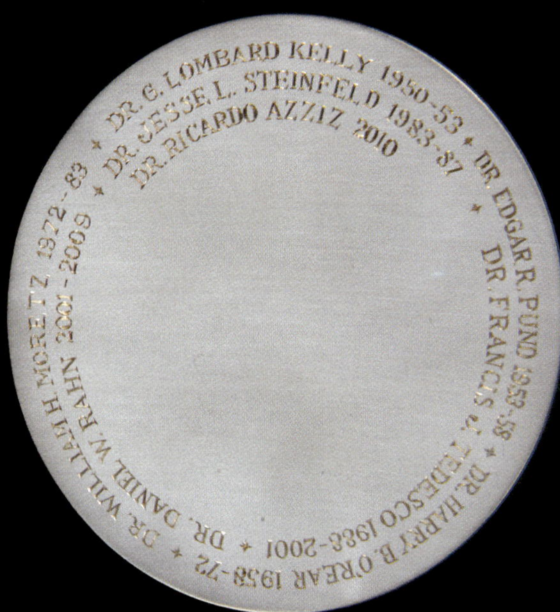
DR. G. LOMBARD KELLY 1950-53
DR. JESSE L. STEINFELD 1983-87
DR. RICARDO AZZIZ 2010
DR. EDGAR R. PUND 1953-58
DR. HARRY B. O'REAR 1958-72
DR. WILLIAM H. MORETZ 1972-83
DR. DANIEL W. RAHN 2001-2009

# AUGUSTA STATE UNIVERSITY

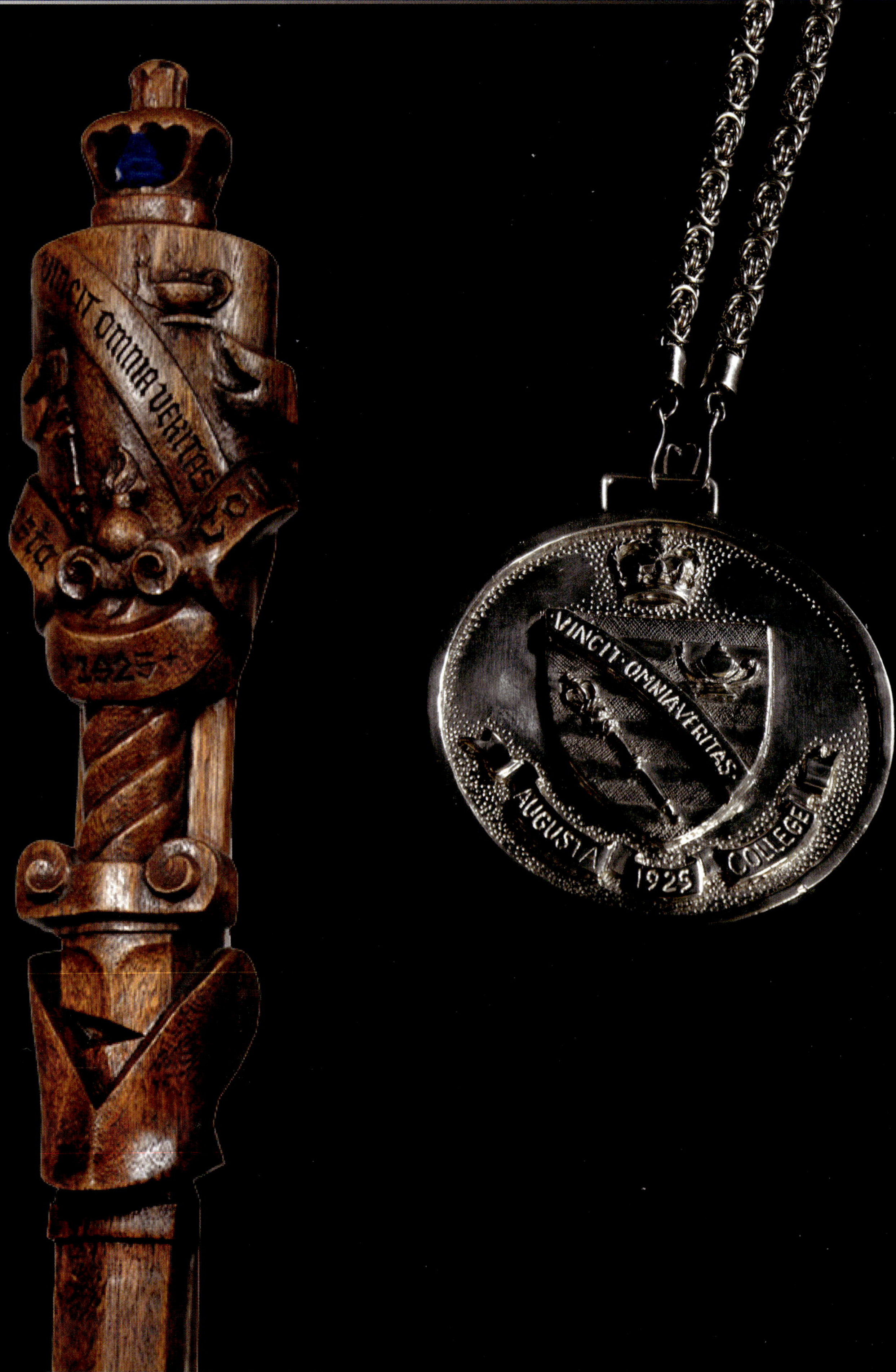

## GEORGE PHINEAS BUTLER (1925–1930)

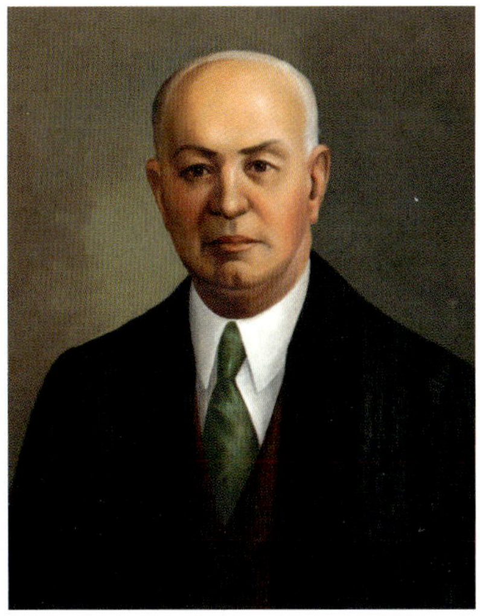

Known as the father of the Junior College of Augusta, Butler was an important figure in Augusta's education in the early twentieth century and a recognized leader in the national two-year college movement. After serving in various positions in post-secondary and higher education, Butler returned to his hometown in 1898 as a professor of mathematics and physics at the Academy of Richmond County. He revitalized the institution's military department, an achievement that earned him the popular title of "Major Butler." Butler became principal of the academy in 1910. During his tenure, he added one year of college to the curriculum, setting the stage for the founding of the JCA in 1925. As its first president, Butler worked tirelessly to make the junior college—the "people's college" as he called it—a success. He envisioned pre-medical courses that would lead students into programs at the Medical College of Georgia, a prophetic aspiration in light of the creation of Georgia Regents University. Butler died of a heart attack in 1933 while duck hunting in North Carolina.

## JAMES LISTER SKINNER (1930–1938)

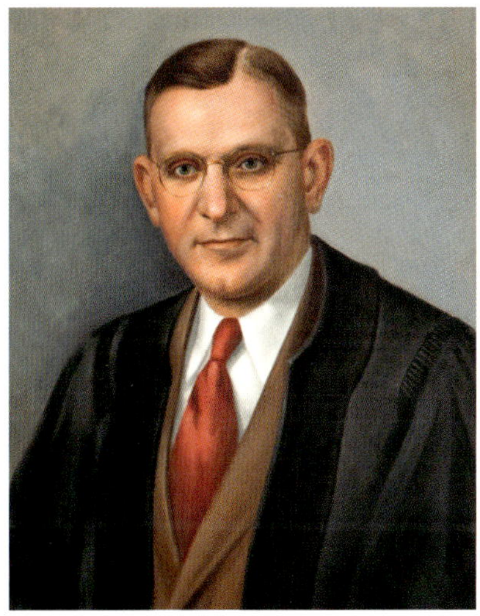

Skinner became the second president of the junior college in 1930, a difficult time to be leader as his years as president coincided with the worst years of the Great Depression. Faculty salaries had decreased and the college's mission, enrollment, and curriculum remained static. It was during these difficult years the college's fledgling football program was discontinued. The college's host institution, the Academy of Richmond County, felt the junior college was crowding out the academy's programs. Skinner postponed a forced departure of the college by securing a grant from the federal government's Public Works Administration to enlarge the premises. The grant was awarded in the fall of 1937. Skinner announced his resignation to be effective January 1, 1938. Skinner left Augusta to assume the presidency of William R. Moore School of Technology in Memphis, Tennessee.

## ERIC WEST HARDY (1938–1954)

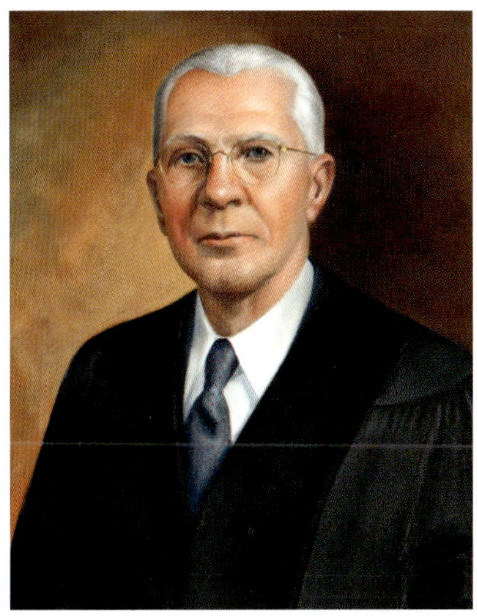

As president of Augusta's junior college, Hardy valued job placement as much as senior college placement. He incorporated vocational training into the college's curriculum. In 1946, he initiated an evening school catering to returning veterans of World War II. GRU's inclusion on Victory Media's Military Friendly Schools List is an accolade of which Hardy would have been proud. Hardy focused the institution's efforts on the needs of the community and it was under his leadership that JCA became a true community college. Hardy retired in 1954, but he did not cease involvement in the college's future. Increasing enrollment threatened the accreditation of both the junior college and the Academy of Richmond County. Hardy was deeply involved in the failed effort to transfer the junior college to the Georgia Baptist Convention. While unsuccessful, the effort did call attention to the issues plaguing the institution—lack of space, no room to grow, and no permanent home.

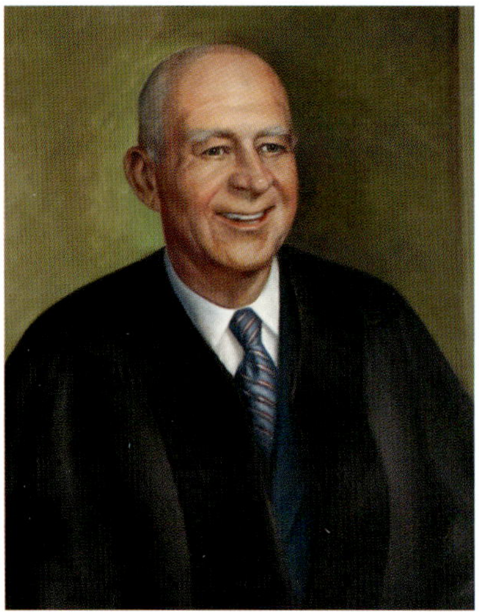

**ANTON PAUL MARKERT (1954–1957)**

Markert, a pioneer of the original faculty of 1926, assumed the presidency of the Junior College of Augusta in 1954. Calm, considerate, and affable, he was a true student's administrator—a major shift in leadership style from the visionary, crusading, and unpredictable Hardy. Markert was president during the prolonged negotiations over the transfer of the Augusta Arsenal property to the Board of Education, but it was his predecessor Hardy who was tapped to oversee the college's move to the historic site in 1957. Although Markert selected the faculty who would transfer to the new campus, he decided to remain at the Academy of Richmond County—his short presidency overshadowed by Hardy's continued involvement in the college.

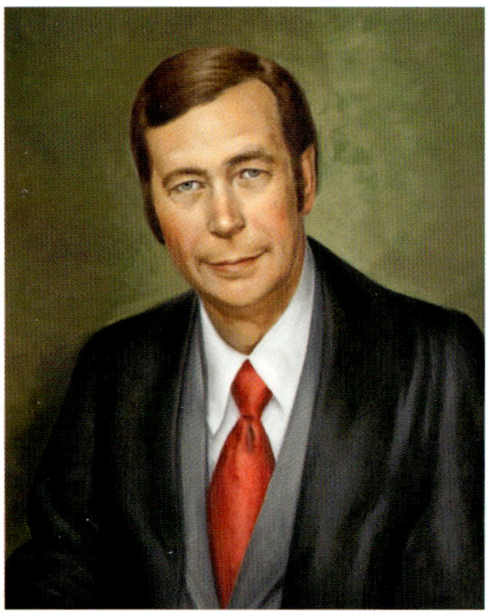

**GERALD BURNS ROBINS (1957–1970)**

Robins began his presidency in 1957, the first year the junior college moved operations to the former site of the Augusta Arsenal. Robins served as president for thirteen years, seeing the name change to Augusta College in 1958, the first baccalaureate degrees conferred in 1967, and WACG—the first noncommercial radio station operated by a University System of Georgia school—go on the air. Robins saw the student body triple in size and worked to transform the campus of warehouses into a collegiate environment. The "expansion years," the transition from a junior to a senior college, were challenging ones for the college and its leaders. In the spring of 1969, a faculty credentials scandal rocked the campus and essentially muzzled the president. Robins (who had served in World War II as a combat navigator) left the presidency in February 1970 after secretly submitting his resignation the previous summer. Robins went on to a faculty position at the University of Georgia, eventually accepting another presidency at a university in Texas.

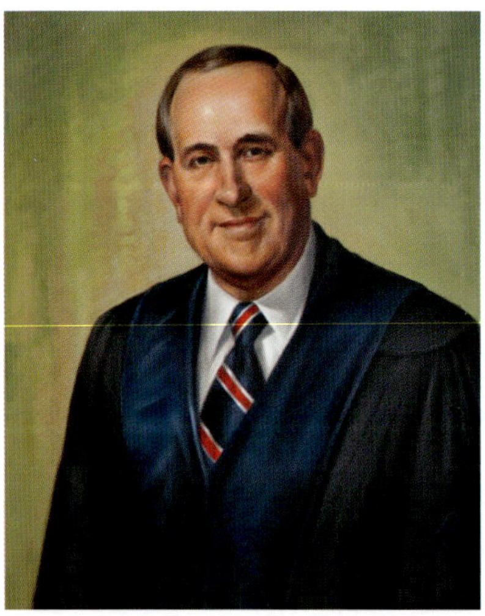

**GEORGE ANDREW CHRISTENBERRY (1970–1986)**

Christenberry was one of the major reasons for the resurgence of public confidence in Augusta College. He was the first of the college's presidents with previous senior college administrative experience having served at Furman and as president of Shorter College. When he assumed the presidency of AC in 1970, the student body was vocal and organized with race relations and the anti-war movement at the top of their agenda. Under Christenberry's leadership the college experienced more growth in both enrollment and faculty than ever before; added master's degrees in business administration, education, and psychology; and reorganized into three schools: Arts and Sciences, Education, and Business. The college also acquired the last five acres of the original arsenal property and secured from the federal government an additional 240 acres in Augusta's Forrest Hills neighborhood. The first president in the institution's long line of leaders to be inaugurated in a traditional academic ceremony, Christenberry retired in 1986. He passed away in 2009 at the age of ninety-three.

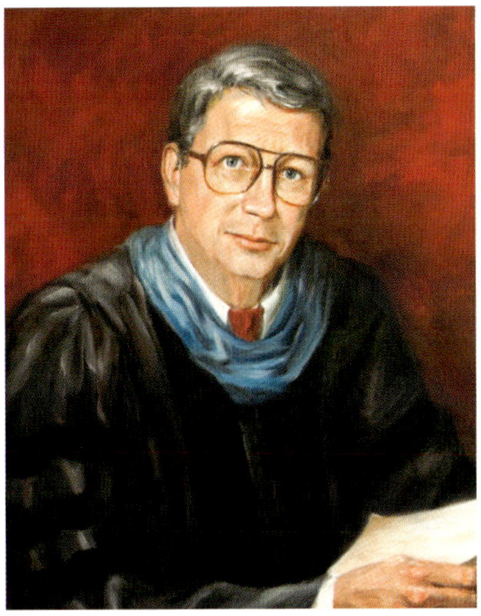

**RICHARD STRONG WALLACE (1987–1991)**

Wallace was named president of Augusta College in 1987 and served in that role until his death from colon cancer in 1991. He joined the college in 1982 as vice president for academic affairs and professor of business administration. During Wallace's tenure, student housing units were constructed near the Forest Hills campus. The next year a physical education/athletic complex (the Christenberry Fieldhouse) was completed on the same property. The university's literacy center, an initiative providing children, adolescents, and adults with high-quality, literacy-related educational experiences, also was created during Wallace's presidency. A carillon was dedicated to the university the year of Wallace's appointment, the ringing of the bells intended to remind the university community of the past and awaken them to the future.

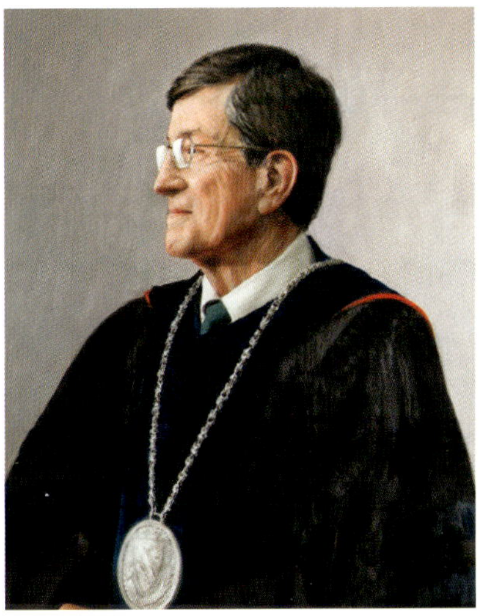

**WILLIAM ANDREW BLOODWORTH JR. (1993–2012)**

Bloodworth's teaching career spanned nearly fifty years, beginning in the public schools of his native Texas and continuing through universities in North Carolina and Missouri. He was serving as provost and vice president for academic affairs at Central Missouri State University when he was named the eighth president of Augusta College, assuming the position in 1993. The institution was elevated to university status in 1996. Bloodworth led ASU through a whirlwind of renovations, new degree programs, national golf championship titles, and expansions. During his tenure, he spearheaded more than $103 million in new construction and renovations and successfully partnered with donors to endow and name two of the college's schools. He moved the university from a commuter, non-residential campus to one offering student housing. After retiring as president in 2012, Bloodworth returned to the classroom and to his lifelong passion for teaching. A first generation college student, Bloodworth was one of the longest serving presidents in the history of the University System of Georgia.

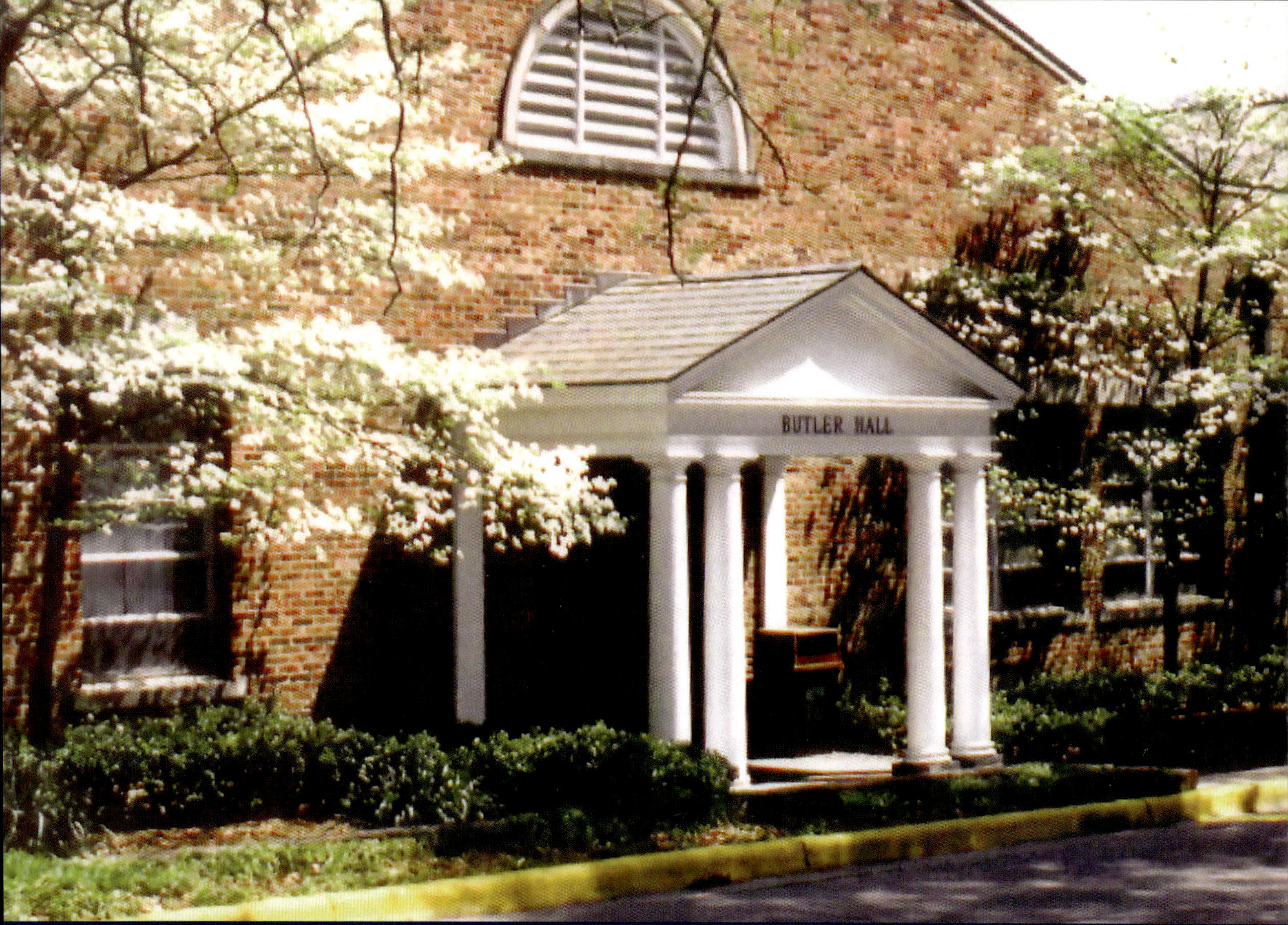


# Campus Development:
## *Growth and Expansion of the Built Environment*

**Founders of the legacy institutions of Georgia Regents University (GRU) would be amazed to see the expansive campuses that now house their educational enterprises. From modest beginnings, the consolidated institution of Augusta State University (ASU) and Georgia Health Sciences University (GHSU) has become the state's fourth research university and its only public academic medical center. On 650 acres of property divided among three Augusta campuses—Health Sciences, Summerville, and Forest Hills—stand over 150 buildings, with additional development being planned.**

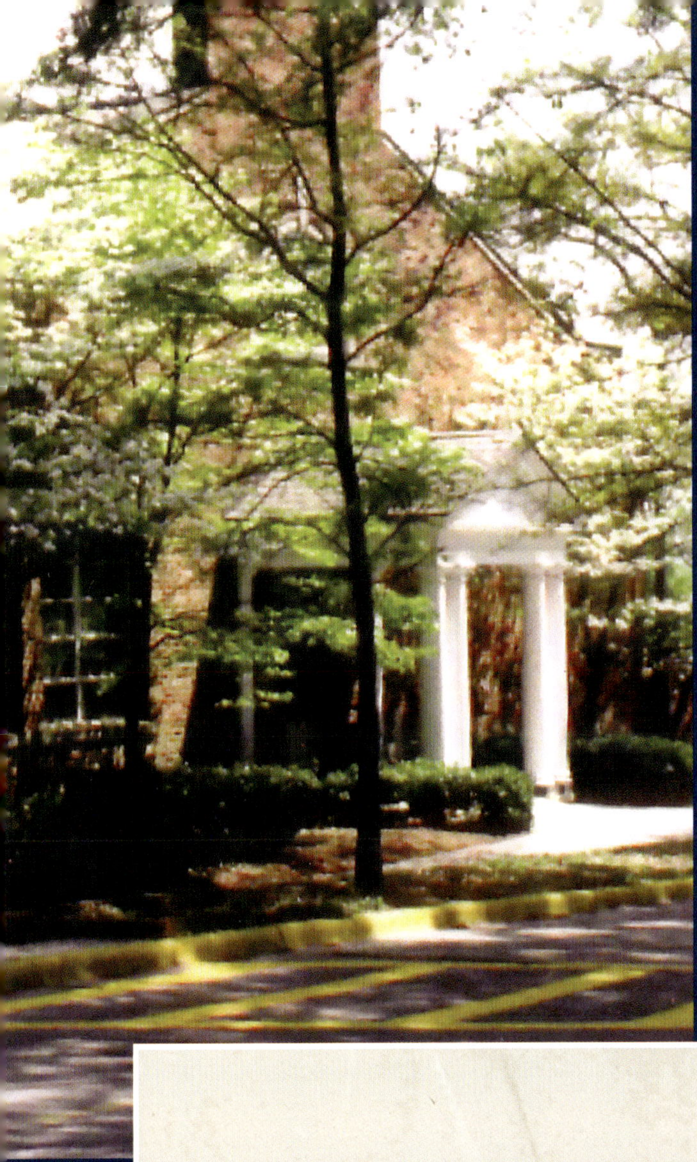

Medical education began in 1826 in two rooms of Augusta's City Hospital. Nine years later the school moved into its new Greek Revival building on Telfair Street. For seventy-seven years, faculty educated new physicians within its walls. Outdated and in disrepair, the building was vacated during the 1912 Christmas holidays. When classes resumed in January 1913, the college had relocated to the former Augusta Orphan Asylum, which later became known as the Newton Building. It housed classrooms, laboratories, an outpatient clinic, a city dispensary, and a library. When a new, modern, city-operated University Hospital opened in 1915, it served as the primary site for the school's clinical training.

*Butler Hall, named after the founding president of the Junior College of Augusta, was one of six classroom buildings on the campus of Augusta State University. The structures were demolished in 2003 to make way for campus growth and development.*

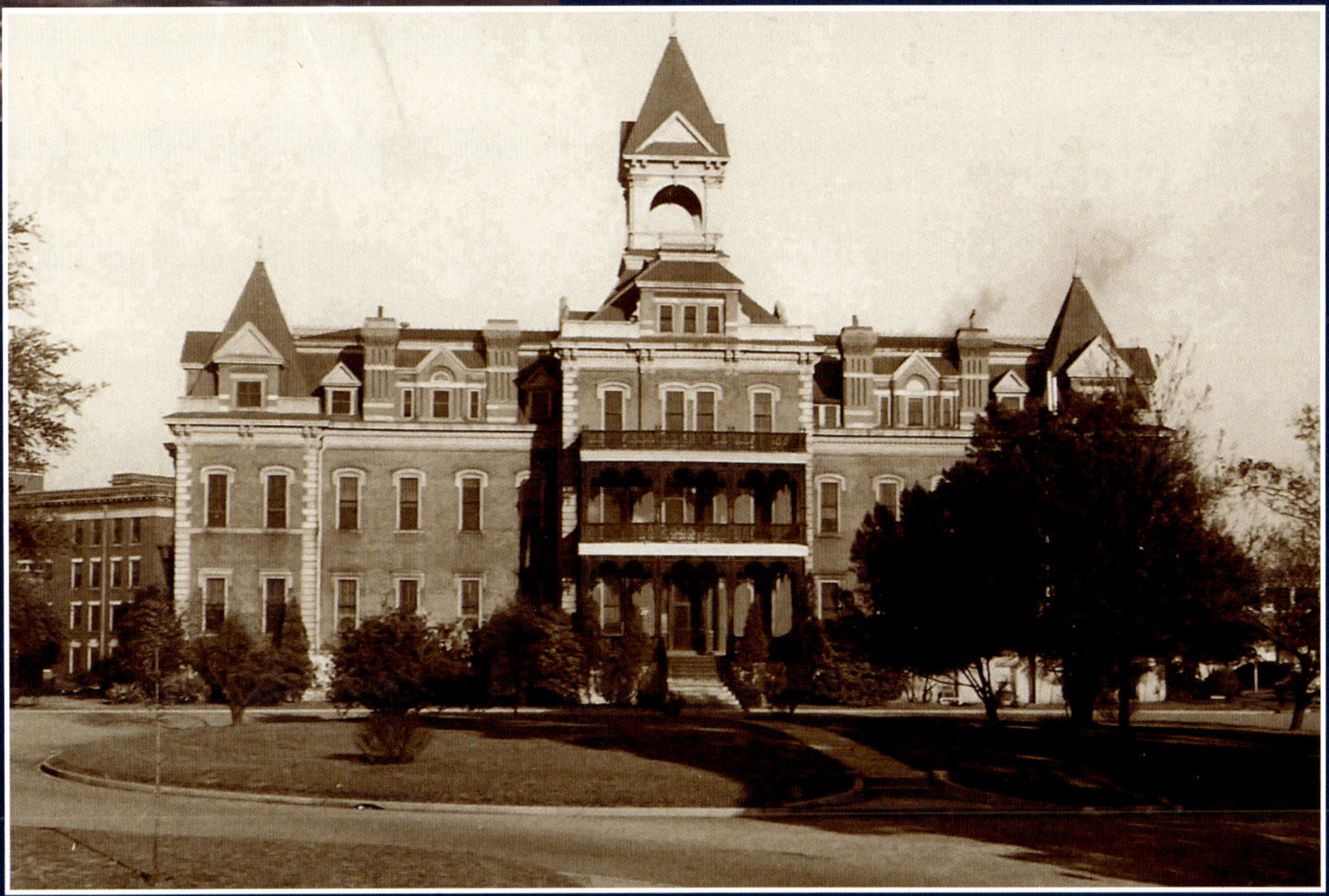

*The Newton Building, formerly the Augusta Orphan Asylum, became the new home of MCG in January 1913. Dr. George Newton and his stepfather, Isaac Tuttle, had founded and funded the orphanage and Newton had served as dean of the medical college in the antebellum era. The building was demolished in 1960.*

The 1937 Dugas Building with both classrooms and laboratories heralded the beginning of the current Health Sciences Campus. Two years later, the Murphey Building, named for prominent Augusta physician and alumnus Eugene Murphey, opened with additional classrooms. Construction of the Kelly Administration Building was completed in 1954, taking some of the functions previously housed in the Newton Building. Used thereafter on a limited basis, the Newton Building was demolished in 1960.

The growing campus and college reached a pivotal moment in its history in 1956 with the construction of its own teaching hospital, the Eugene Talmadge Memorial Hospital, now Georgia Regents Medical Center. Dr. Rufus Payne, a close associate of Kelly's and superintendent of Battey State Tuberculosis Hospital in Rome, Georgia, was recruited to MCG to supervise construction of the facility. When the hospital opened, Payne was the first superintendent. Dr. Lois Ellison, GRU medical historian-in-residence, noted, "At that time, we became a true academic

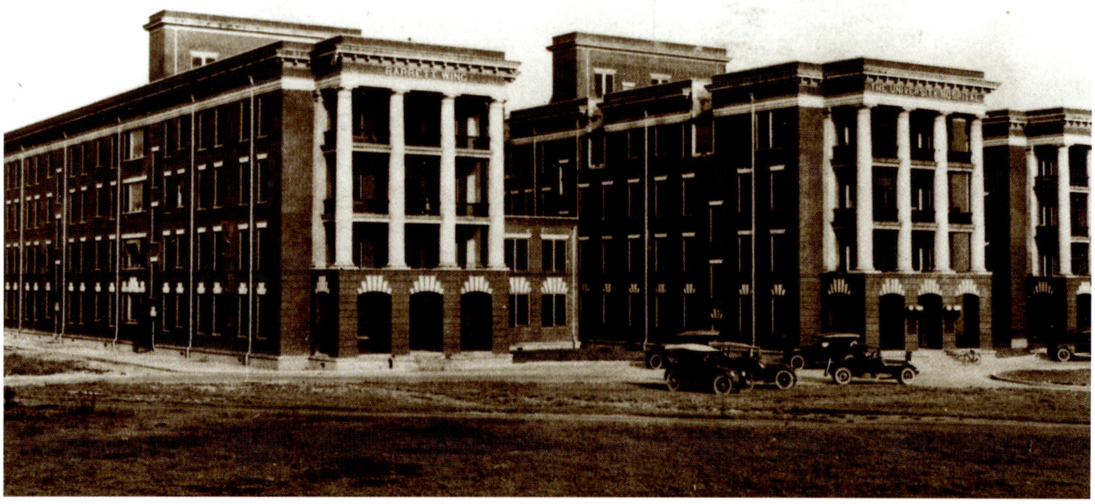

*Left: University Hospital opened in June 1915 between Gwinnett (Laney Walker Boulevard) and Harper Streets. The 275-bed structure contained a center administrative section and two four-story wings. The original structure was demolished in the early 1990s.*

*Below: Named in honor of early faculty member Dr. Louis Alexander Dugas, the 1937 Dugas Building was the first new construction on campus in over one hundred years. The structure housed basic science classrooms and laboratories and was funded by the Public Works Administration.*

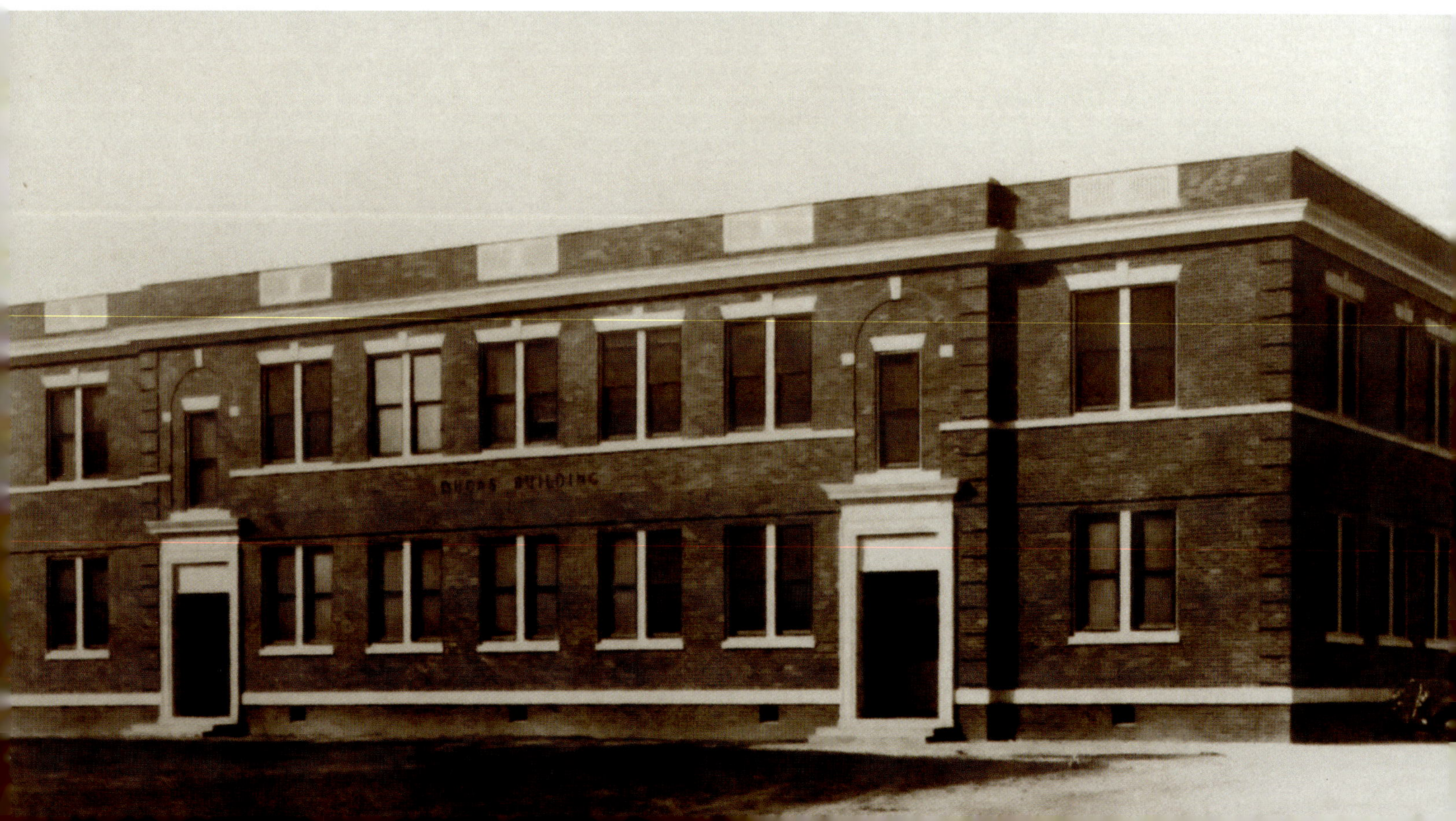

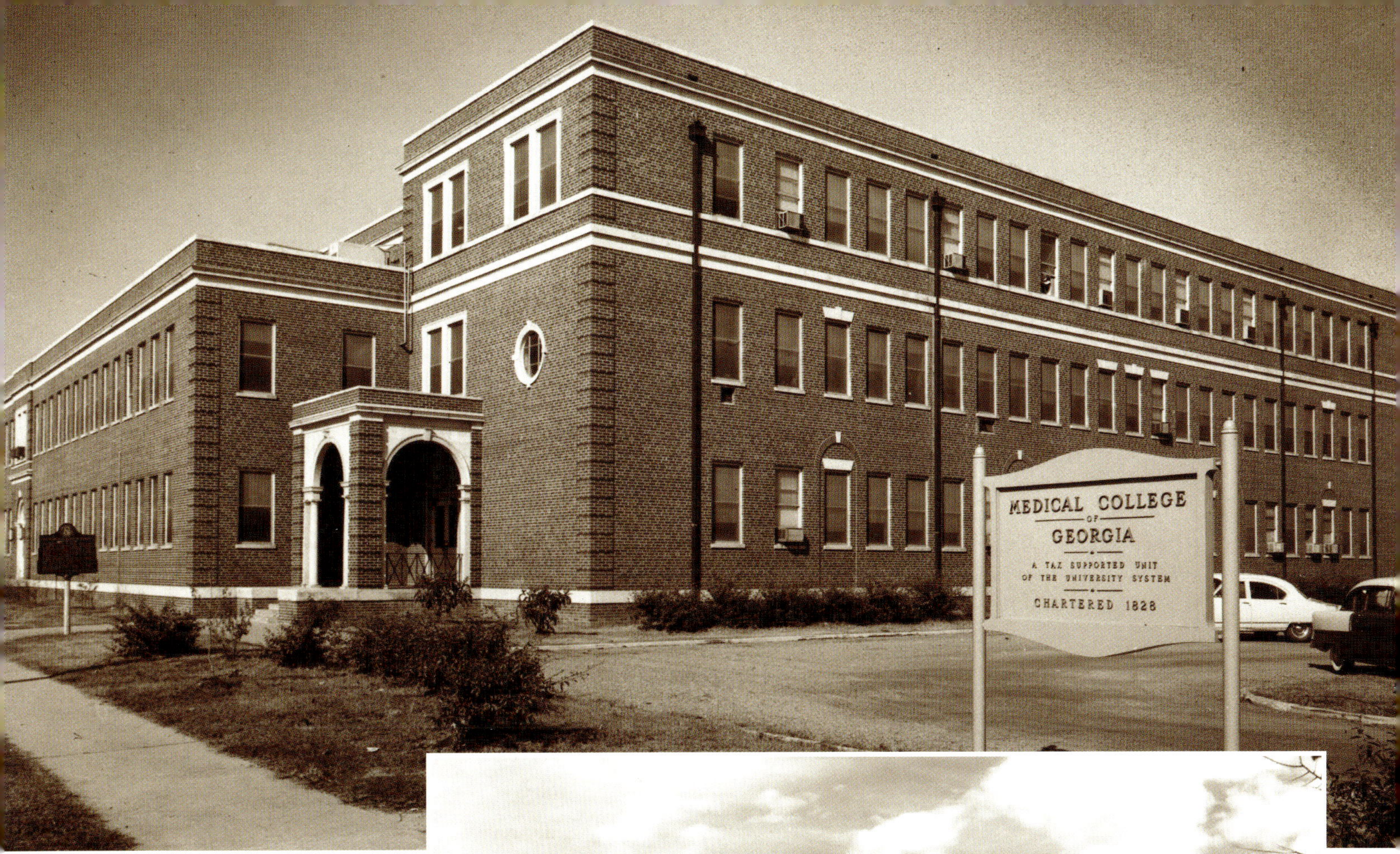
MEDICAL COLLEGE
OF
GEORGIA
A TAX SUPPORTED UNIT
OF THE UNIVERSITY SYSTEM
CHARTERED 1828

*Above: The Kelly Administration Building was named for MCG's last dean and first president, Dr. G. Lombard Kelly. Occupied in 1954, the building originally housed administrative offices, the anatomy department, library, and dog laboratory, which were moved from the Newton Building. The building has undergone several additions and renovations.*

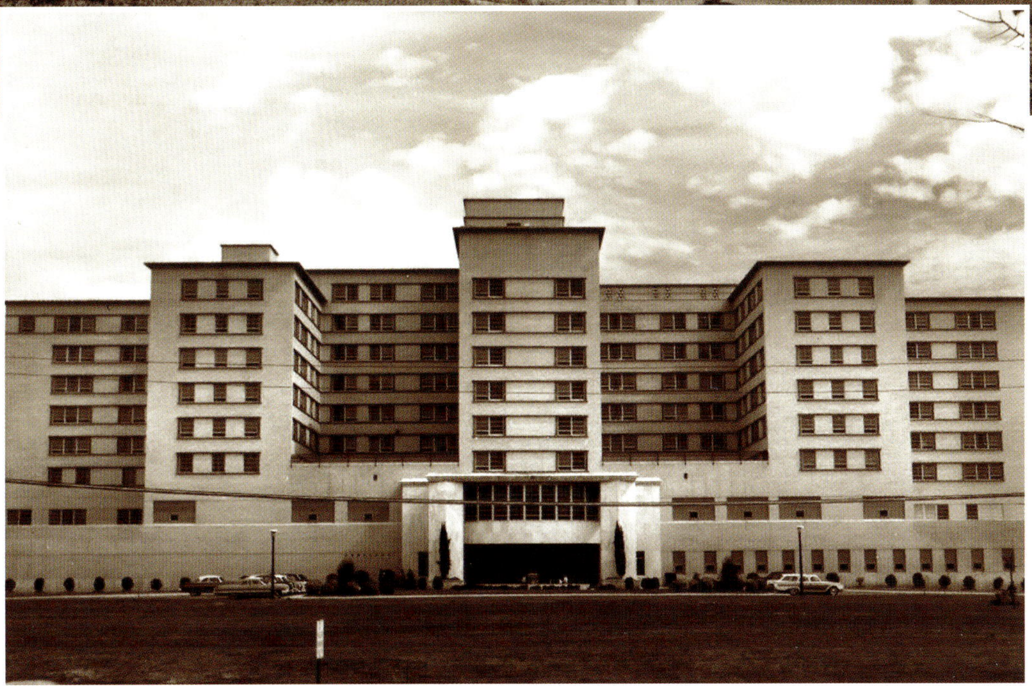

*Right: The Georgia General Assembly named MCG's new teaching hospital the Eugene Talmadge Memorial Hospital for the former governor prior to its construction and opening in 1956.*

medical center." A clinical research wing was added to the back of the hospital in 1961.

In 1962, the school purchased twenty-five acres of land on present-day Laney Walker Boulevard. The first buildings to open on the new property included the Student Center in 1967 and the campus' first student housing, Village Apartments, in 1968. Meanwhile, the Robert B. Greenblatt, MD, Library opened in 1963, the first freestanding library in the school's 135-year history.

The early 1970s saw two major additions. The University System of Georgia record for largest instructional building was broken in 1970 when the Carl T. Sanders Research and Education Building opened on Laney Walker Boulevard. The 303,000-square-foot building was designed for basic science instruction. The next year the first permanent home for the School of Dentistry was opened at the corner of Fifteenth Street and Laney Walker Boulevard. For the previous seven years, classes had been taught in two small buildings the faculty

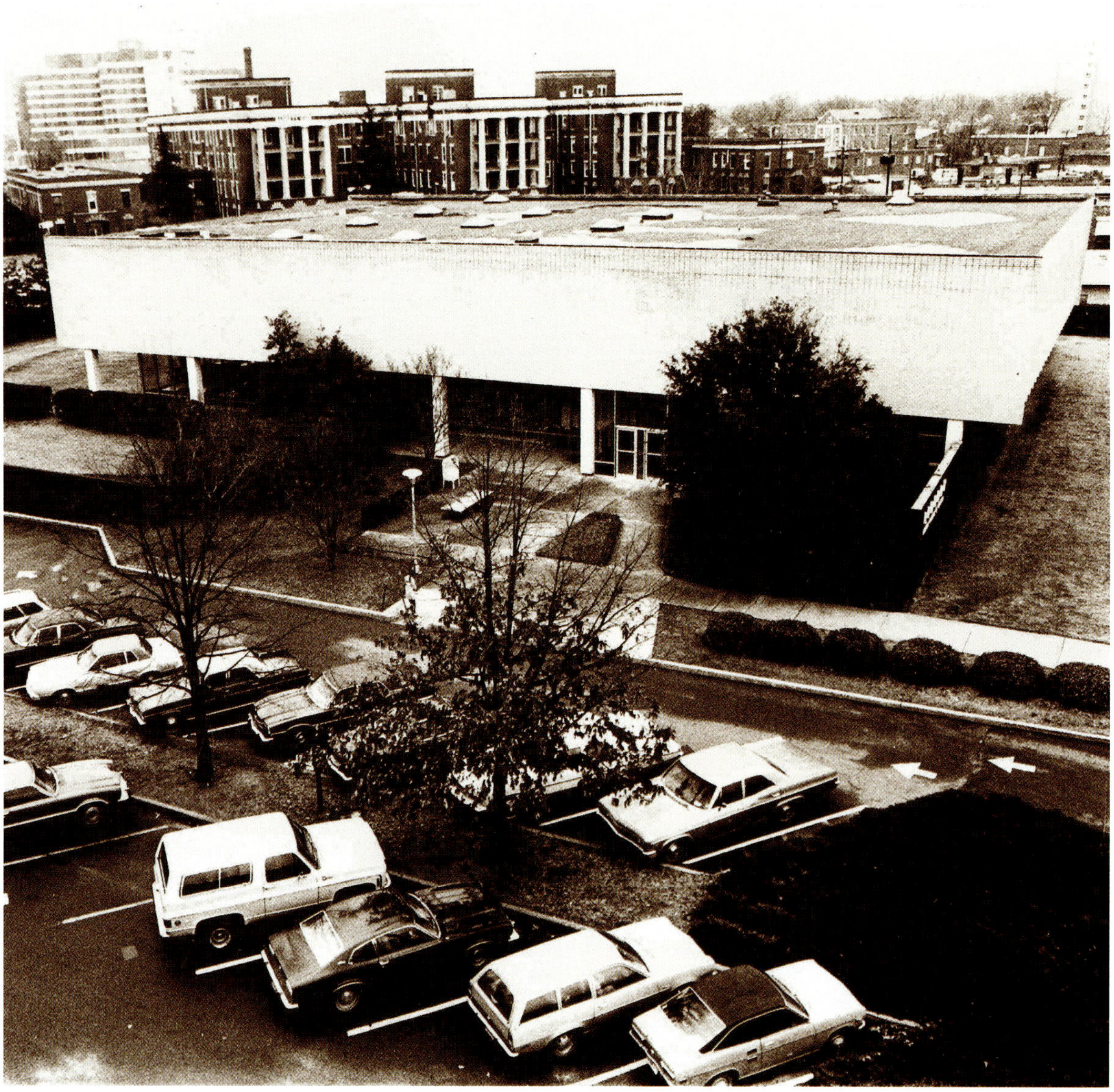

*When the building opened in 1963, it was the first in the school's history to be devoted solely to a library. Later it was expanded and named in honor of Robert B. Greenblatt, MD, eminent physician, scholar, and researcher. In addition to the regular holdings are the historical manuscripts, books, and artifacts in Historical Collections and Archives.*

affectionately called "trailers." In 1973, the City of Augusta sold the old University Hospital facility to MCG. While the majority of the complex was demolished, two wings were saved and renovated: the Milton Antony Wing, which became the Walter L. Shepeard Building, and the Jennings Wing, which became the Jennings Building, named for William D. Jennings Jr., a 1902 graduate who also served as Augusta's mayor.

The late 1970s and early 1980s saw several notable campus additions. The 1976 opening of the hospital's Virgil P. Sydenstricker Wing added 240 beds and doubled the hospital's research potential. The William F. Hamilton Wing was added to the Sanders Research and Education Building in 1979. A year later, an addition was made to the library, increasing its size and enabling computer-aided instruction.

Growth continued unabated in the 1990s. The Ambulatory Care Center and Specialized Care Center, which included the hospital's emergency room and intensive care units, were added to the

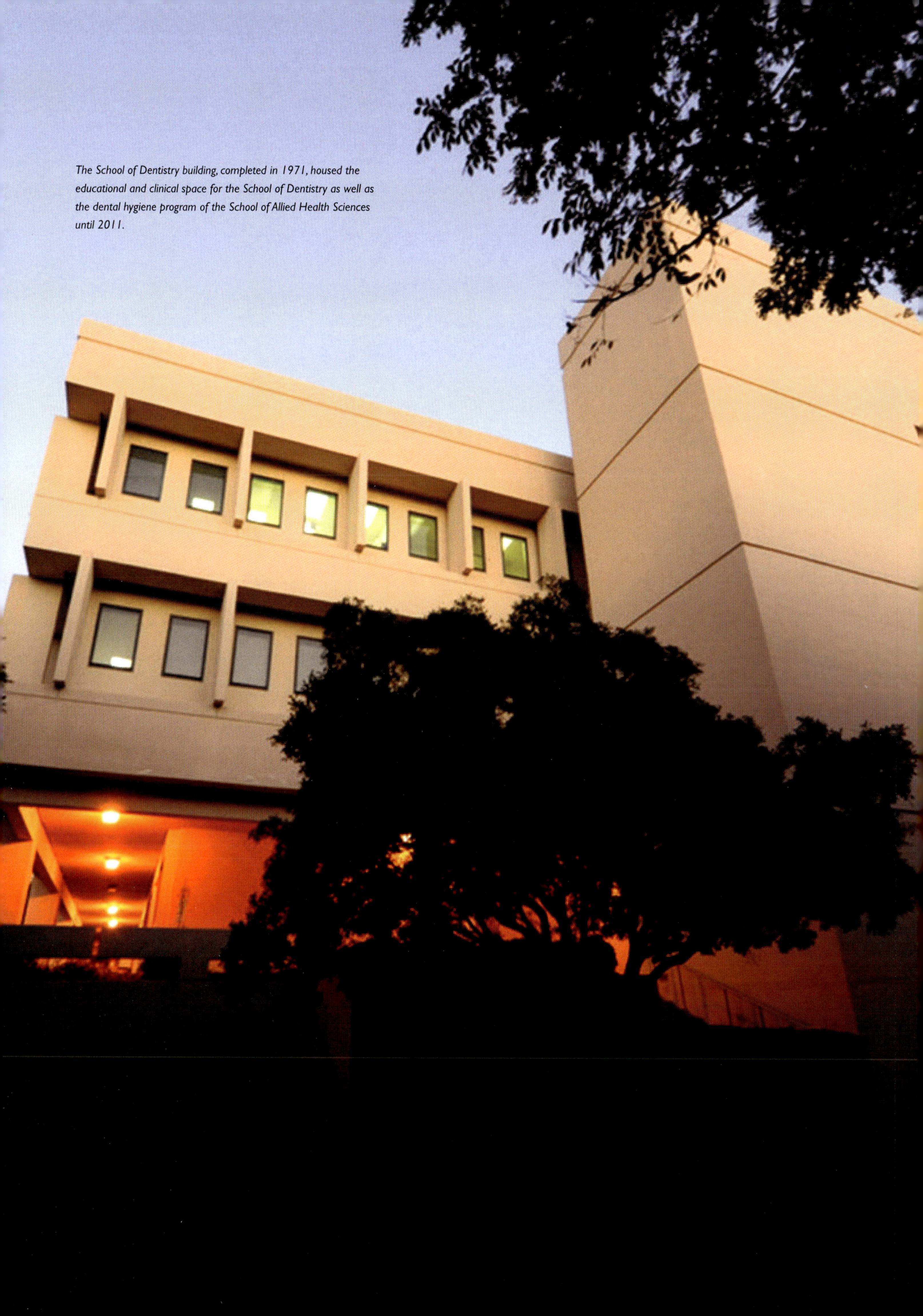

*The School of Dentistry building, completed in 1971, housed the educational and clinical space for the School of Dentistry as well as the dental hygiene program of the School of Allied Health Sciences until 2011.*

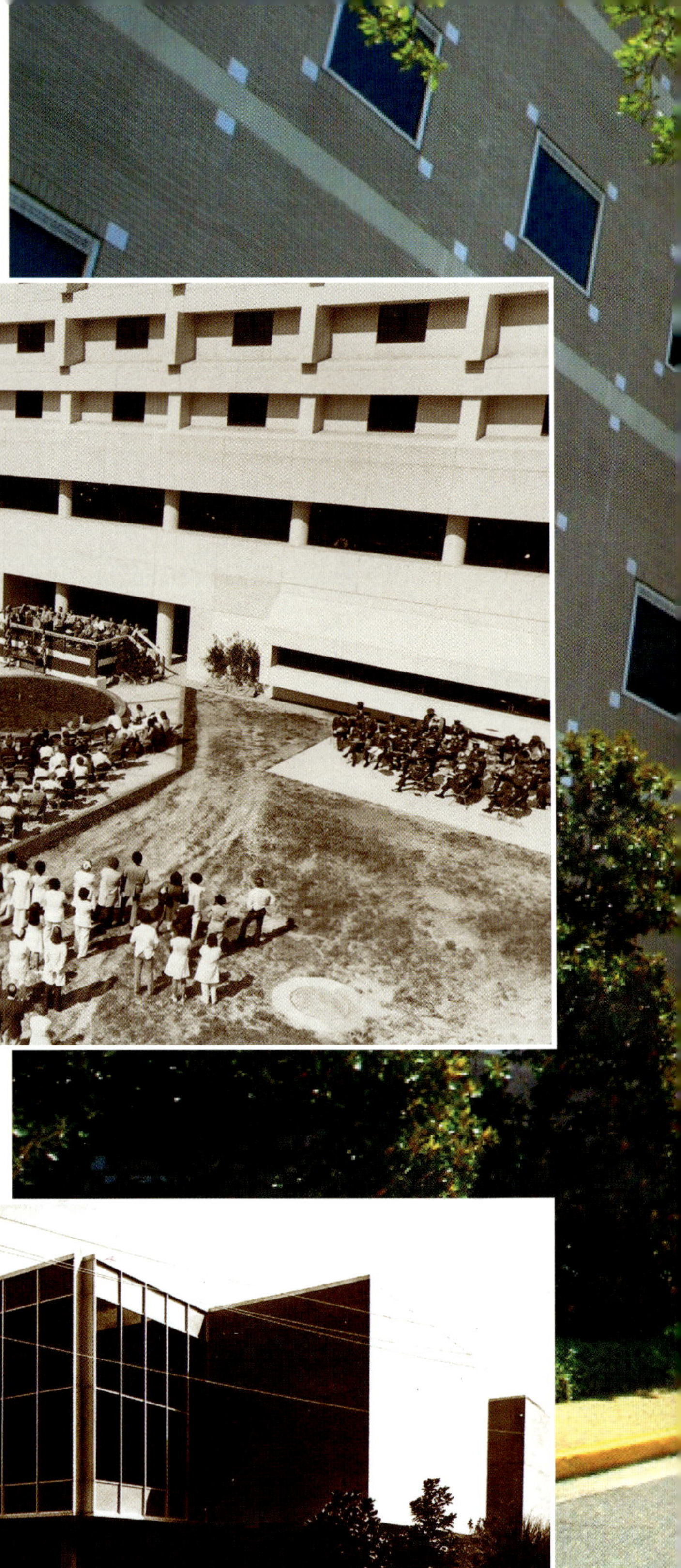

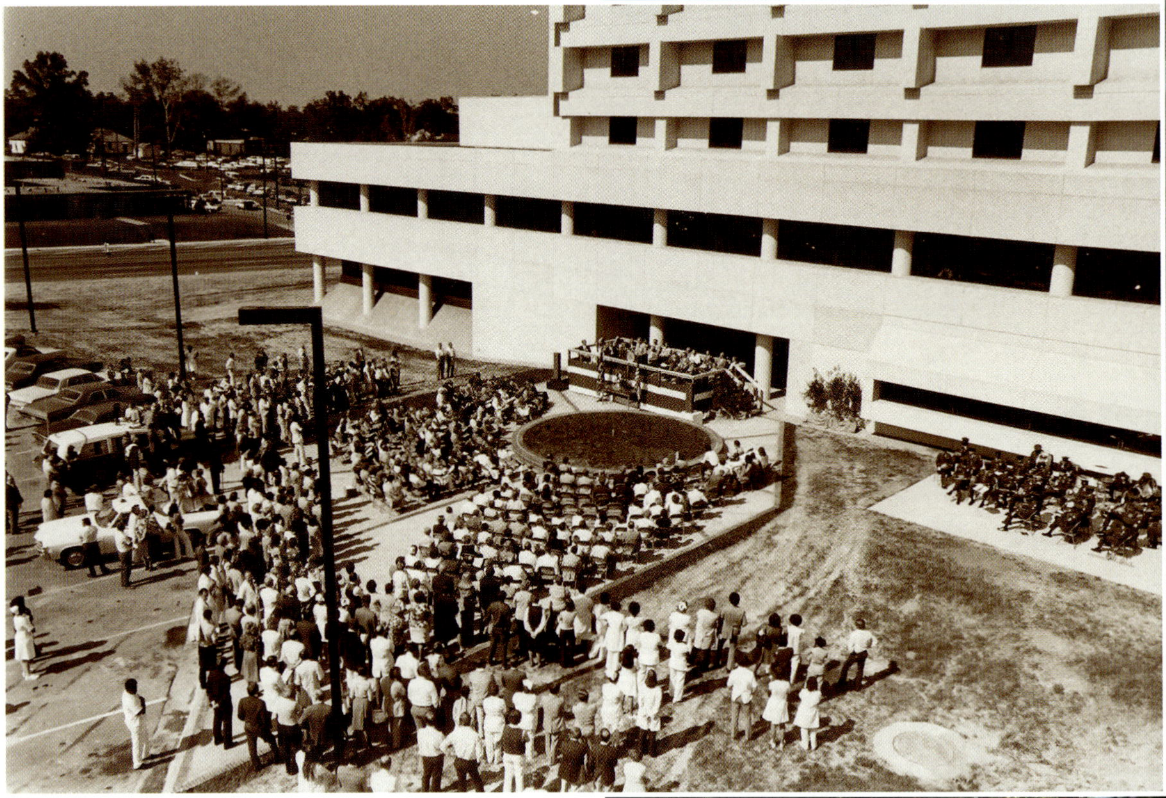

*The Sydenstricker Wing, opened in 1976, was named in memory of Dr. Virgil P. Sydenstricker. The eight-story building increased the patient bed capacity by over two hundred.*

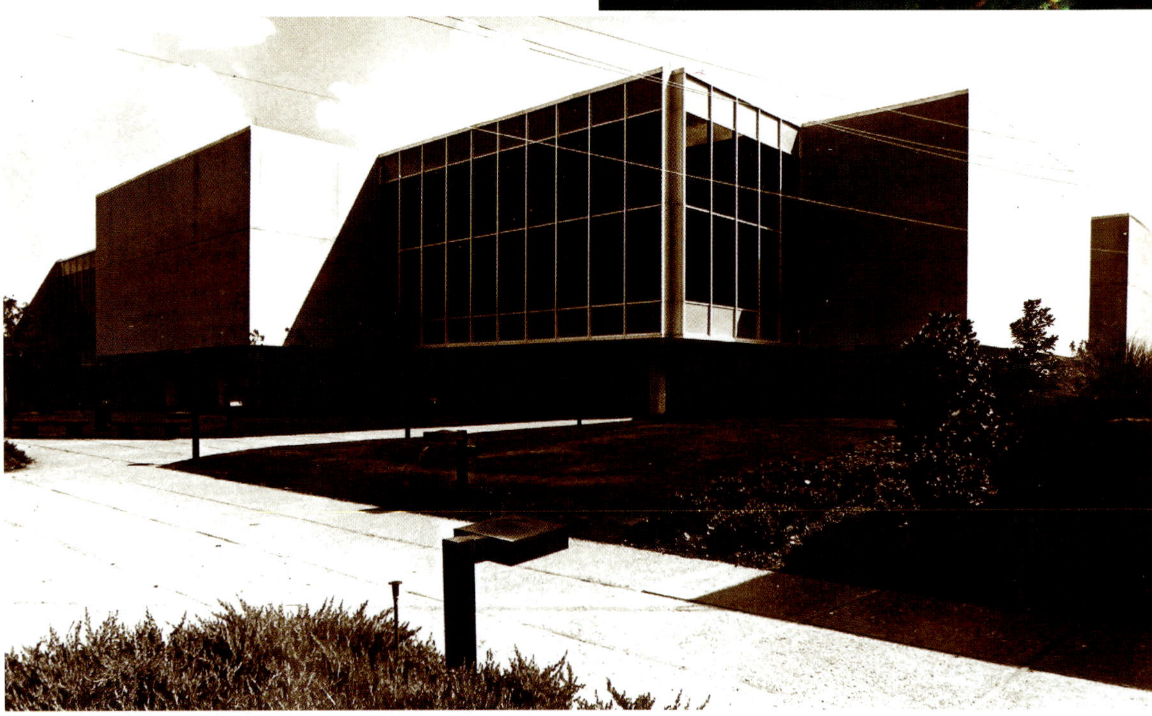

*Named for the father of seventy-fourth Georgia governor, Carl E. Sanders, the Carl T. Sanders Research and Education building became home to basic sciences and associated research departments, as well as modern classroom space for medical students.*

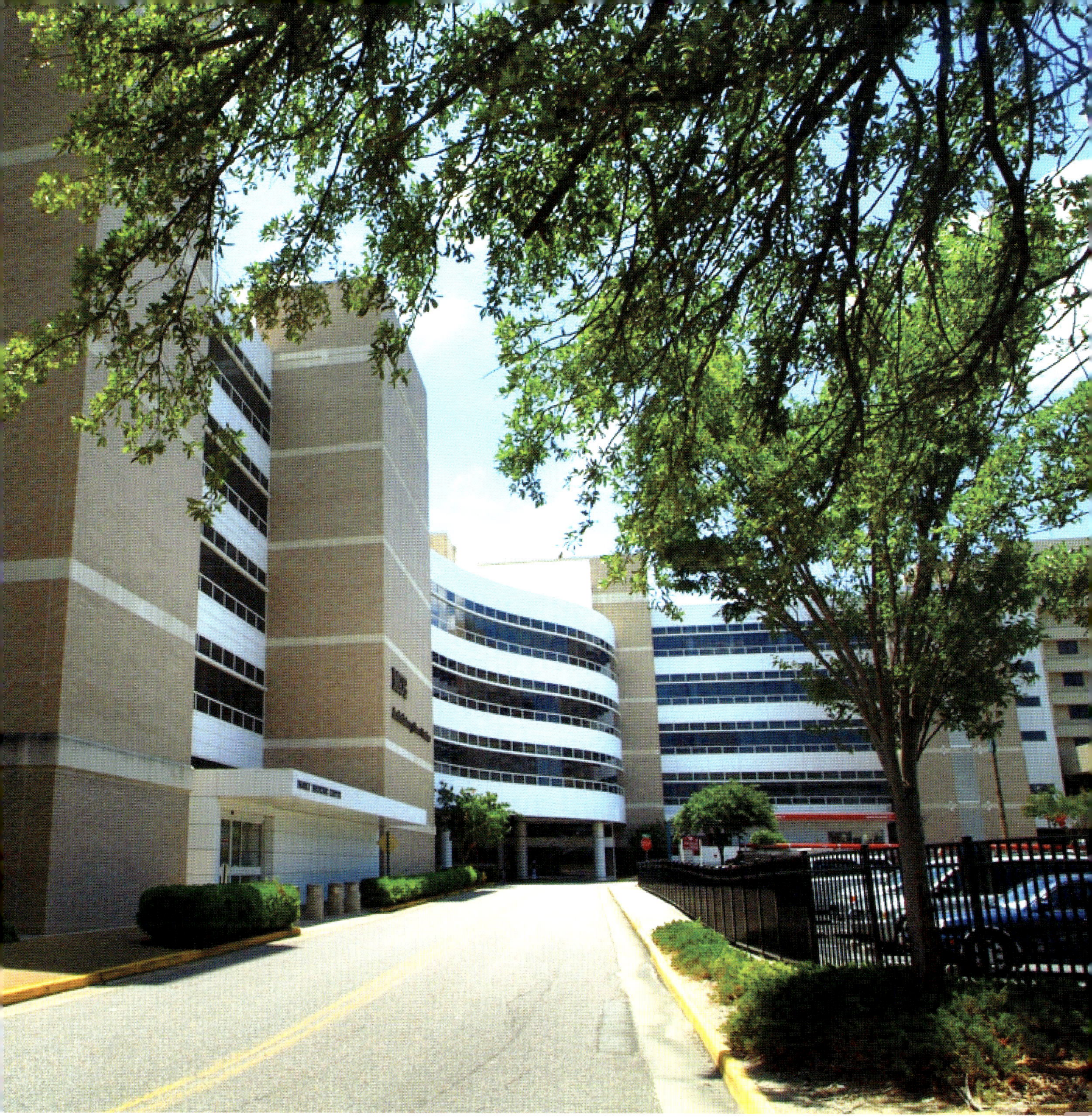

*The Ambulatory Care and Specialized Care Centers opened in 1992–1993, adding over 365,000 square feet to the patient-care complex. An emergency room, trauma center, outpatient clinics, and four twelve-bed intensive care units were added to the Specialized Care Center in December 1992. The ACC, which consolidated over eighty-eight outpatient clinics, was occupied in 1993.*

hospital in 1992–1993. Additionally, the Children's Medical Center (now Children's Hospital of Georgia) was opened to focus on children's needs while providing family-centered care. As research programs grew, the Interdisciplinary Research Building opened in 1995 to supplement existing facilities. The original facility featured an adaptable design to meet the university's changing needs.

In its last decade before the consolidation, the medical college added several significant structures to its campus. The Wellness Center, a 2003

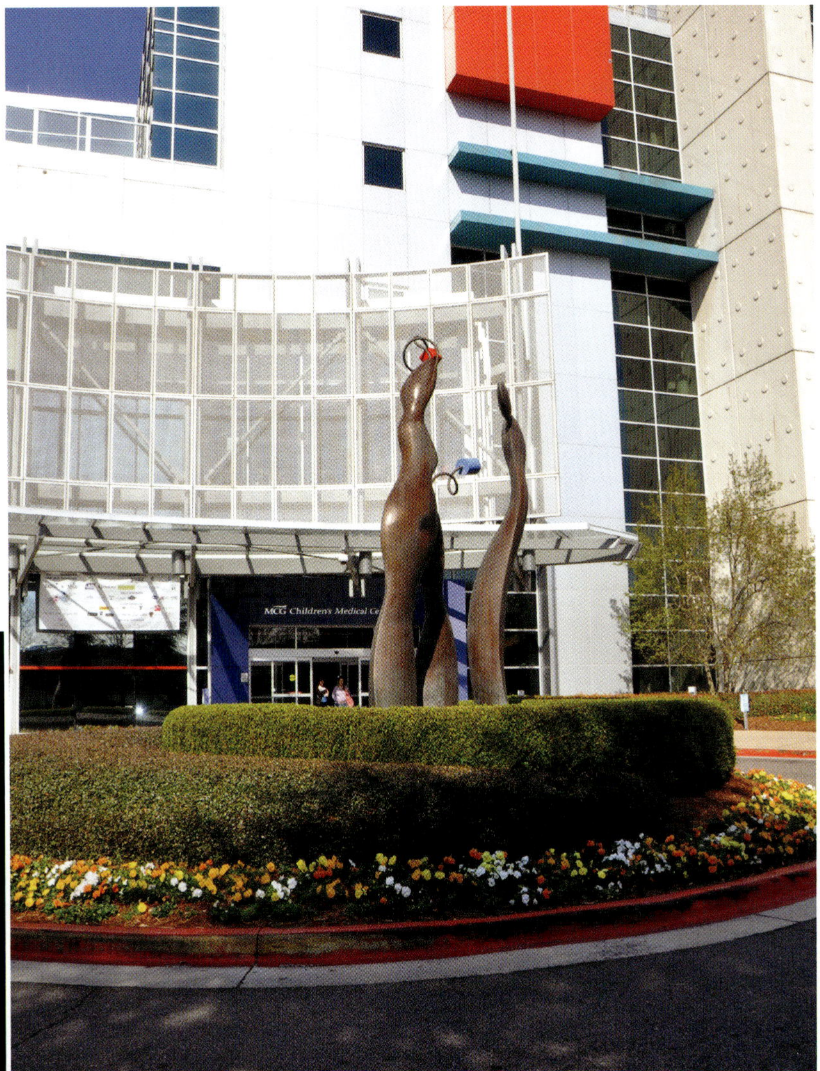

*Left: The Children's Medical Center (now the Children's Hospital of Georgia) opened in 1998. With over 150 beds dedicated exclusively to children from birth through adolescence, the hospital is focused on patient family-centered care. It houses the area's only pediatric trauma center.*

*Below: The Interdisciplinary Research Building, opened in 1995, included thirty research laboratories and office support space. The 2004 addition, which almost doubled the building's size, included biotechnology incubation, additional research laboratories, and the Department of Physiology.*

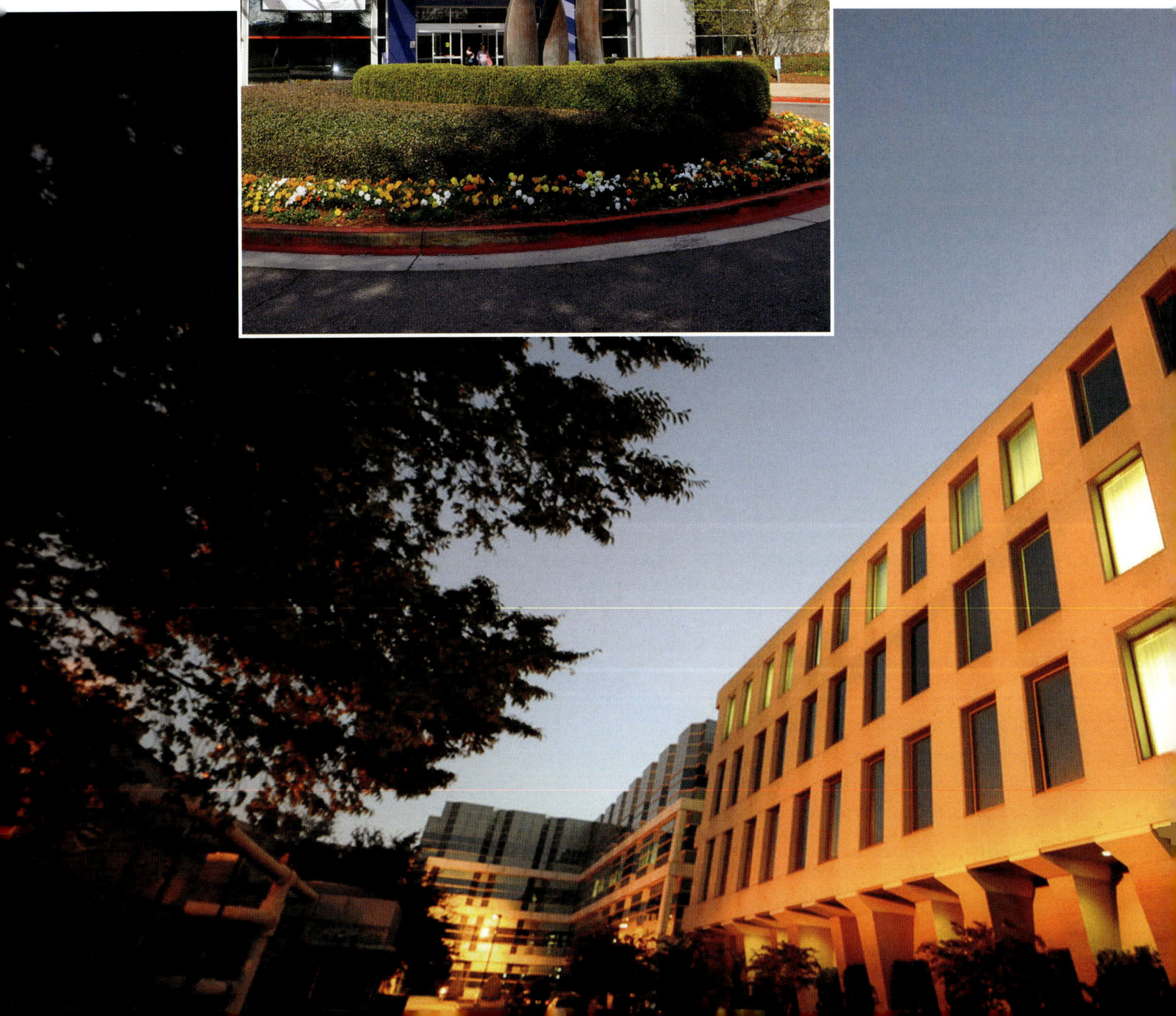

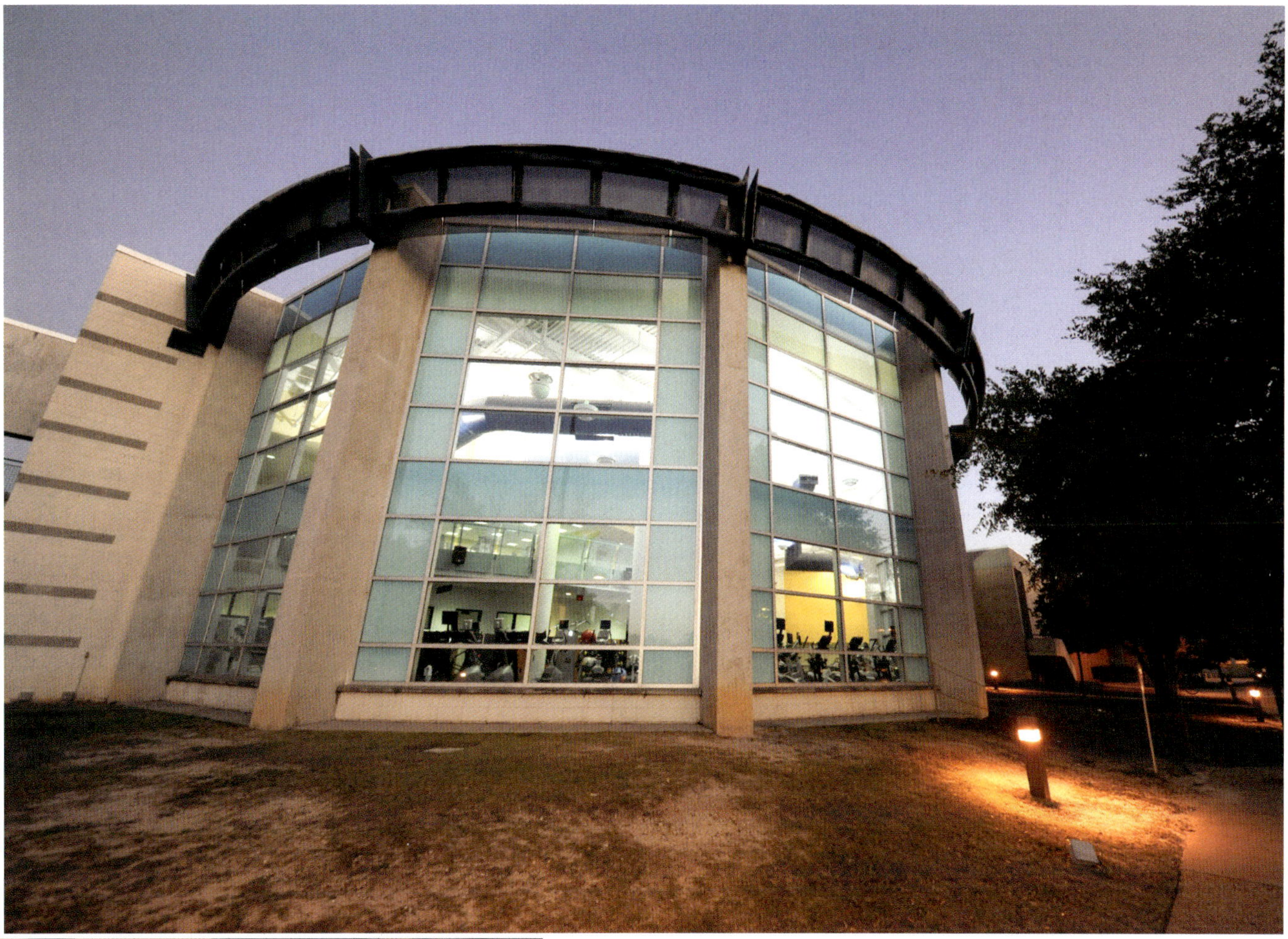

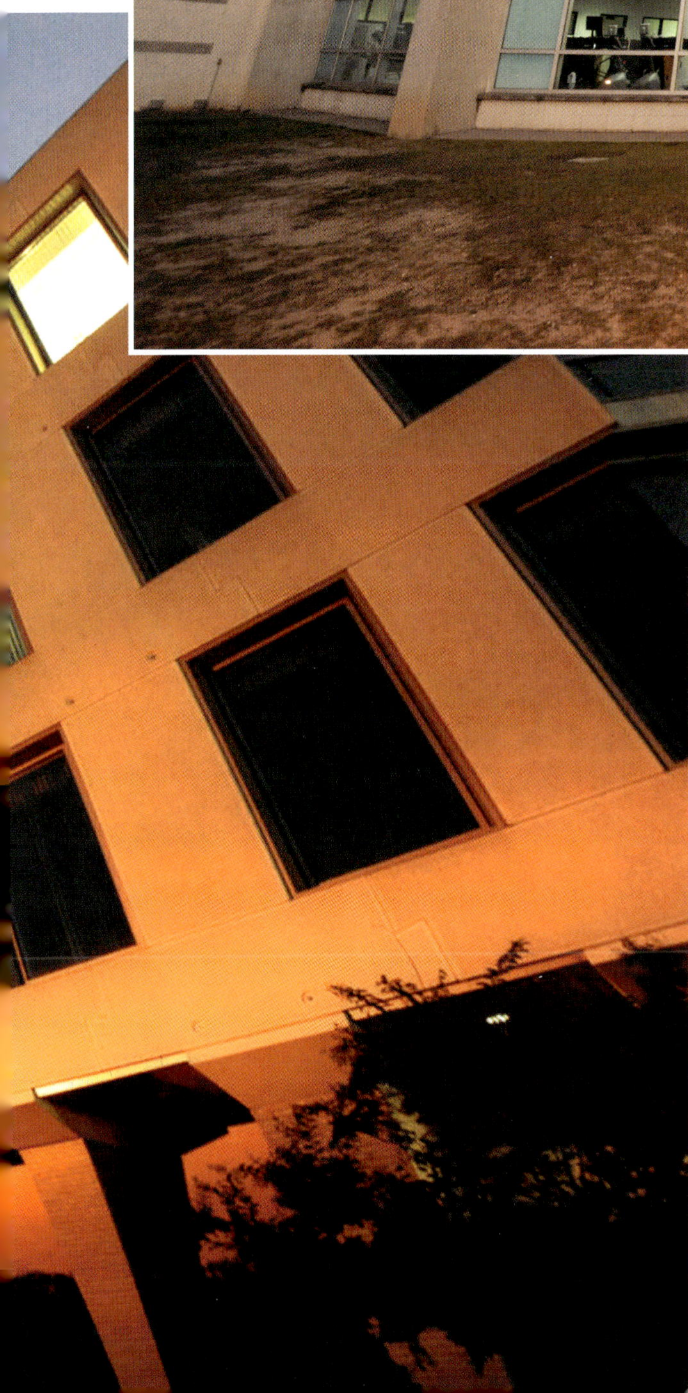

*The Wellness Center was a welcome addition to the Student Center in 2003. With state-of-the-art fitness equipment, as well as basketball courts, weight rooms, and a walking/jogging track, the center is open to all students, faculty, staff, and their families.*

addition to the Student Center, featured basketball courts, weight rooms, and a jogging track. During the 2004 Homecoming festivities, the four-story Interdisciplinary Research Building Phase II opened. The Cancer Research Center and the Health Sciences Building opened in 2006 and 2007, respectively. The GRU Cancer Center, a treatment facility designed with participation from cancer survivors, opened in 2010.

With $10 million from the City of Augusta for the purchase and clearing of the land, MCG acquired an adjoining fifteen-acre Gilbert Manor public housing complex for a new College of Dental Medicine

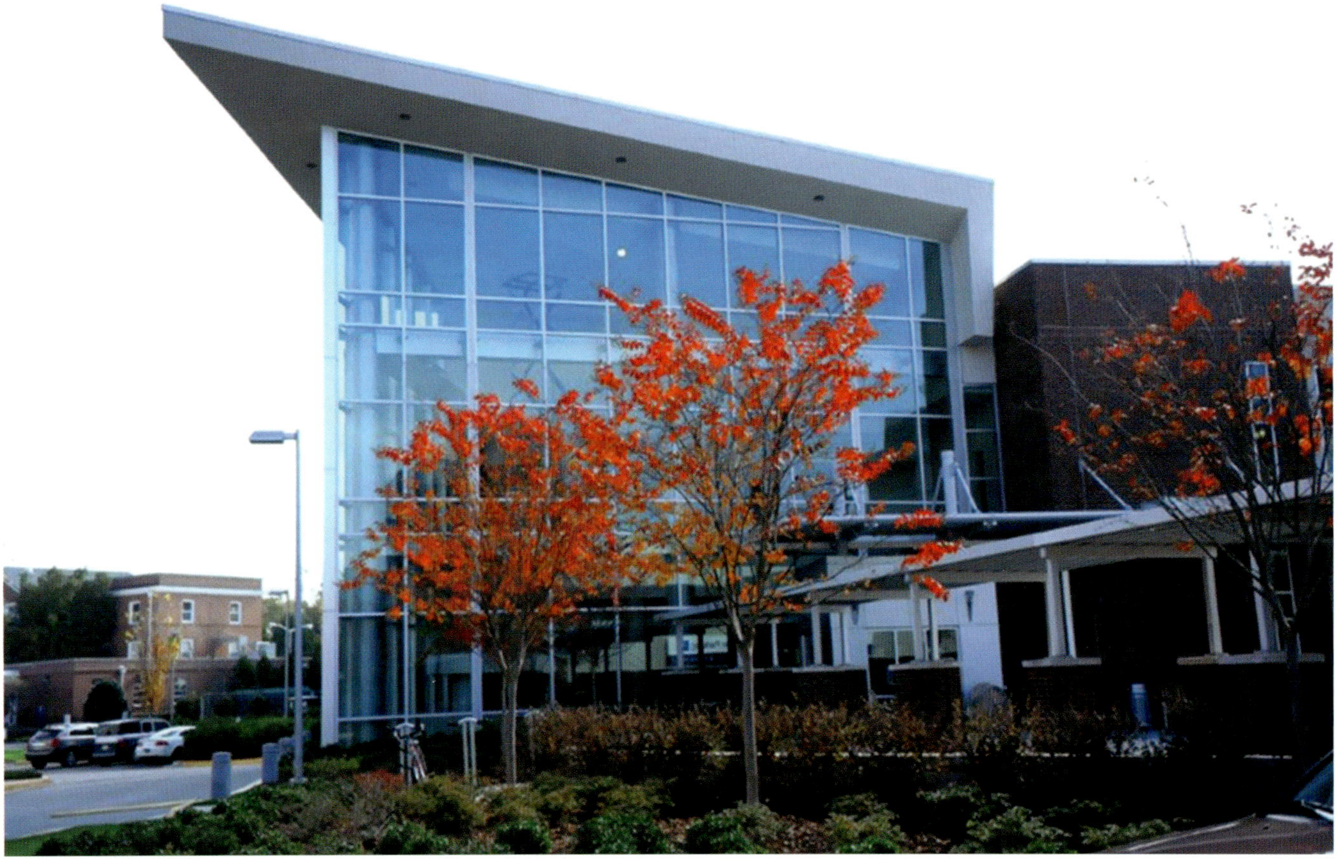

*The Cancer Research Center opened in 2006 and four years later was joined by the Cancer Treatment Center. Developed with input from cancer survivors, the treatment center features a patient-focused, multi-disciplinary team approach.*

*The new College of Dental Medicine building opened in 2011 accommodating approximately 350 dental students and sixty dental residents per year.*

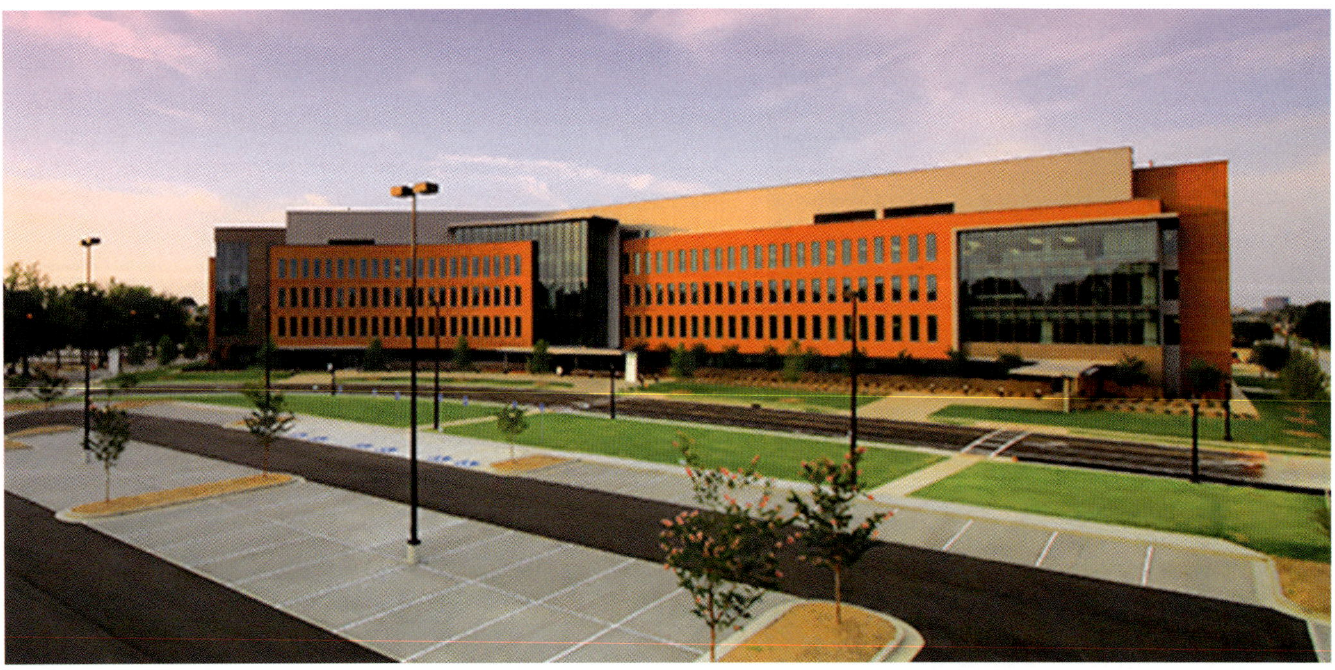

building, which opened in 2011. Construction began in November 2012 on a three-story, interdisciplinary academic building and simulation center named the J. Harold Harrison, MD, Education Commons Building, located on a portion of the former Gilbert Manor property.

Augusta State University also experienced remarkable growth from its more humble start in 1926 when the Junior College of Augusta (JCA) and the Academy of Richmond County (ARC) jointly moved into a new facility on Baker Avenue. In 1957, the junior college, having outgrown its space, moved to the former Augusta Arsenal property on Walton Way.

Purchased from Freeman Walker in the mid-1820s, the property had been home to the arsenal since its move, brick by brick, from the Savannah River in 1827. The seventy-two-acre arsenal had been

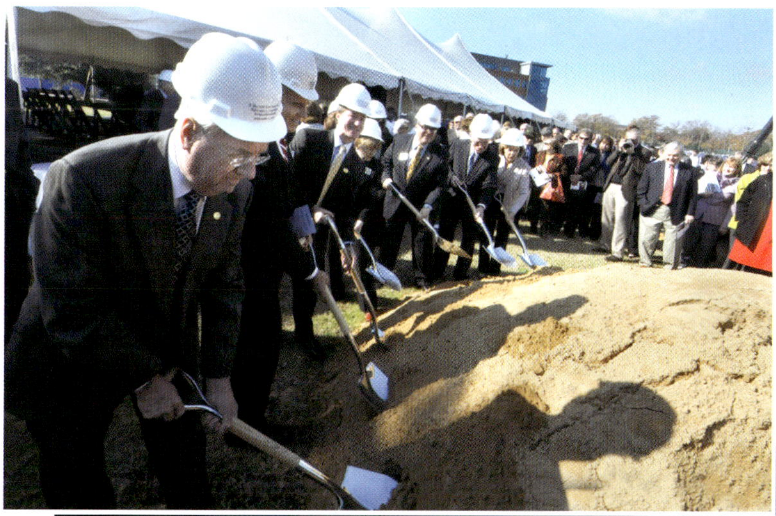

*Left: In November 2012, construction got underway on a 172,000-square-foot building to house facilities for the medical and dental colleges. The J. Harold Harrison, MD, Education Commons is named in honor of the late Dr. Harrison, a renowned vascular surgeon.*

*Below: Four original 1827–1829 arsenal buildings became the home to the JCA in 1957. Benet House (pictured) is a National Historic Landmark, recognizing its importance as the boyhood home of Pulitzer Prize-winning poet laureate Stephen Vincent Benet, whose father commanded the arsenal in the early twentieth century. Rains Hall bears the name of George Washington Rains, arsenal commandant during the Civil War, and after the war, regent at ARC, MCG faculty member, and dean.*

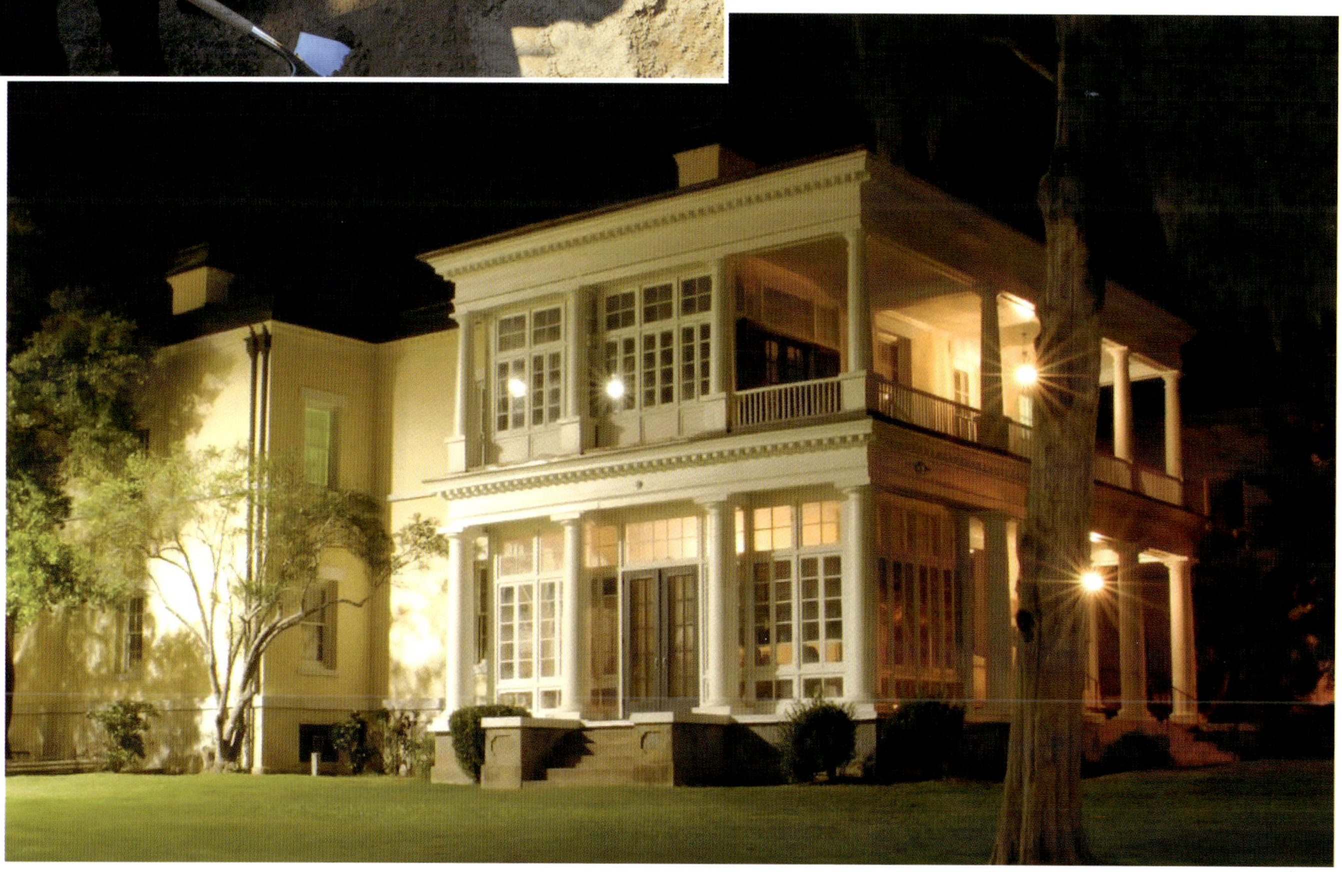

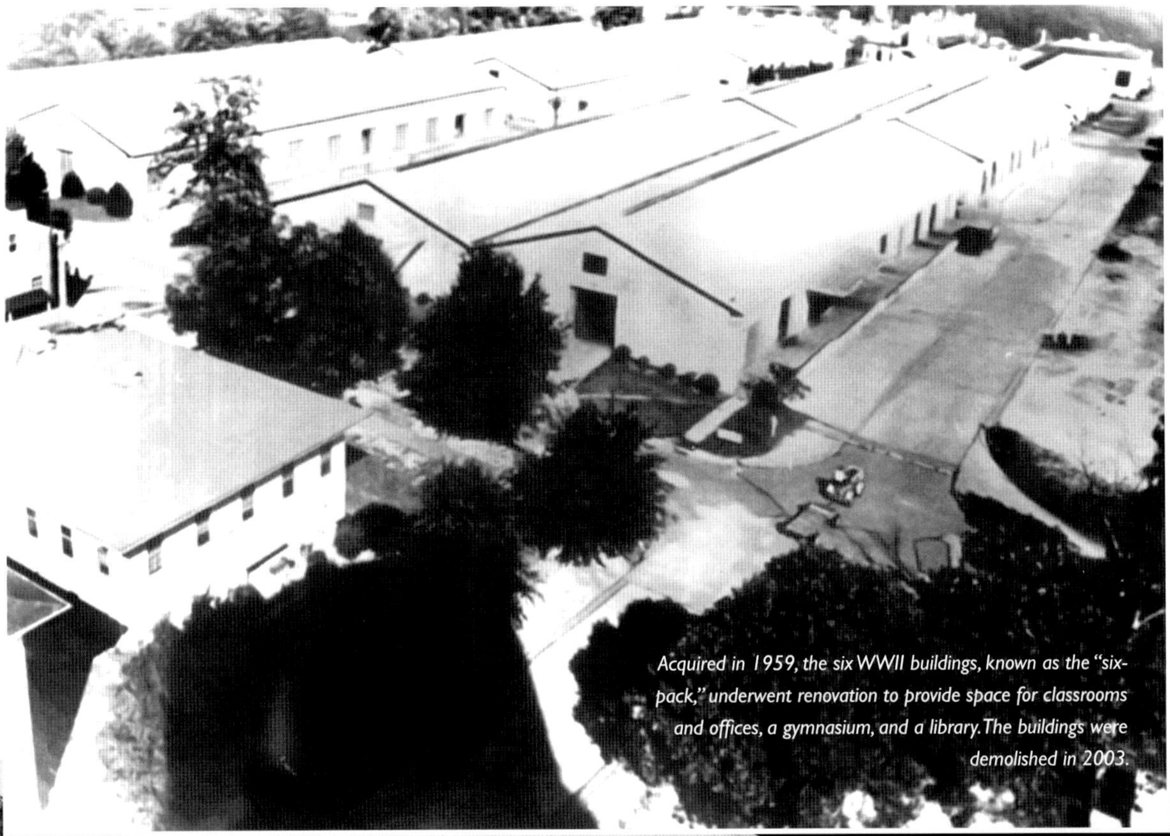

Acquired in 1959, the six WWII buildings, known as the "six-pack," underwent renovation to provide space for classrooms and offices, a gymnasium, and a library. The buildings were demolished in 2003.

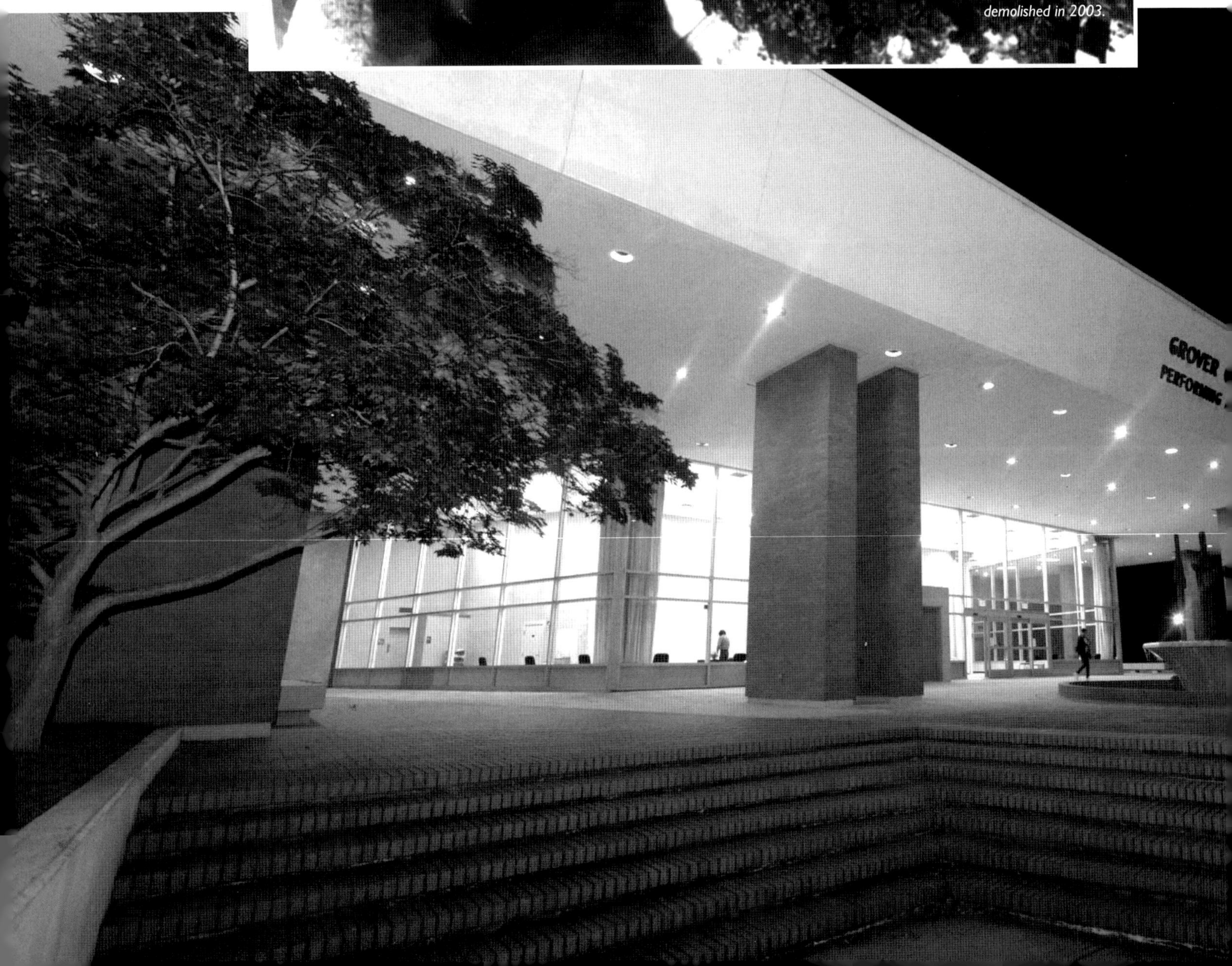

decommissioned in 1955. With help from then State Senator Carl Sanders and other political leaders, negotiations with the federal government led to the acquisition of the property for the JCA. Initially, only a 38.21-acre parcel holding forty-six buildings was transferred, including the four original 1827–1829 arsenal buildings, which were transformed for college use. Before classes began, nine additional acres had been acquired.

In 1958, the JCA joined the University System of Georgia and became Augusta College (AC). The following year AC acquired a fifteen-acre parcel containing six large World War II-era warehouses which, after renovations, provided most of the academic space for nearly fifty years. Three of the warehouses opened in 1960 housing the student center, library, and science facilities. A fourth warehouse became the long-awaited gymnasium in 1962. In 1965, the fifth warehouse was transformed into a classroom building and a second floor was added to the library. Renovations on the sixth warehouse were finally completed in 1975.

The 1960s saw the first new construction when, in 1968, the Fine Arts Center and the Performing Arts Theatre were the first buildings constructed specifically for academic use. Also in 1968, work began on the conversion of the large arsenal optic shop into a four-story student center (now Washington Hall) as well as on a 1941 warehouse to house a swimming pool.

In the early 1970s, AC received two important property donations: the 1900 home of Georgia Supreme Court Justice Boykin Wright, a gift from

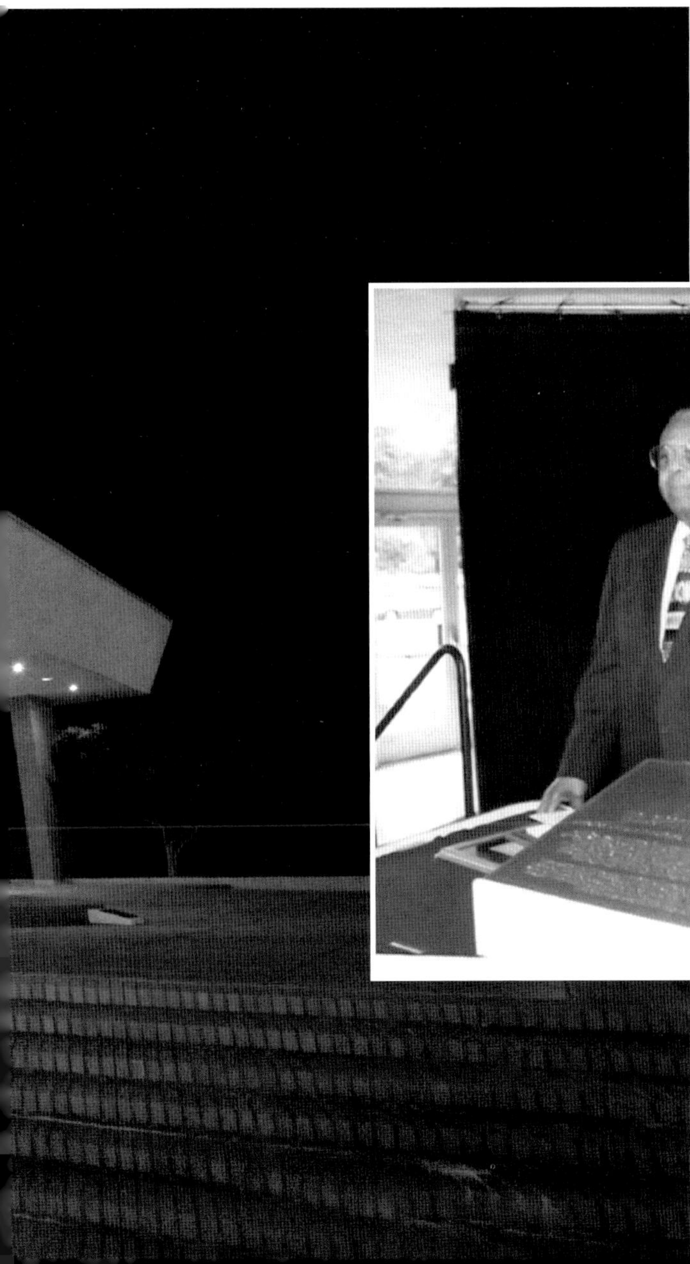

*Left: The 1968 Performing Arts Theatre was named in honor of Grover C. Maxwell in 1983. It provides over seven hundred seats for concerts, lectures, and theatrical performances.*

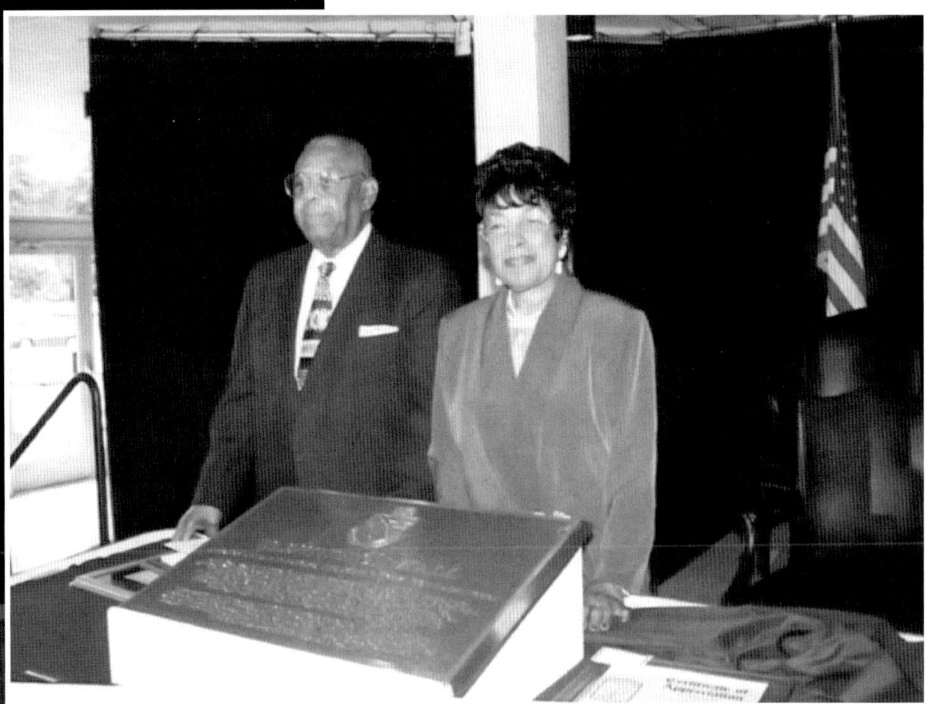

*Below: The College Activity Center opened in 1968 following conversion from the arsenal optic shop into a student center with support offices. In 1997, it was renamed Washington Hall to honor community educators and leaders Drs. Isaiah and Justine Washington.*

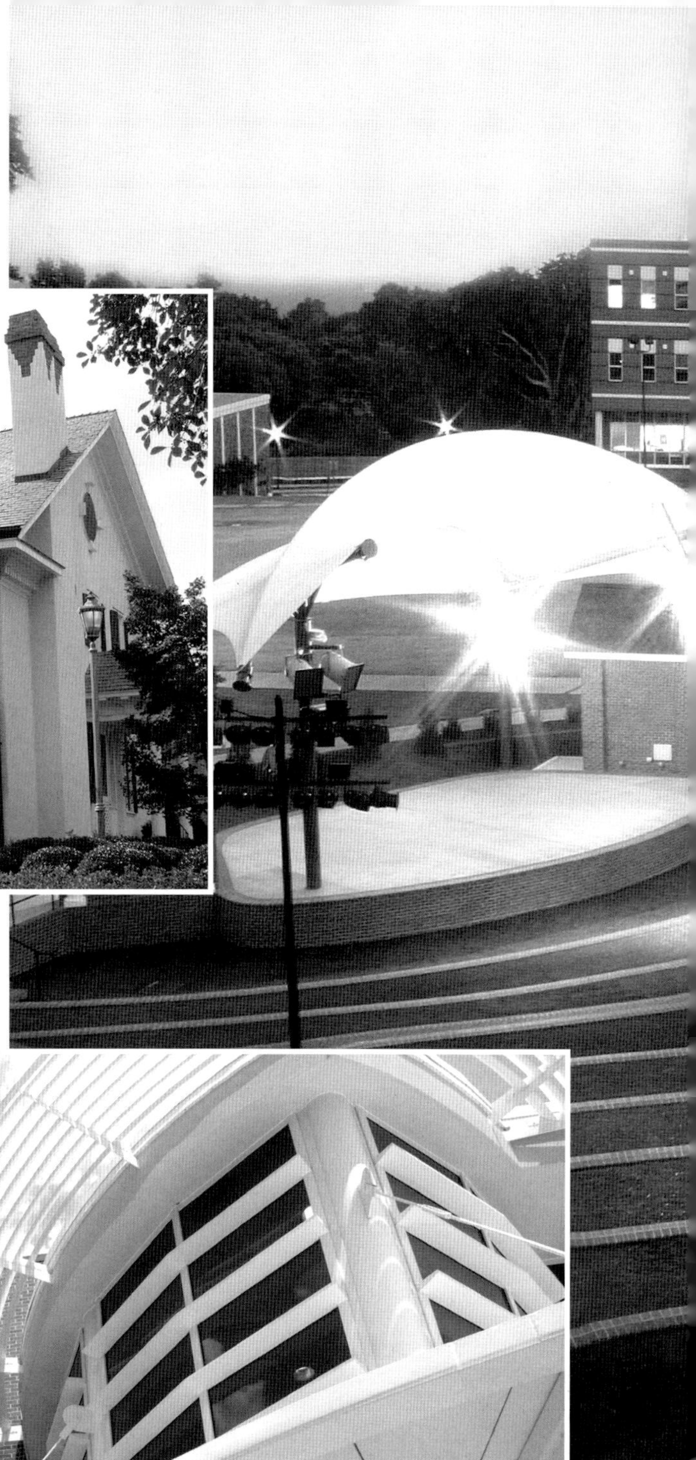

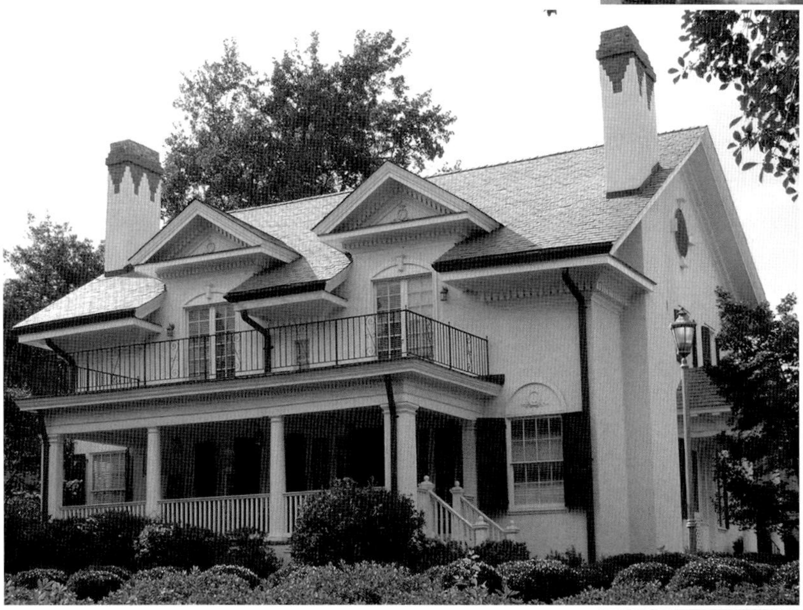

*In the early 1970s, the estate of Jefferson Maxwell donated his home to Augusta College. Among other things, it served for years as the alumni house and hosted many alumni, university, and community events.*

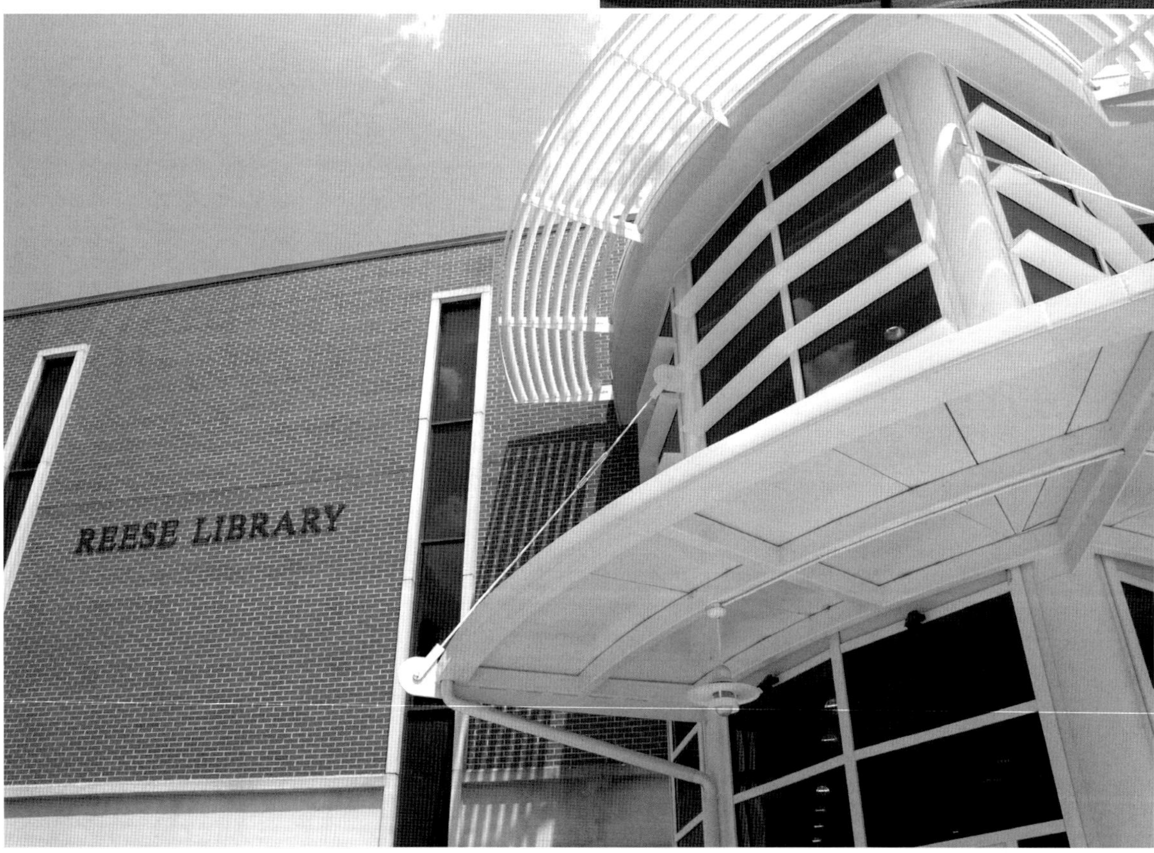


*The Reese Library opened in 1977 representing a significant expansion of space for both library resources and study space for students. In 2006, the Jaguar Student Activities Center opened, housing dining facilities, a fitness center, meeting rooms, lounges, and a ballroom. Because of the uniquely designed atrium that connected the two buildings, the following year the university received the University System's Real Estate Award.*

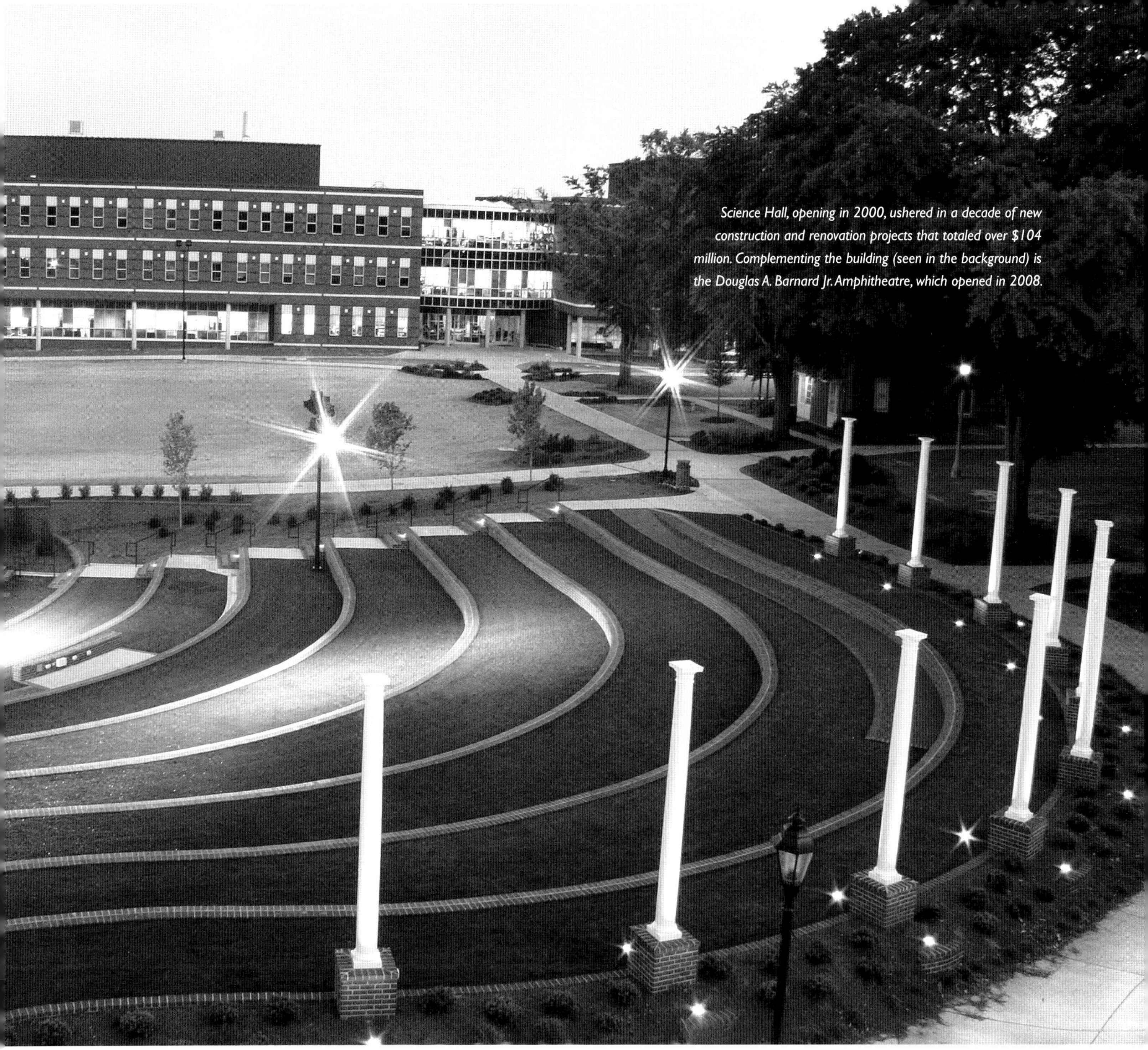

*Science Hall, opening in 2000, ushered in a decade of new construction and renovation projects that totaled over $104 million. Complementing the building (seen in the background) is the Douglas A. Barnard Jr. Amphitheatre, which opened in 2008.*

Marguerite Wright Hillman in memory of her father, and the 1917 home of Jefferson Maxwell, a gift of his estate. In the '70s, campus buildings received names—academic buildings were named in honor of former college presidents and the four original arsenal buildings honored former commandants. The college had long needed a larger library and in 1977 the Reese Library opened, named in honor of the parents of alumna and benefactor Katherine Reese Pamplin. That same year the college acquired the last tract and building (now Galloway Hall) of the arsenal property, then in use by the U.S. Army Reserve Training Center.

For twenty years there was no new construction on the Walton Way campus of AC. Then in 1997 the Board of Regents authorized construction of a new science building. The building was the first in what would be over $104 million in new construction and renovations occurring over the next decade. While the Science Building was under construction, a highly publicized account of the asbestos roofs on the six warehouses-turned-academic buildings led to the Board of Regents fast-tracking two new classroom facilities to replace the old structures. The first, Allgood Hall, opened in 2002, followed by University Hall in 2004.

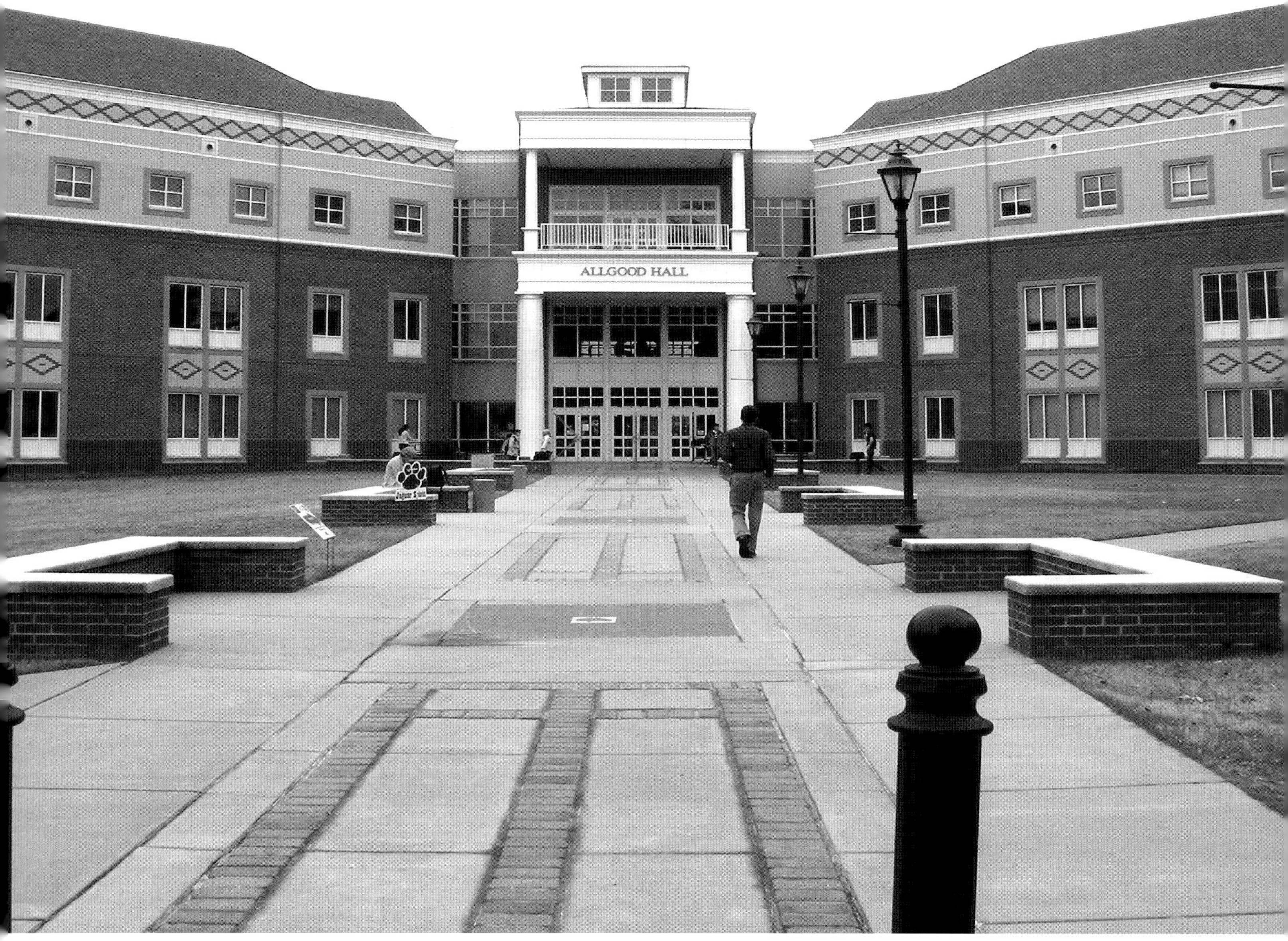


*Allgood Hall, named for alumnus, former state senator, and member of the Board of Regents Thomas F. Allgood and his wife Thelma "T", opened in 2002, providing classrooms, study spaces, and faculty offices.*

In addition to classroom and faculty office space, the early twenty-first century brought other improvements to campus. University Hall's funding package also included demolition of the six-pack academic buildings, as well as a new, redesigned Walton Way campus entrance, featuring an arch and a nineteen-foot-tall, three-tier, wrought-iron fountain. In 2003, the first of four phases of a History Walk opened, anchored by an 1870 guardhouse that underwent renovation into a museum. The year 2006 brought the addition of Jaguar Student Activities Center (JSAC), and two years later the D. Douglas Barnard Jr. Amphitheatre opened in the center of campus, providing an outdoor space for concerts and other activities. Both provided spaces for students to congregate, study, and relax between classes. The final phase of the History Walk through the center of campus was completed in 2011.

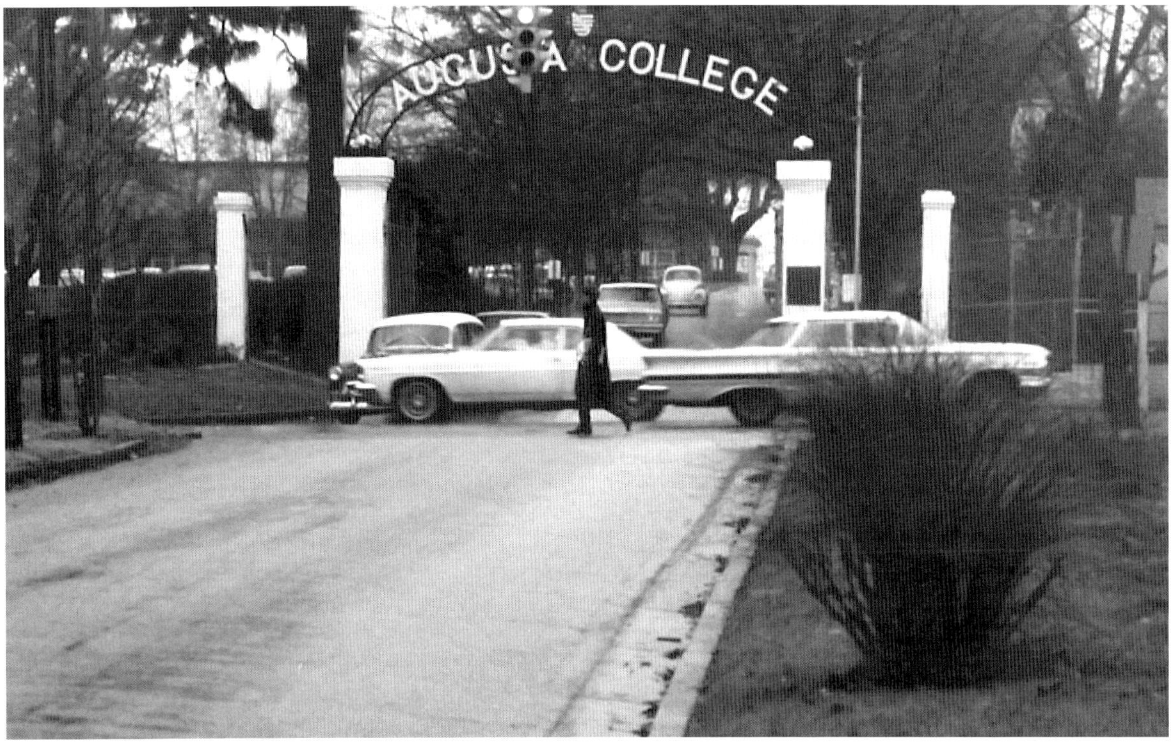


The narrow Walton Way entrance (above) was redesigned in 2002 featuring an arched entry and a three-tier fountain named in honor of Russell Blanchard, alumnus and founder of the AC Foundation (see image below).

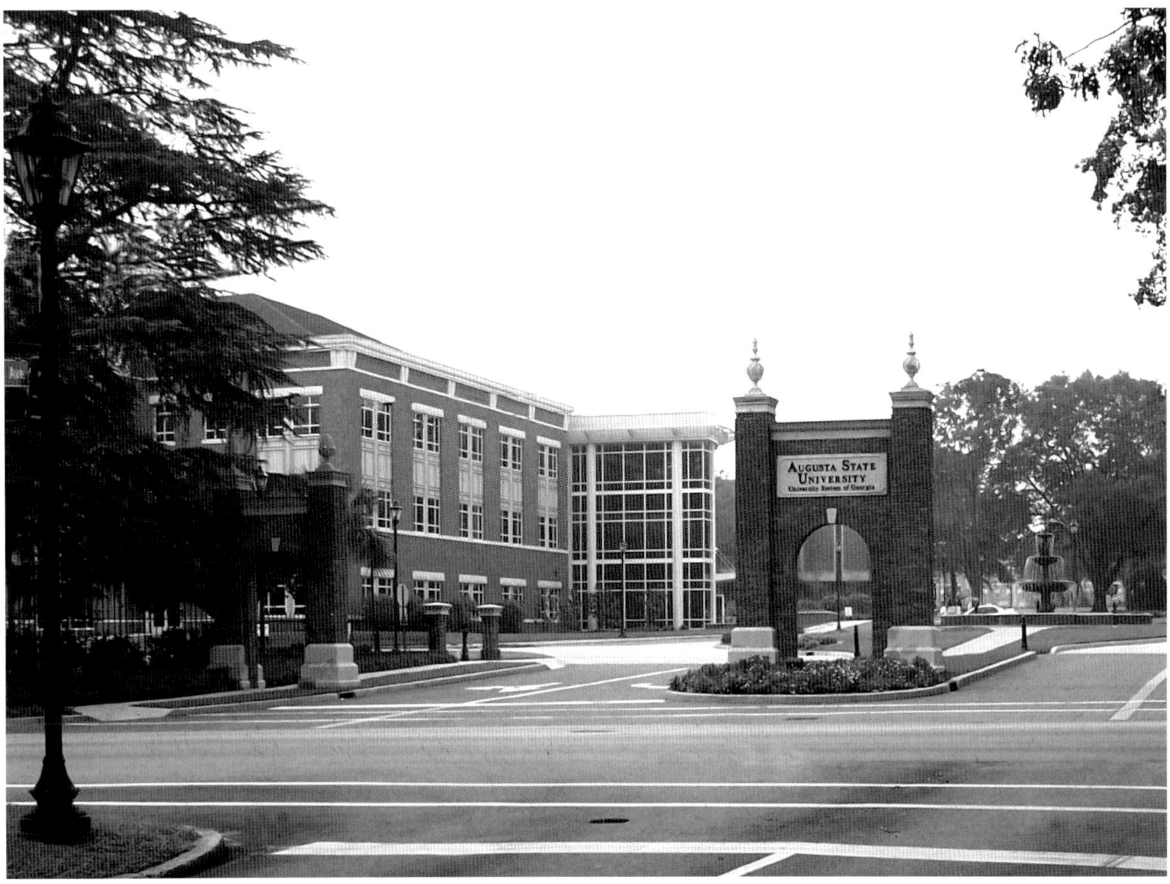

The Forest Hills campus, acquired in the 1970s, led to a second location for ASU. Originally the home of World War I's Camp Hancock until deactivation in 1918, a large tract became the site of the luxury Forrest Ricker Hotel in 1926. One of the hotel's amenities was an eighteen-hole golf course designed by famed architect Donald Ross. A tournament win there in 1930 by golfing great Bobby Jones began his famed Grand Slam of Golf, a feat later recognized with a historical marker at the course.

Confiscated by the federal government during World War II, the hotel was converted into Oliver General Hospital for wounded soldiers and later veterans; the adjoining course became the Armed Forces Golf Course. In 1977, the college acquired a portion of the property including the course, renaming it the Forest Hills Golf Club. The course adjoins the Physical Education/Athletic Complex, which opened in 1990, with an arena, walking track, weight room, classrooms, and offices. The complex was later renamed the Christenberry Fieldhouse in honor of former AC president George Christenberry. In 2005, a golf pavilion was added and two years later, a golf practice facility and the J. Fleming Norvell Collegiate Golf House. In front of the golf course on Magnolia Avenue is the university's Literacy Center.

The university also obtained additional property on the south side of Wrightsboro Road, along Damascus Road. Here a gated, twenty-four-acre, apartment-style complex known as University Village opened in 2005 to provide housing and amenities, including a swimming pool, walking trails, and a clubhouse.

The outlook for the continued growth of Georgia Regents' campuses in Augusta is bright and the university will soon expand beyond its current footprint. In 2012, Georgia Governor Nathan Deal approved the transfer of the Augusta Golf and Gardens property on the Savannah River in downtown Augusta to the University System of Georgia. Other locations in the downtown area are also being proposed for future development. All offer exciting possibilities for the future.

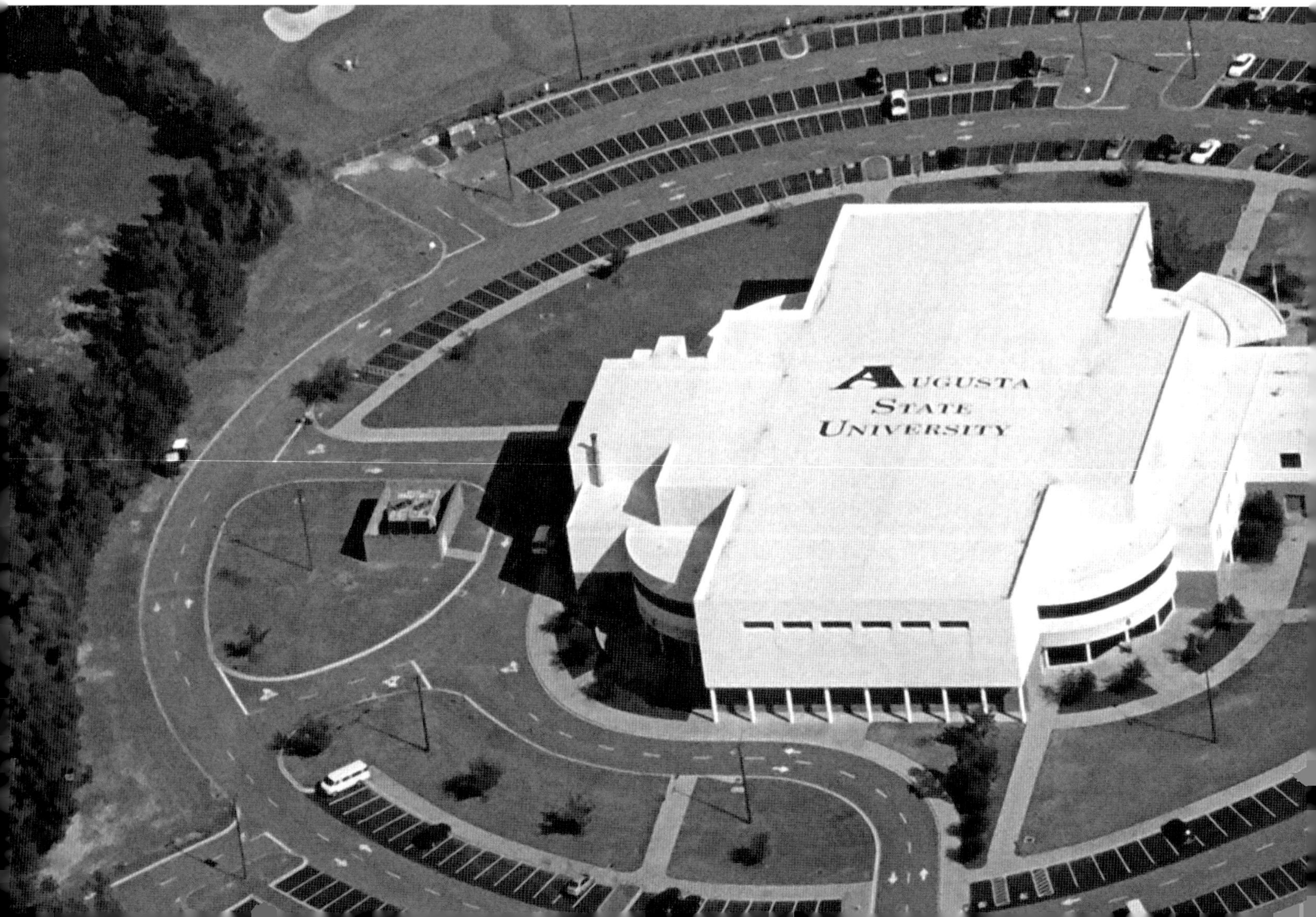

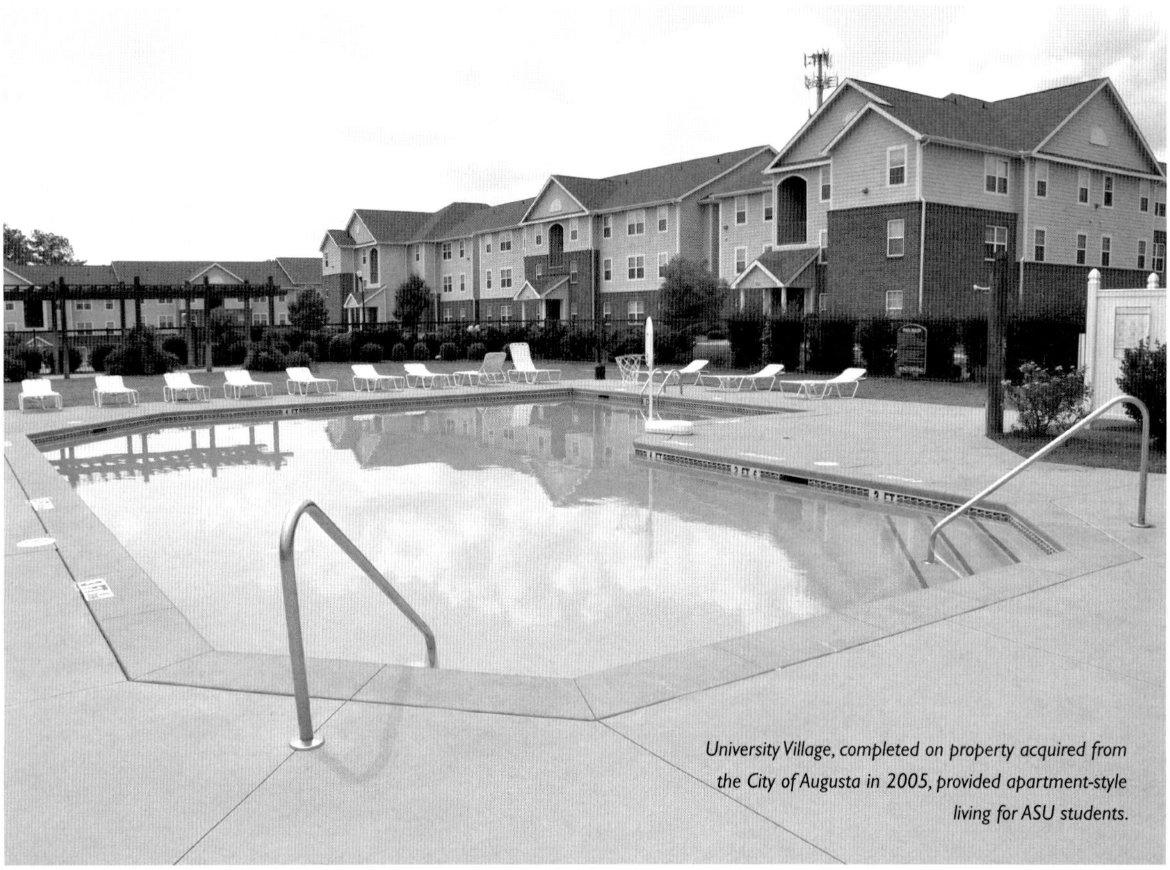

*University Village, completed on property acquired from the City of Augusta in 2005, provided apartment-style living for ASU students.*

*Left: The 1990 Physical Education/Athletic Complex was renamed Christenberry Fieldhouse in 2003 to honor former AC president George Christenberry. It holds a 3,026-seat arena, walking track, weight room, and a human physiology lab as well as space for kinesiology faculty and athletics staff. The complex also includes playing and practice fields.*

*Below: Named for ASU golf benefactor J. Fleming Norvell, the Collegiate Golf House and Practice Facility opened in 2007 on the Forest Hills Campus. Professional golfer Henrik Norlander (pictured in the foreground) was a member of the national championship Division I golf team.*

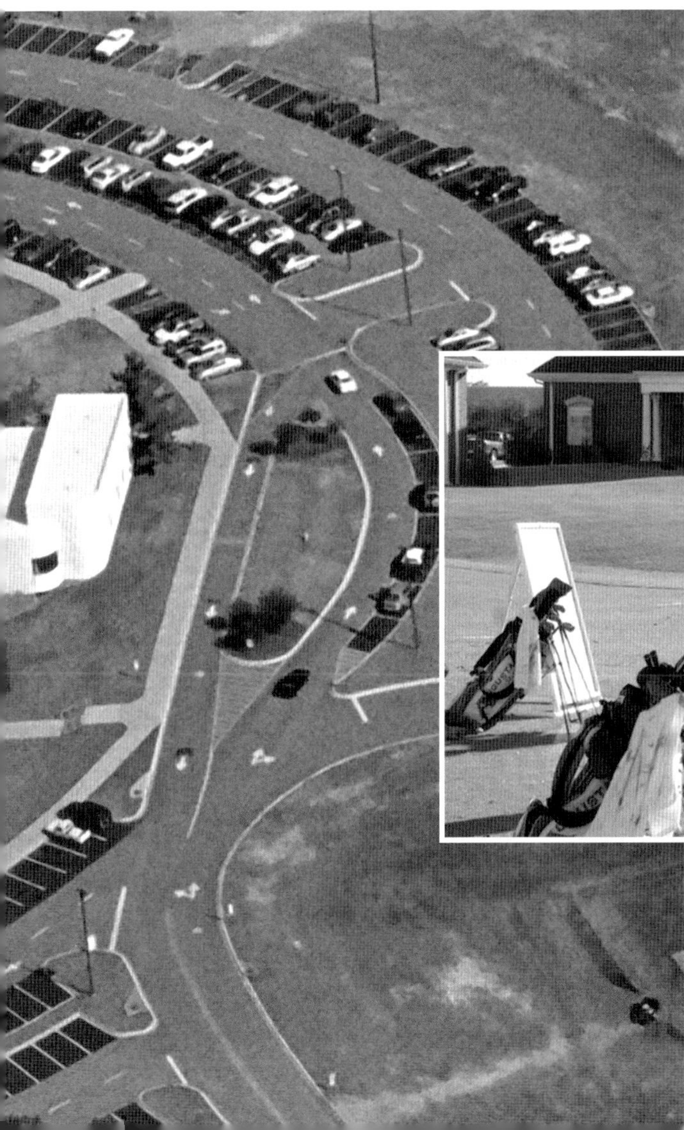

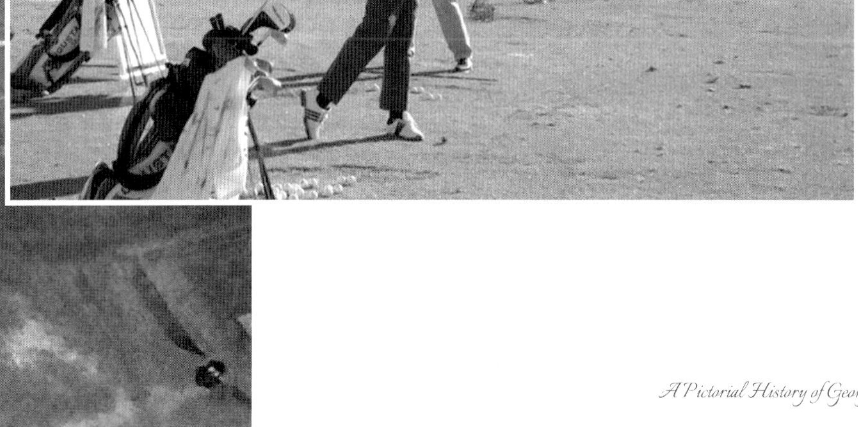

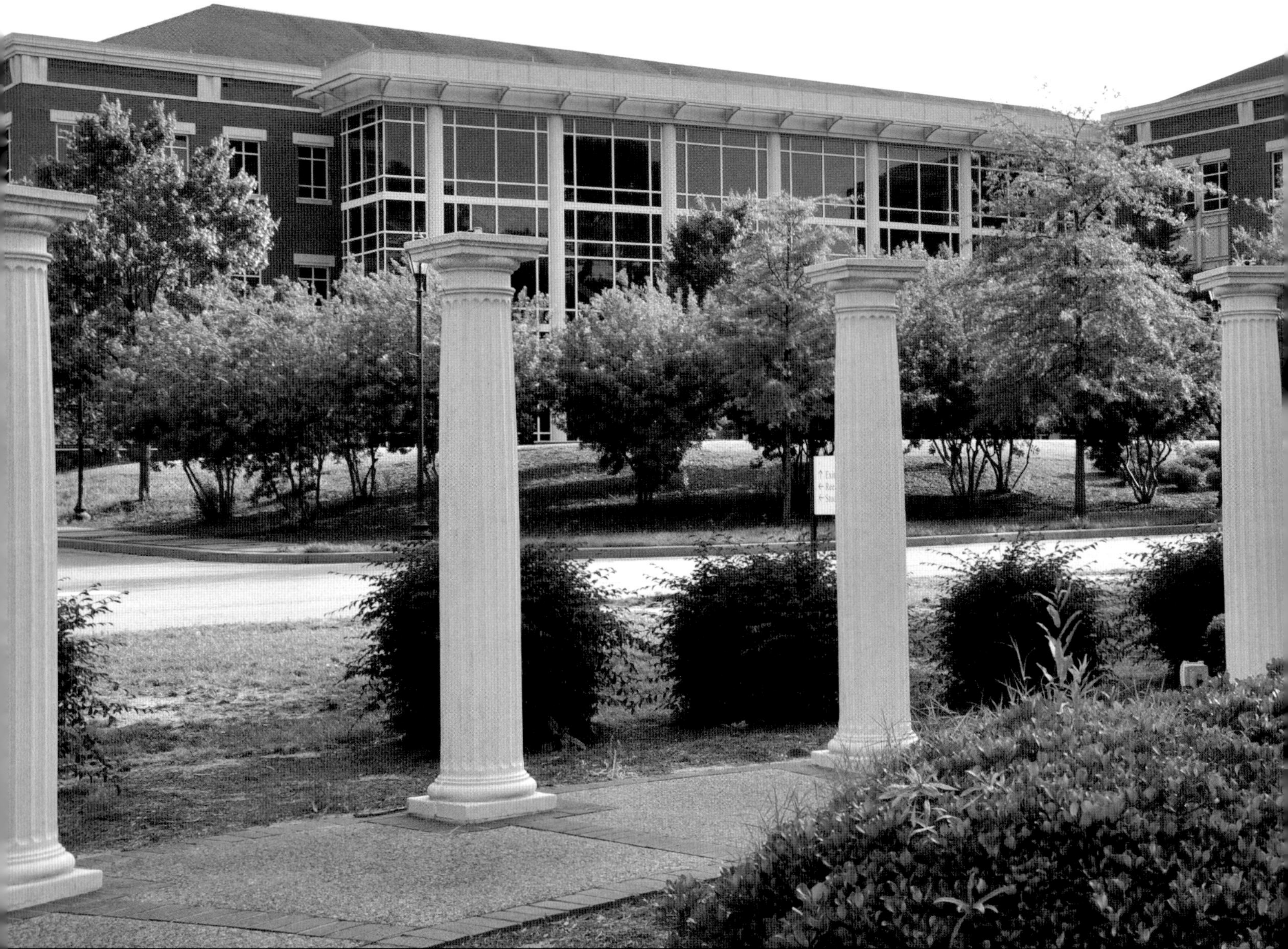

# ACADEMICS:

## *A Tradition of Excellence in Teaching and Learning*

The Medical Academy of Georgia opened in 1829 with seven students and three faculty members. Dr. Lewis D. Ford was the dean and taught material medica, chemistry, and pharmacy. Dr. Milton Antony, the school's founder, taught the practice of medicine and midwifery and diseases of women and children and Dr. Ignatius P. Garvin taught anatomy and surgery. A one-year course, which included lectures and clinical training under established physicians, led to a bachelor of medicine degree. Students could then go on to another

In December 1829, changes in the school's charter expanded the curriculum to a second year, doubled the size of the faculty to six, and allowed the school to grant the doctor of medicine degree. That year the name became the Medical Institute of Georgia. In 1833, it changed to the Medical College of Georgia (MCG), the same year it awarded its first four MD degrees. In 1838, because competition from other medical colleges with shorter terms was eating into the school's enrollment, MCG reluctantly abandoned its six-month term and reduced it to the standard four.

In its early years, there were no rigid entrance requirements. Students were admitted on letters of recommendation from medical professionals. Basic preclinical subjects were anatomy, physiology, and chemistry. Advanced and clinical subjects included surgery, medicine, pharmacy, therapeutics, material medica, obstetrics, and the diseases of women and children. Students attended six lectures a day. Until 1877 students had to write a thesis, usually in Latin, to graduate.

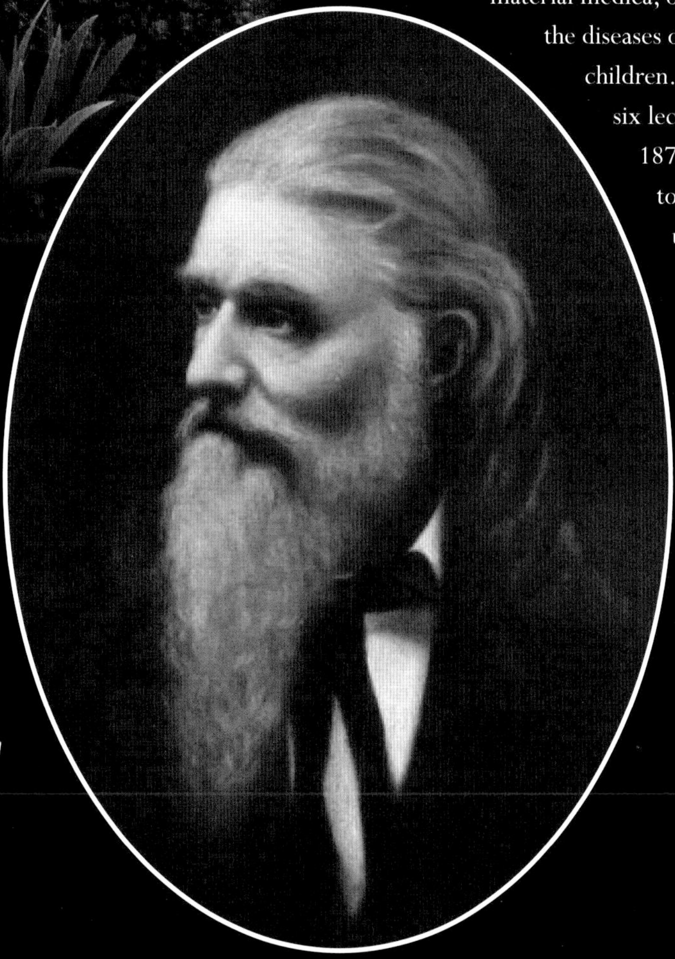

*The first dean, Dr. Lewis DeSaussure Ford, taught material medica, chemistry, and pharmacy to the young men who studied at the medical college. An early advocate of medical reform, he was one of the founders and the first president of the Medical Association of Georgia. He remained on faculty for over fifty years.*

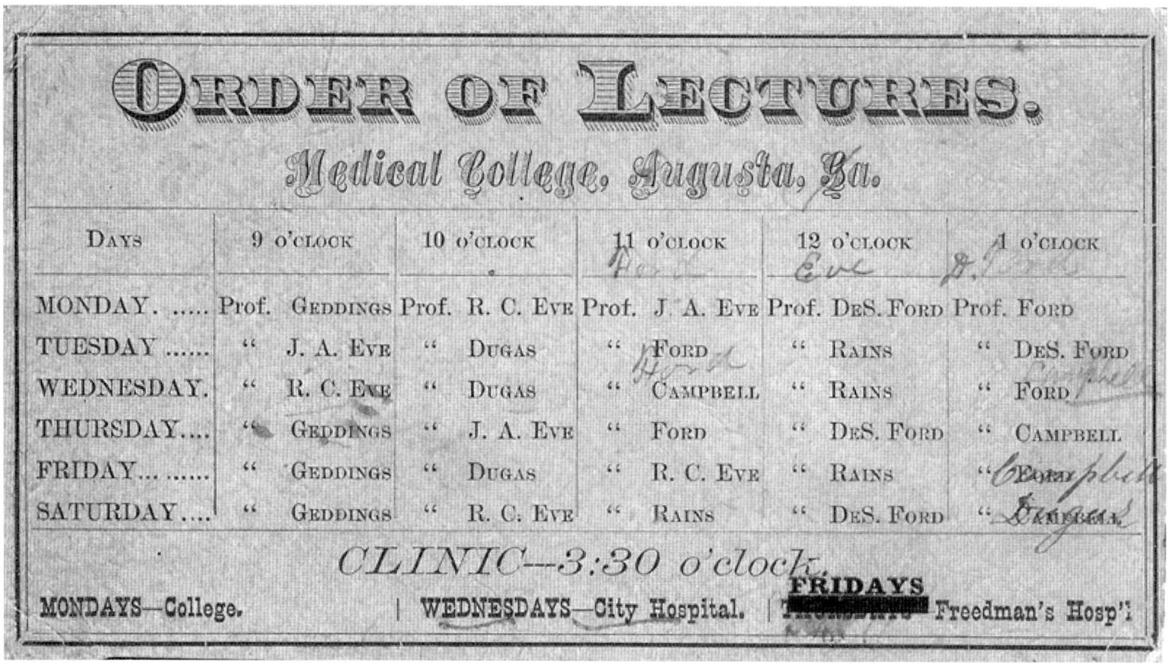

# ORDER OF LECTURES.

## Medical College, Augusta, Ga.

| DAYS | 9 O'CLOCK | 10 O'CLOCK | 11 O'CLOCK | 12 O'CLOCK | 1 O'CLOCK |
|---|---|---|---|---|---|
| MONDAY. ..... | Prof. GEDDINGS | Prof. R. C. EVE | Prof. J. A. EVE | Prof. DES. FORD | Prof. FORD |
| TUESDAY ...... | " J. A. EVE | " DUGAS | " FORD | " RAINS | " DES. FORD |
| WEDNESDAY. | " R. C. EVE | " DUGAS | " CAMPBELL | " RAINS | " FORD |
| THURSDAY.... | " GEDDINGS | " J. A. EVE | " FORD | " DES. FORD | " CAMPBELL |
| FRIDAY... ...... | " GEDDINGS | " DUGAS | " R. C. EVE | " RAINS | " FORD |
| SATURDAY.... | " GEDDINGS | " R. C. EVE | " RAINS | " DES. FORD | " CAMPBELL |

*CLINIC—3:30 o'clock.*

MONDAYS—College. | WEDNESDAYS—City Hospital. | FRIDAYS [redacted] Freedman's Hosp'l

*This early schedule details the lectures given by faculty and the clinical practice expected of students in the antebellum era.*

The institution grew and by the 1850s had reached a matriculation over 150, with about fifty MDs awarded each year. During the Civil War, MCG closed and was reopened in November 1865. Enrollment reflected the impoverishment and desolation of the post-bellum South and numbers rebounded slowly.

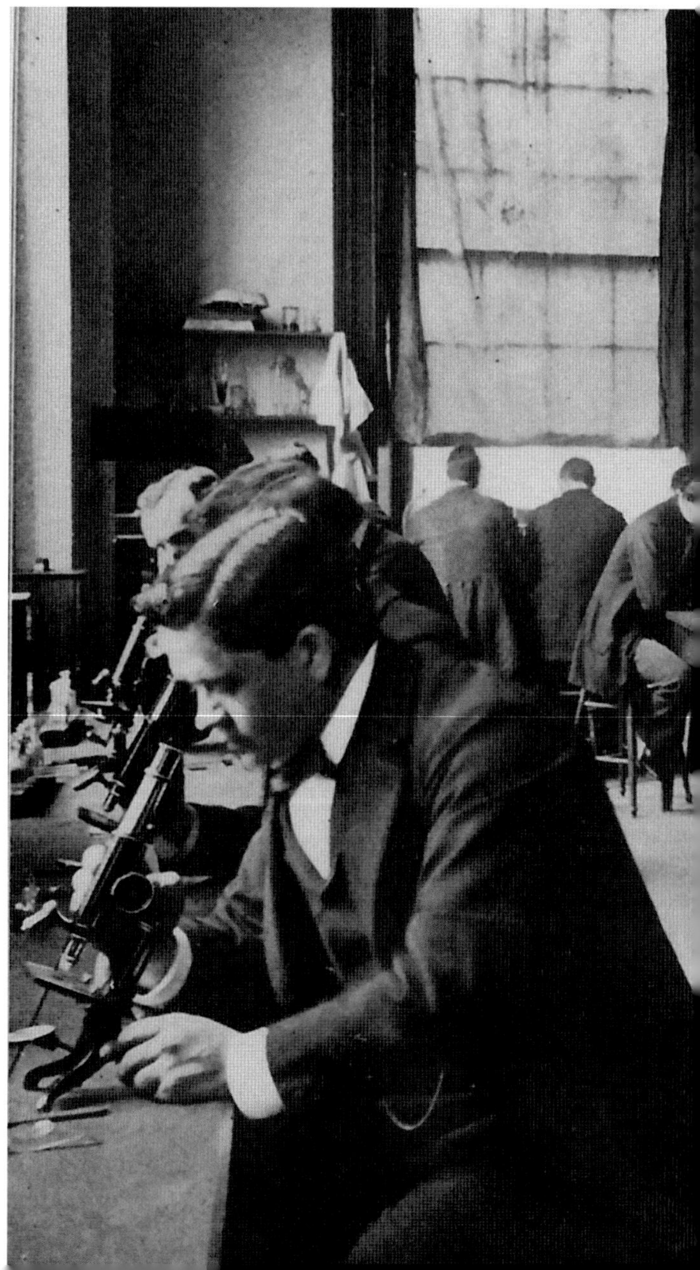

In the late nineteenth century, medical education and graduation requirements were strengthened. Residency training began at City Hospital in 1888. MCG added a third year in 1893 and extended all terms to six months. Beginning in 1896, the State Board of Medical Examiners required graduates to pass a state exam before they could practice medicine. MCG added a chair of pathology in 1897 and courses in bacteriology and histology in 1898, the same year it instituted an optional fourth year. In 1900, the fourth year became a requirement. Medical education then consisted of the first two years of basic science instruction, followed by two years of clinical training.

In 1909, at the behest of the Council on Medical Education and Hospitals, Abraham Flexner of the Carnegie Endowment inspected MCG and wrote a devastating report on what he found. The dissecting

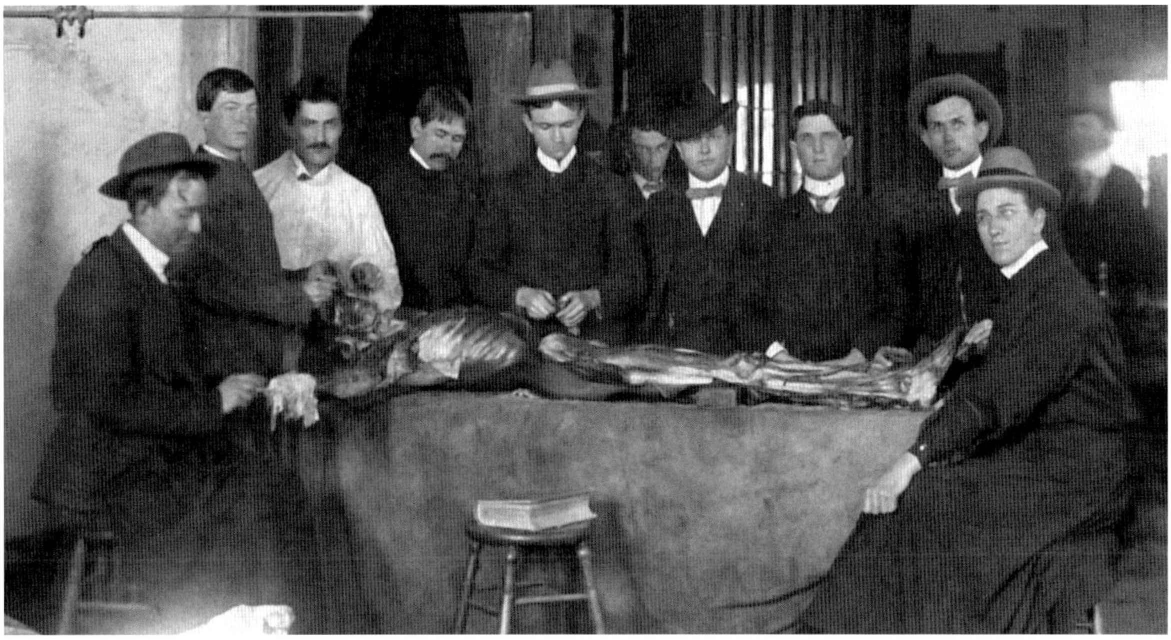

*As is the practice today, students in the nineteenth century learned anatomy firsthand working with cadavers. Most were provided through purchase but some came from being "resurrected" from local cemeteries, mainly Cedar Grove.*

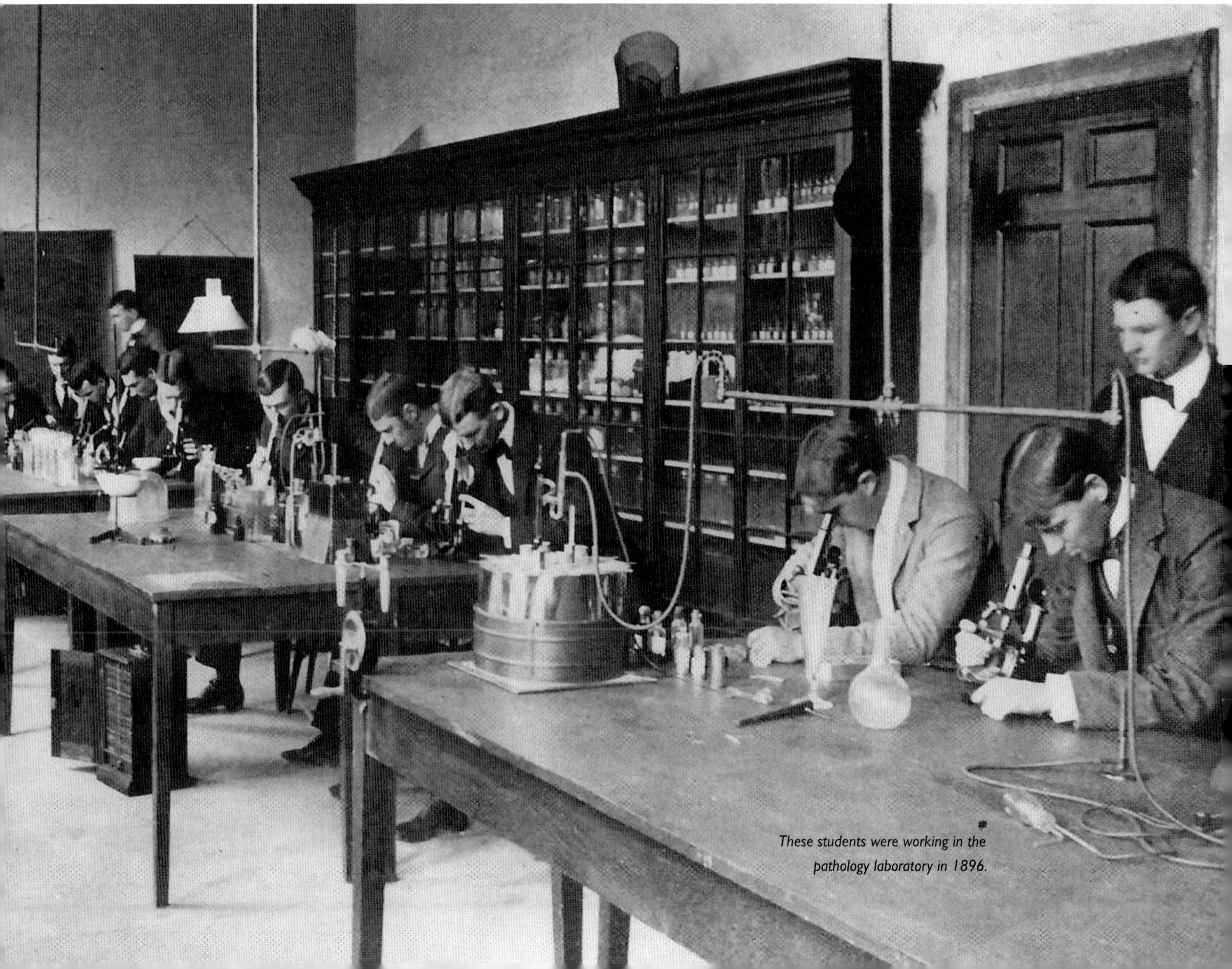

*These students were working in the pathology laboratory in 1896.*

room was dirty; equipment was meager for chemistry, fair for histology and pathology, but practically non-existent for bacteriology; clinical facilities were poor; students received little obstetrical training and no clinical laboratory work. Entrance requirements were nominal. He recommended the University of Georgia sever its loose ties with the institution and let it die.

The institution responded with major reforms that included a curriculum revision, a clear definition of faculty responsibilities, and improved pedagogy. The school added new fields in dermatology and therapeutics, as well as an obstetrical clinic. Pursuant to the legislative act of 1911, a more formal relationship with the University of Georgia was established in 1912, and a year later entrance requirements were upgraded. Beginning in 1918, candidates needed at least two years of college to be admitted. Admission numbers initially dropped, but program improvements continued. A residency program with University Hospital began in 1919 and two years later with the Department of Public Health. Enrollment began to climb steadily in the new MCG, reaching 102 in 1922.

With Georgia hit hard by the Great Depression, the 1930s were years of challenges, but there were accomplishments. Starved for funding, the University System of Georgia eliminated eight schools in 1933, including MCG. Public outcry, however, led to a quick reinstatement. In 1934, the Association of American Medical Colleges revoked MCG's "A" rating, but restored it two years later, much to students' relief. Bright spots in the decade included distinguished teaching and research in the Departments of Obstetrics, Orthopedics, Pediatrics, Neurosurgery, Endocrinology, and Gynecology. In 1937, Departments of Neuropsychiatry, Tuberculosis, and Anesthesiology were established.

With World War II came a major involvement between the medical college and the U.S. government, as they implemented new programs to meet the nation's need for more doctors.

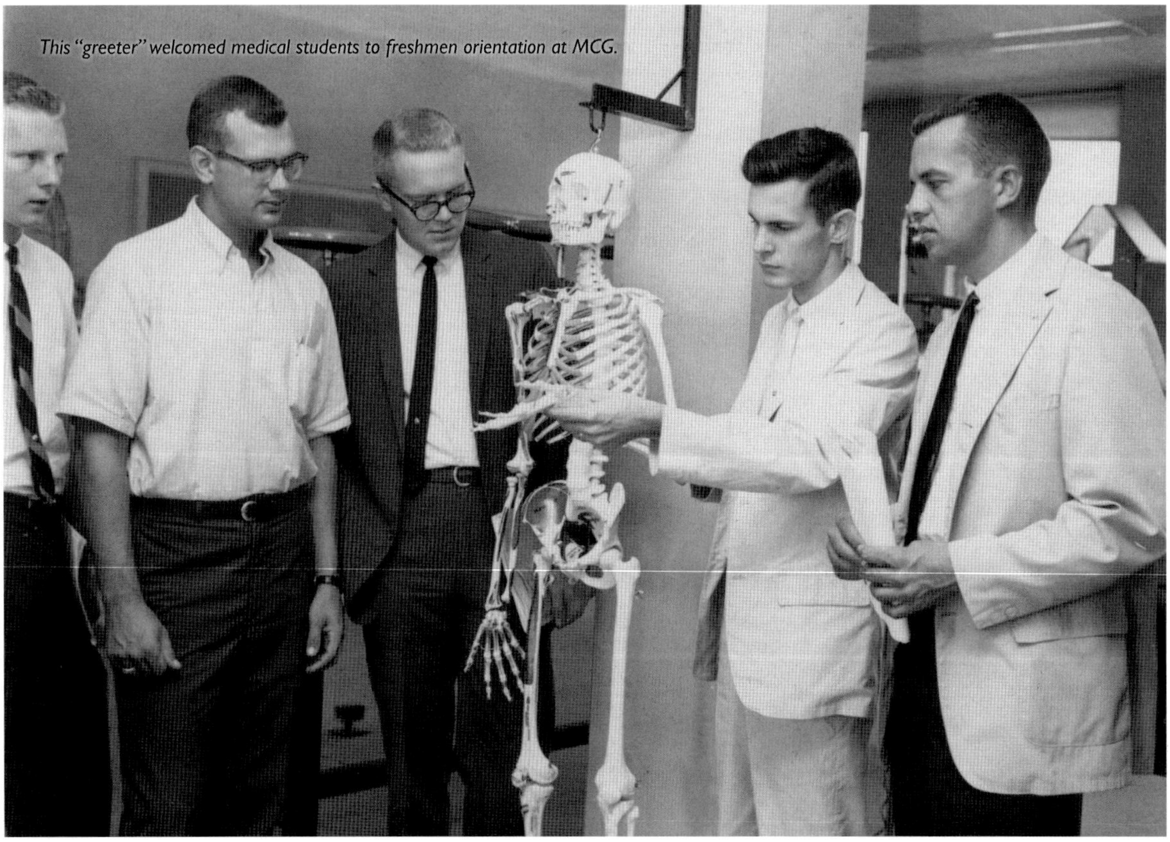
*This "greeter" welcomed medical students to freshmen orientation at MCG.*

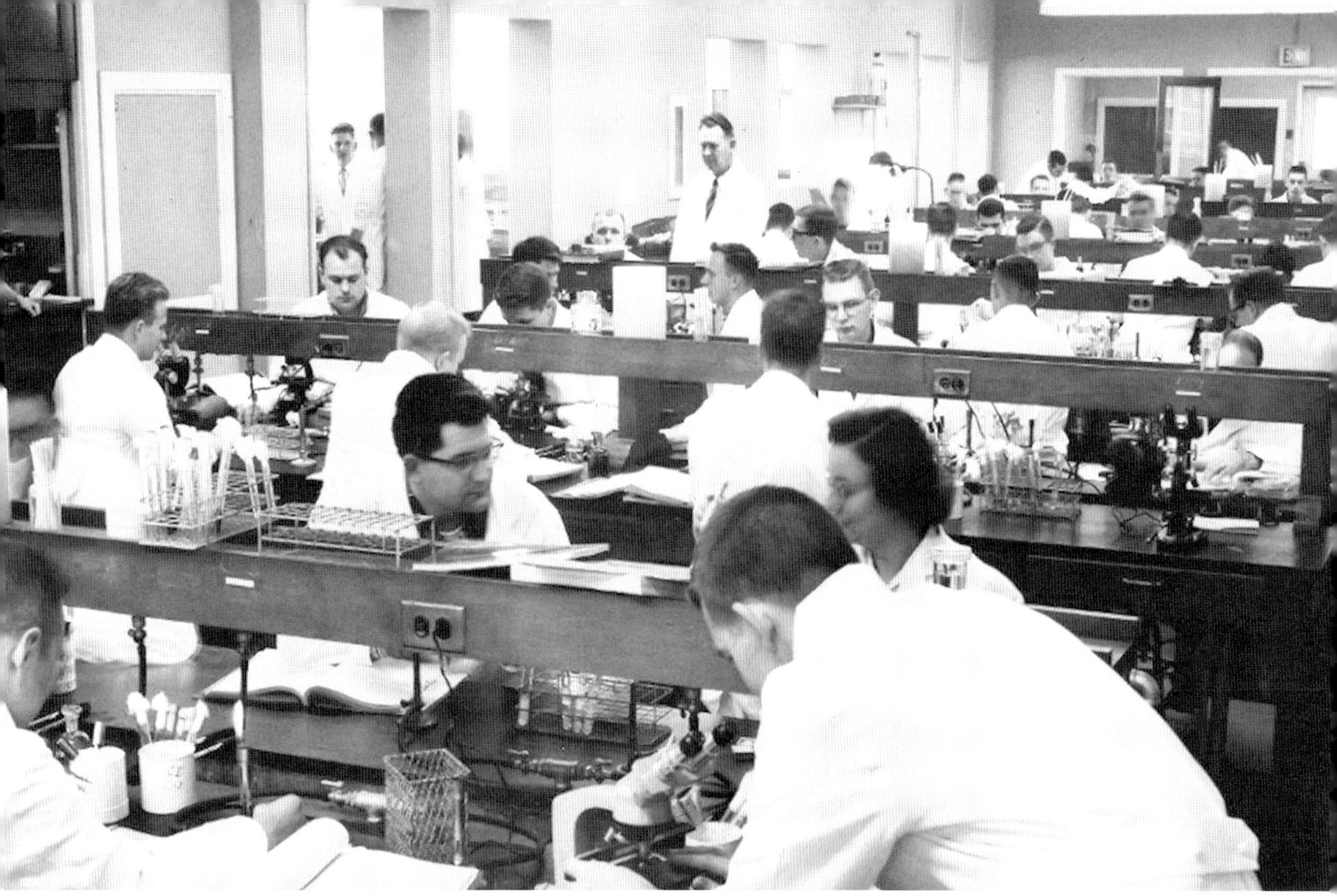

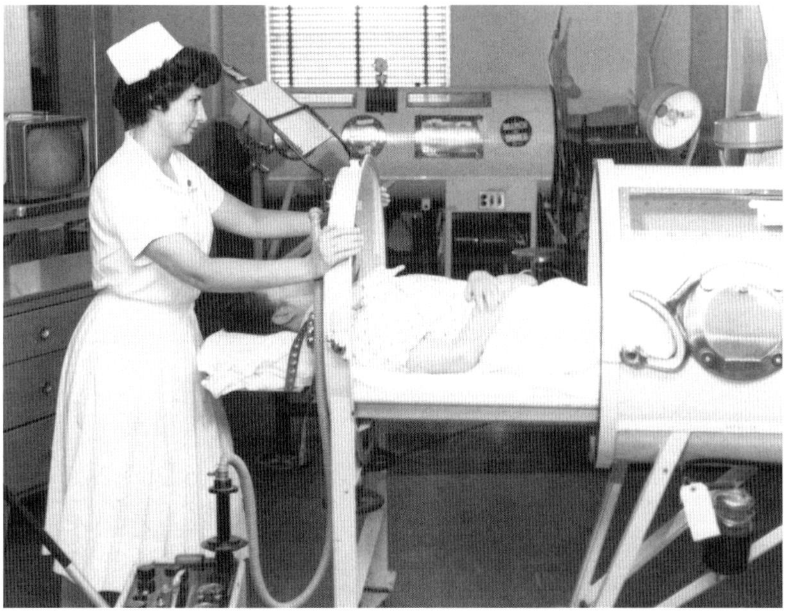

*Above: Students study in a microbiology laboratory in the 1950s.*

*Left: Talmadge Hospital housed the Southeastern Respiratory Care Center for the treatment of polio patients. When the unit closed, the iron lungs were stored in a building at AC.*

After the war, curricular expansion continued with new Departments of Medical Art and Oncology and the opening of a cancer clinic at University Hospital. Especially significant was the college's coming of age as an autonomous institution. In 1950, the medical school separated from the University of Georgia and became a freestanding institution reclaiming its old name, the Medical College of Georgia. In 1951, a new graduate division awarded its first master of science degrees in medical art and medical microbiology. By 1962, when the School of Graduate Studies was created, the PhD was offered in five areas.

In 1956, UGA's nursing program transferred to MCG and became the School of Nursing, offering a baccalaureate degree. That same year, the MCG-owned Eugene Talmadge Memorial Hospital opened for patient care, giving the institution its own teaching hospital.

MCG's School of Dentistry opened in 1967 for dental hygiene students. Doctoral students were admitted two years later, with the first DMD degrees awarded in 1973. The college organized the School of Allied Health Sciences in 1968 to house radiologic technology, physical therapy, and medical illustration. By the end of the 1960s, five schools within MCG offered education in a wide variety of health sciences fields.

With all the new opportunities for study, enrollment almost doubled from 1964 to 1971. In addition to more medical students, more students enrolled in other areas, including dentistry, allied health sciences, graduate

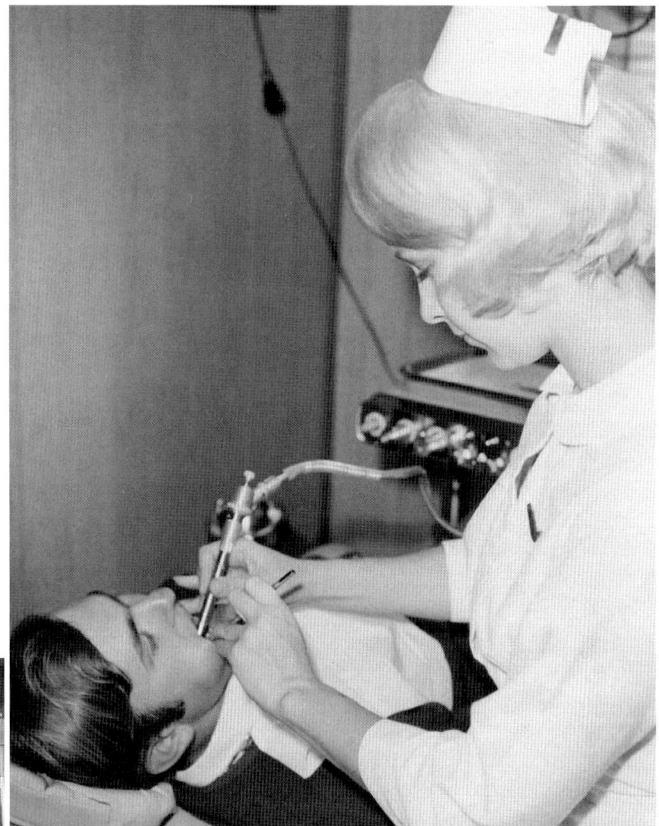

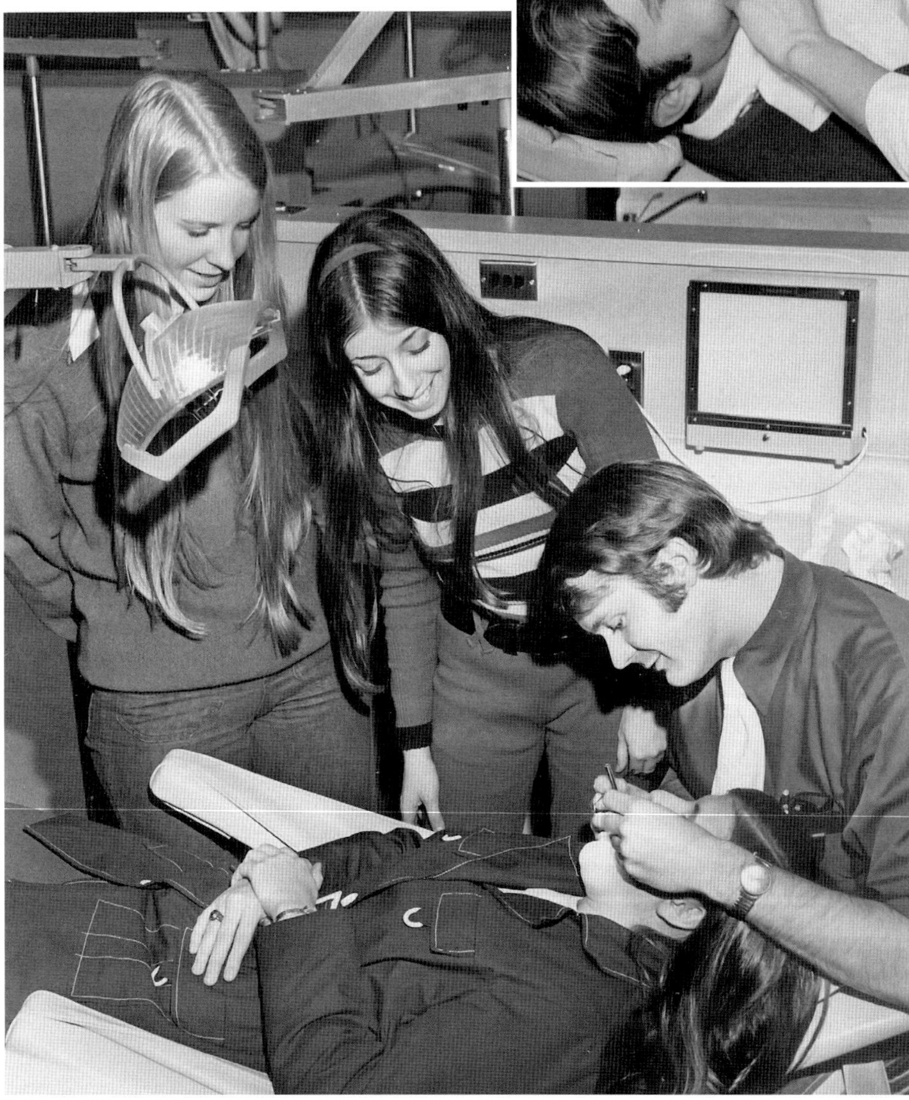

*Above: This dental hygiene student provided supervised oral care for a patient.*

*Left: Dentists-in-training worked with patients under the supervision of dental faculty.*

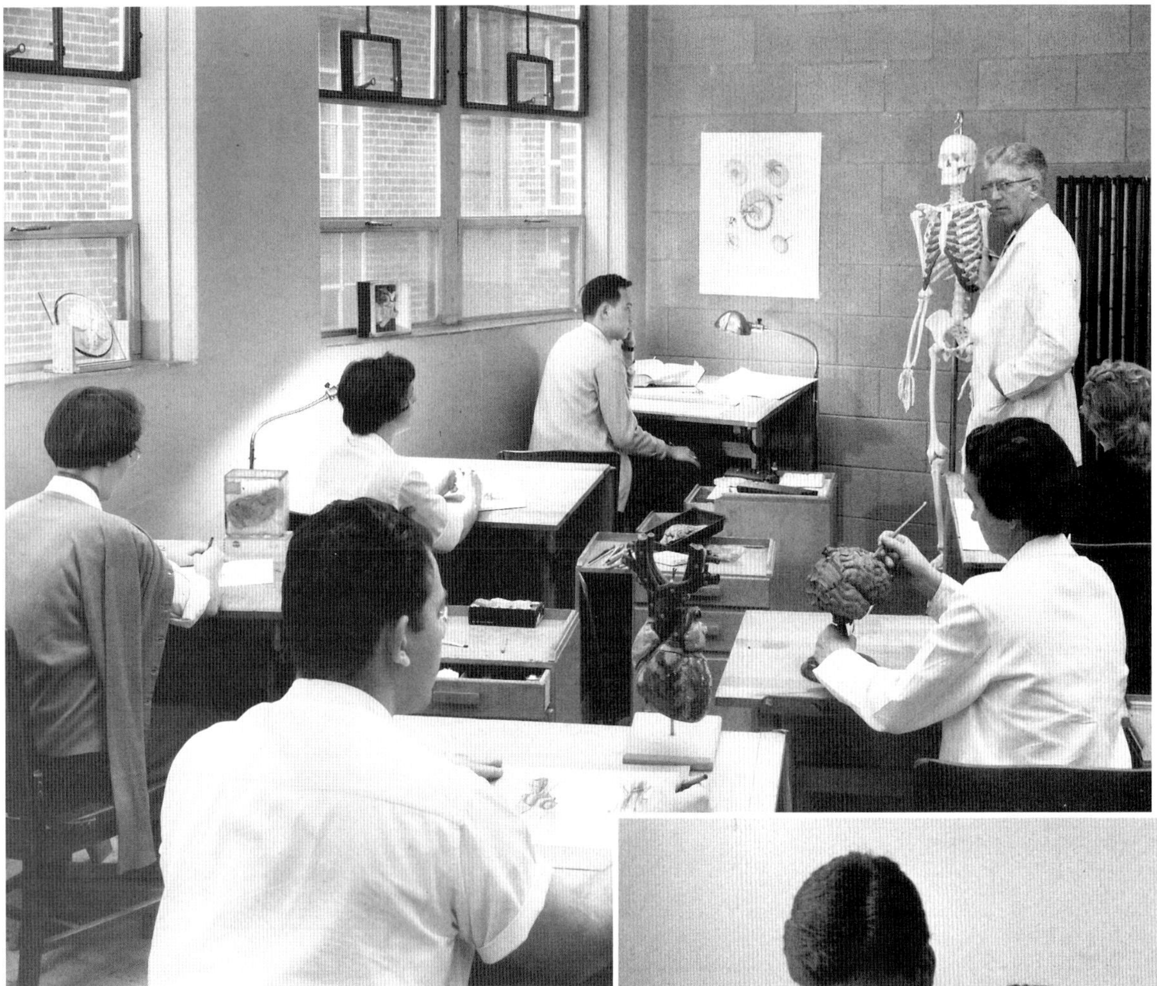

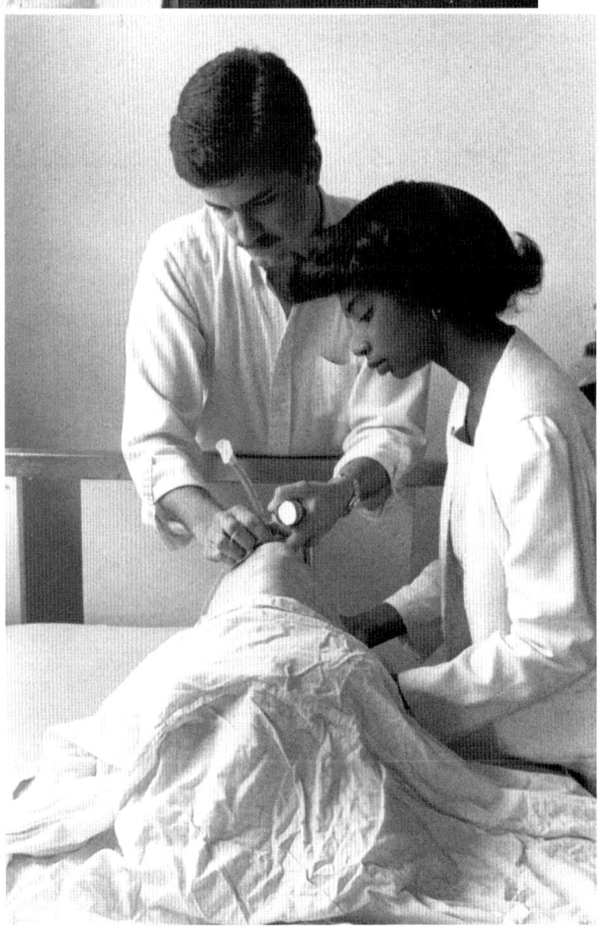

*Above: Medical illustration students practiced their craft under the supervision of Professor Orville A. Parkes.*

*Right: Respiratory therapy students practiced their techniques on a mannequin.*

studies, and nursing. Growth in the School of Nursing was phenomenal; in 1975, enrollment passed one thousand, nursing faculty had grown to fifty-six, and nursing students had twelve different paths to a degree. In 1980, MCG had 488 faculty members and awarded 685 degrees.

Expansion continued in the next three decades. Baccalaureate and certificate programs in diagnostic sonography began in 1981–1982. An associate degree program in occupational therapy began in 1984. In the 1990s, advances in distance learning in allied health sciences enabled non-traditional students to work on

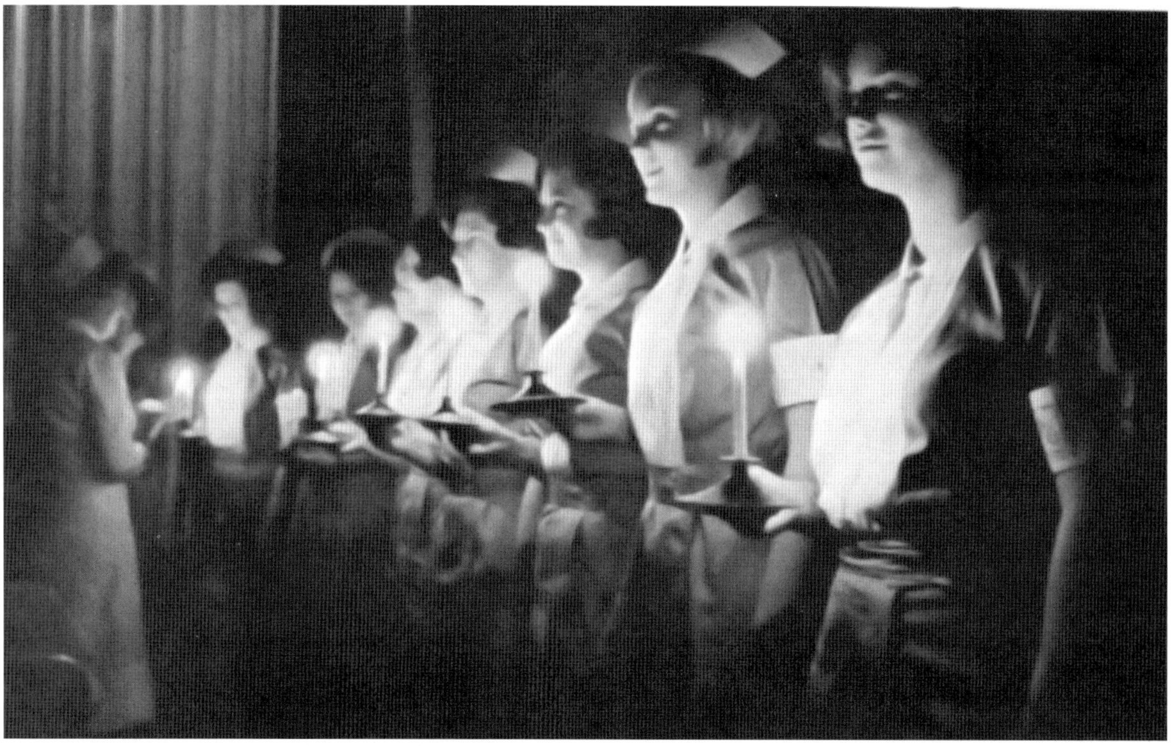

*In the Capping Ceremony, MCG nursing students pledged to wear their caps in a manner that brought distinction to their alma mater and to the nursing profession. This ceremony incorporated the "Florence Nightingale lamp" represented by a candle.*

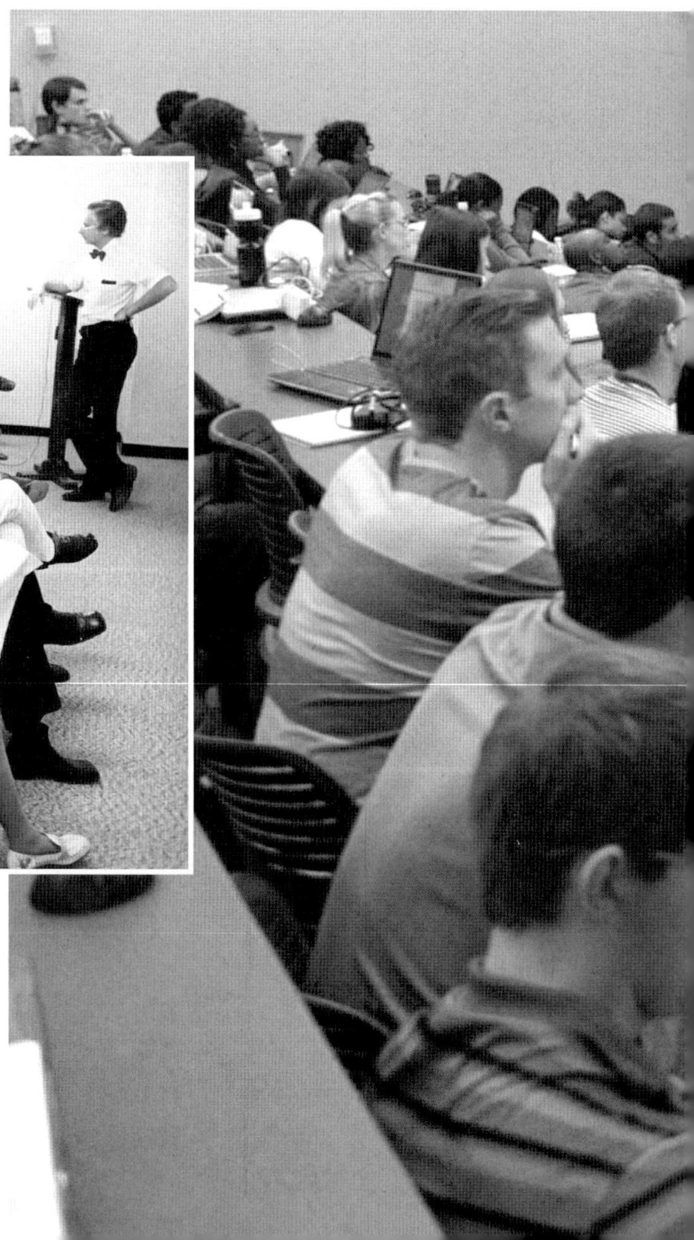

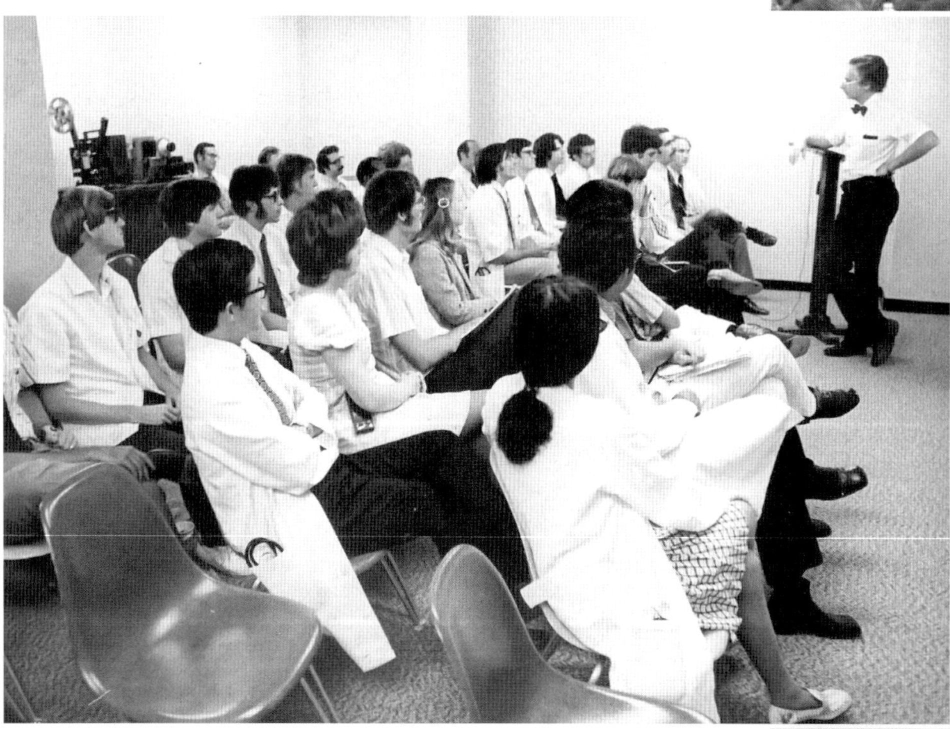

*Students' clinical education has long included rounds made with medical faculty. These residents prepared for grand rounds.*

their degrees even miles from Augusta. The School of Nursing was one of the first to open a patient simulation lab. The 1990s also saw the opening of centers in sports medicine, vascular biology, telemedicine, and senior health. A distance-learning program leading to a baccalaureate in medical technology began in 1993. Along with the rest of the University System of Georgia, in 1998 MCG converted to the semester calendar.

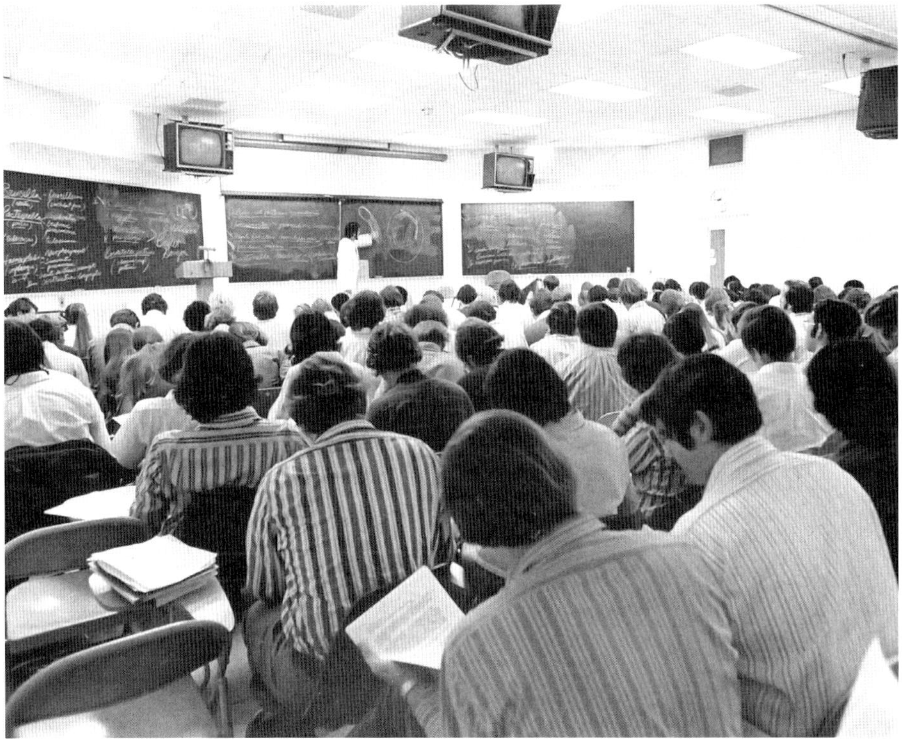

*Right: In this 1979 class, students made notes as the faculty member lectured and shared information on the blackboard.*

*Below: MCG students and faculty members use sophisticated technology to convey information in more recent classes.*

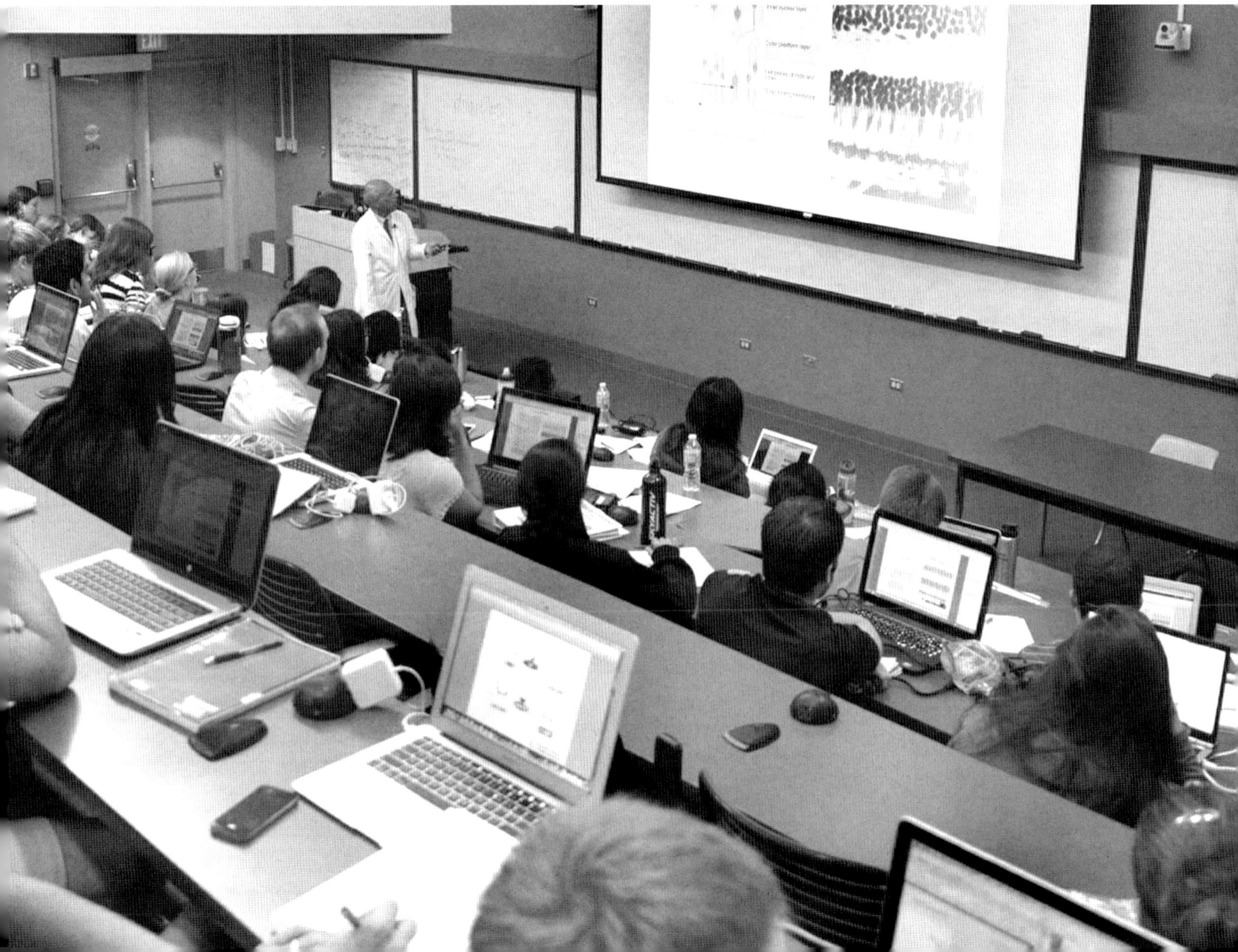

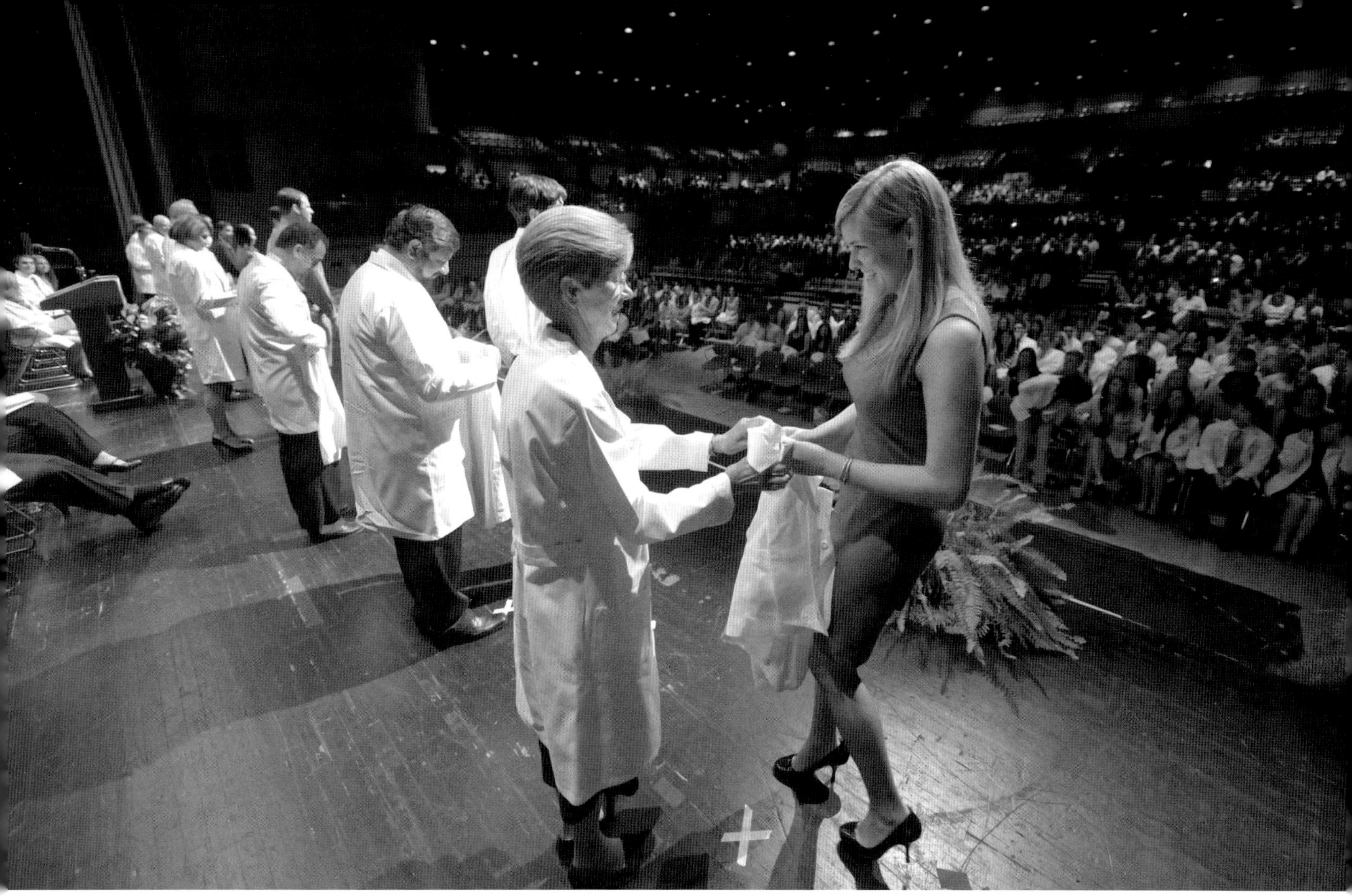

*Early in their freshman year, all medical students receive a white coat to symbolize their entry into physician training. Initiated in 1996, MCG's White Coat Ceremony was among the first in the nation.*

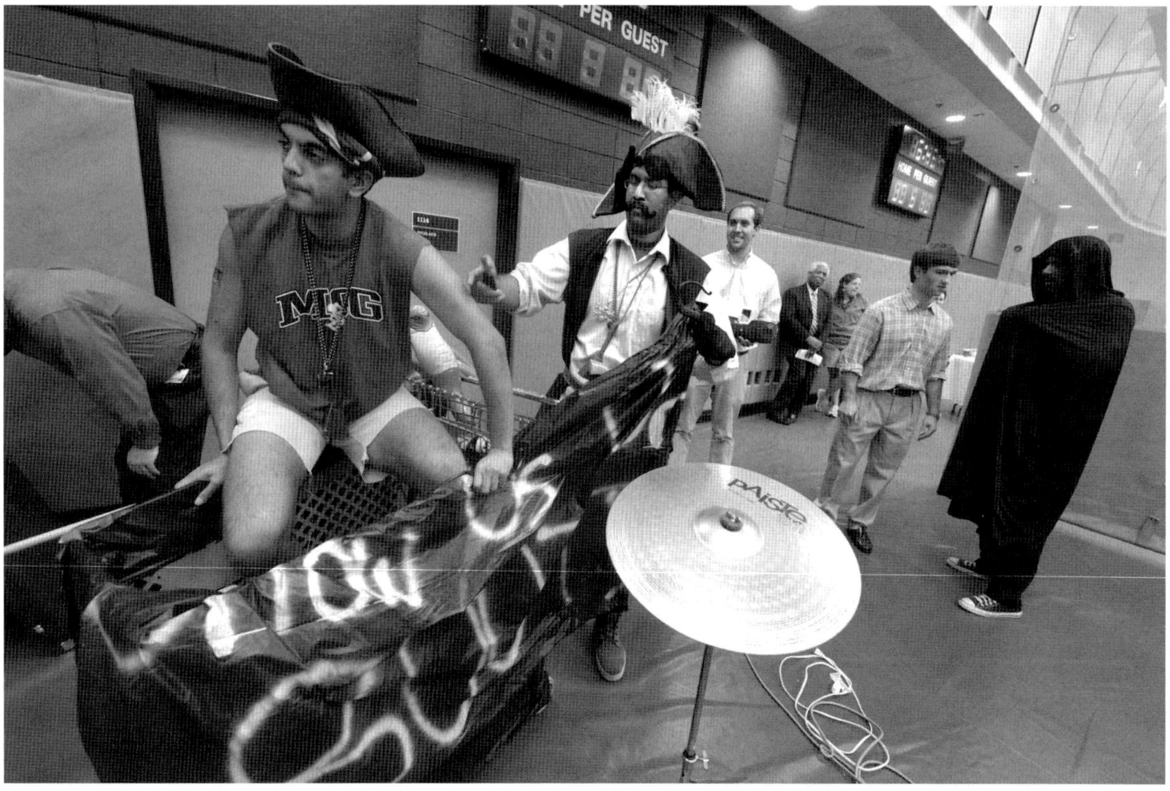


*Since 2002 medical students have participated in the annual Raft Debate involving an ethical dilemma for students to decide.*

In 2011, the institution's name changed to Georgia Health Sciences University (GHSU) and its schools were elevated to colleges; dentistry changed to dental medicine and the name of the Medical College of Georgia was retained for medicine. Its role with the Medical Center and the Physician's Practice Group realigned to better reflect its complex mission and its role in the state.

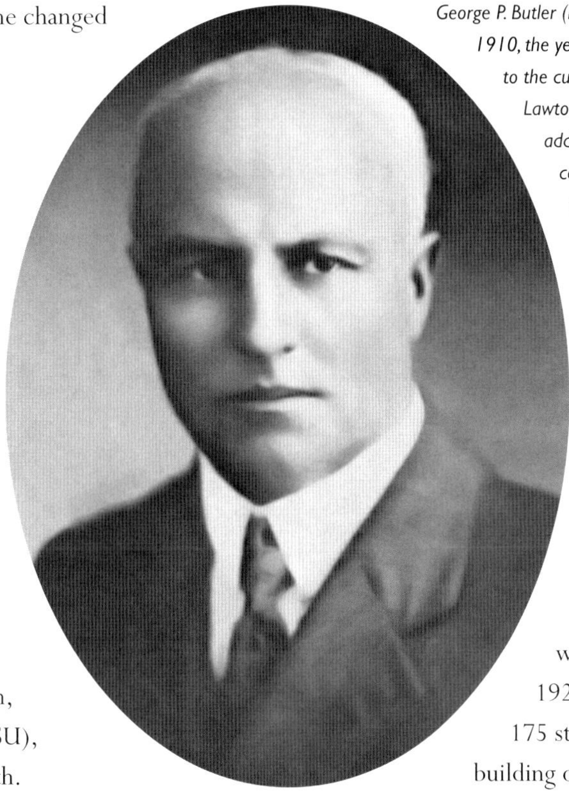

*George P. Butler (left) became principal of ARC in 1910, the year college work was formally added to the curriculum as a fifth year designed by Lawton B. Evans. Butler helped turn this additional year into a full-fledged junior college and later became known as the "father of the Junior College of Augusta."*

The second legacy institution, Augusta State University (ASU), also underwent steady growth. Its parent institution, the Academy of Richmond County (ARC), chartered in 1783 and opened two years later, offered post-secondary courses intermittently from the late eighteenth century on. In 1872, for example, fifty to sixty students at ARC were doing college-level coursework. In 1910, a year of college work was formalized, offering Latin, German, English, trigonometry, algebra, geometry, chemistry, physics, biology, bookkeeping, some industrial courses, and pre-medical courses.

Thus when the Junior College of Augusta (JCA) was formally chartered in 1925 with eleven faculty and 175 students, sharing ARC's new building on Baker Avenue, it already had 140-year-old roots. It was the first and, for a while, only public junior college in Georgia and it grew quickly. By 1933, the JCA had 250 students who paid $100 a year in tuition. ROTC, teacher training, and pre-med supplemented the liberal arts curriculum. The American Association of Junior Colleges named the Junior College of Augusta one of the ten best in the United States.

*The first class of the U.S. Cadet Nurses entered JCA in January 1944, and two other classes started each seventeen weeks for the duration of the war.*

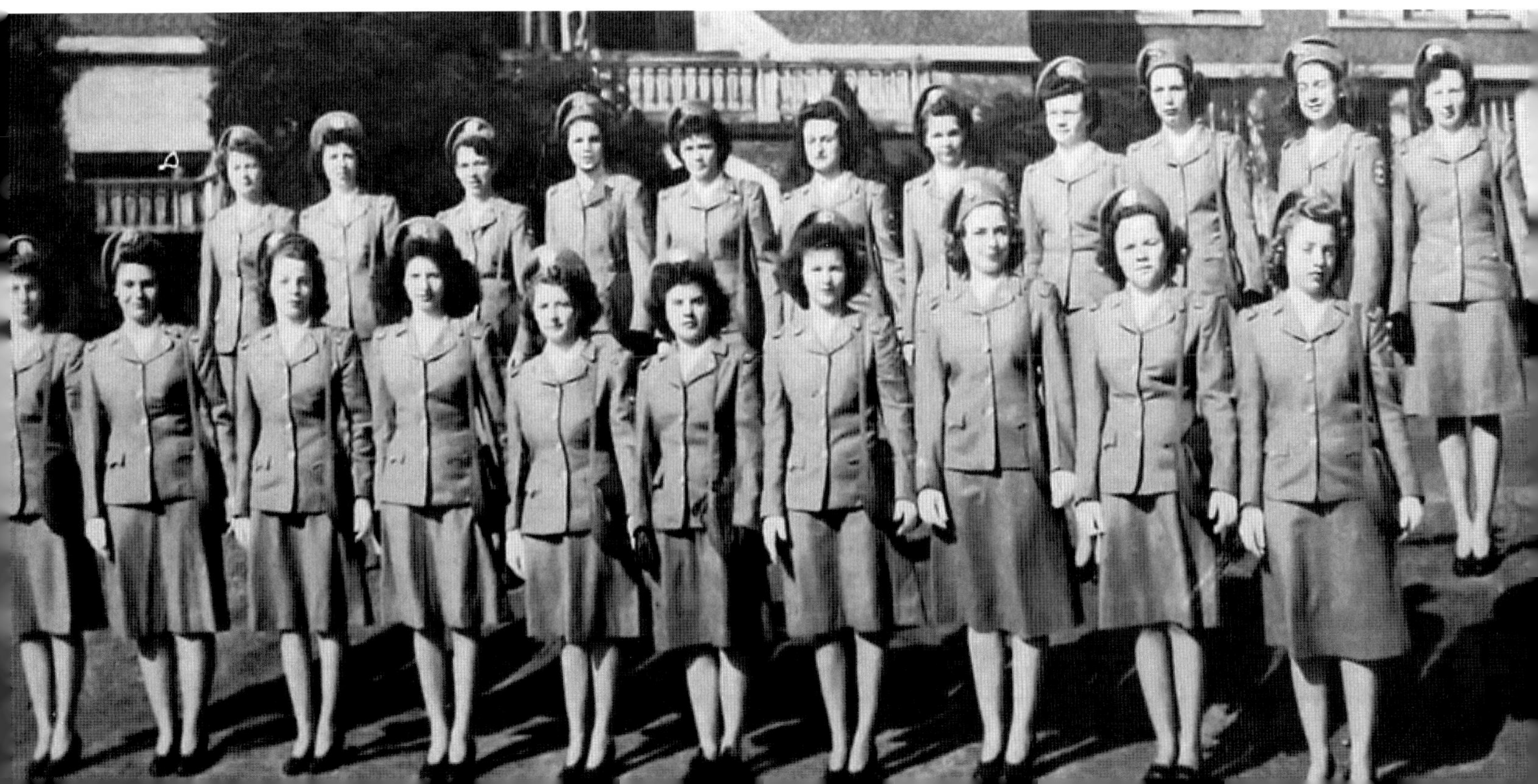

In 1952, the college was reorganized into four fields: liberal arts, vocational education, pre-professional training, and fine arts. The JCA became Augusta's community college. To accommodate the flood of returning veterans after the war, the college also established a hugely successful evening division. But the growth of JCA created a crunch for space in the ARC building. In 1946, enrollment reached a record 363. After the introduction of vocational courses in 1952, more than one thousand students were enrolled in those courses alone, either full or part time. Another 160 were in the commercial night school and over four hundred in extension courses. The Baker Avenue facility was bursting. If JCA were to survive, it would need a new home.

The institution found a solution when the U.S. Arsenal property on Walton Way became available in 1955 after being decommissioned. Eighteen faculty members from the old Junior College of Augusta-Academy of Richmond County made the move to its new campus in 1957. The following year the board of education turned the institution over to the University System of Georgia. Its name changed to Augusta College (AC), although it remained a two-year college until 1963, when the Board of Regents granted four-year status, approving programs leading to bachelor's degrees in arts, business administration, and science. The college would also be required to earn accreditation from the Southern Association of Colleges and Schools (SACS).

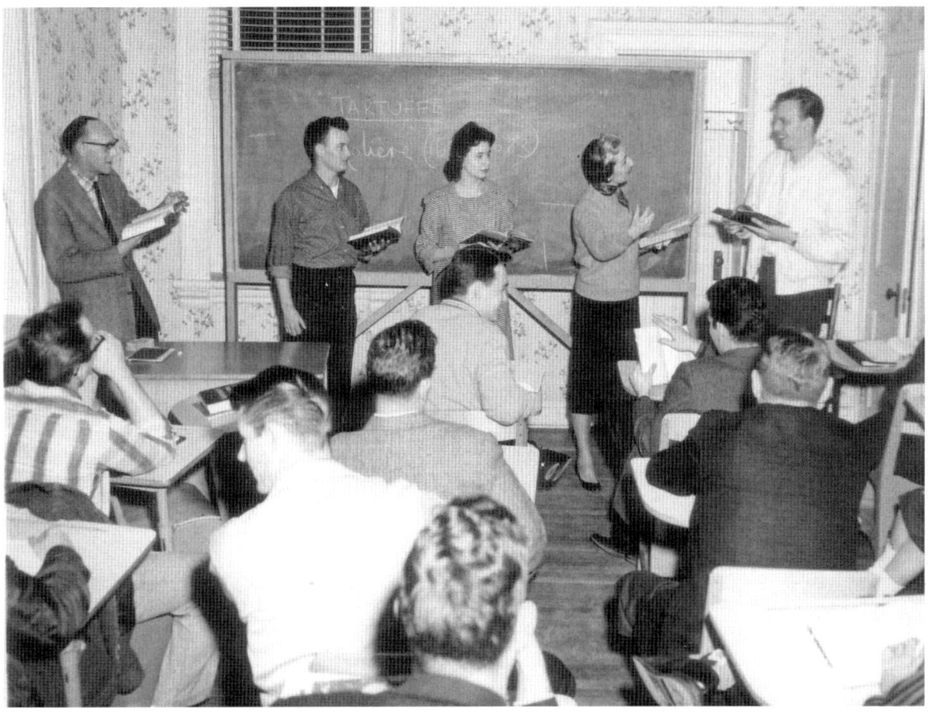

*Left: After the move to the arsenal site, U.S. Army buildings were adapted for college use. These students attended a World Literature class in a room in the former officers' quarters.*

*Below: This undated photograph shows an early graduation outside on the Walton Way campus.*

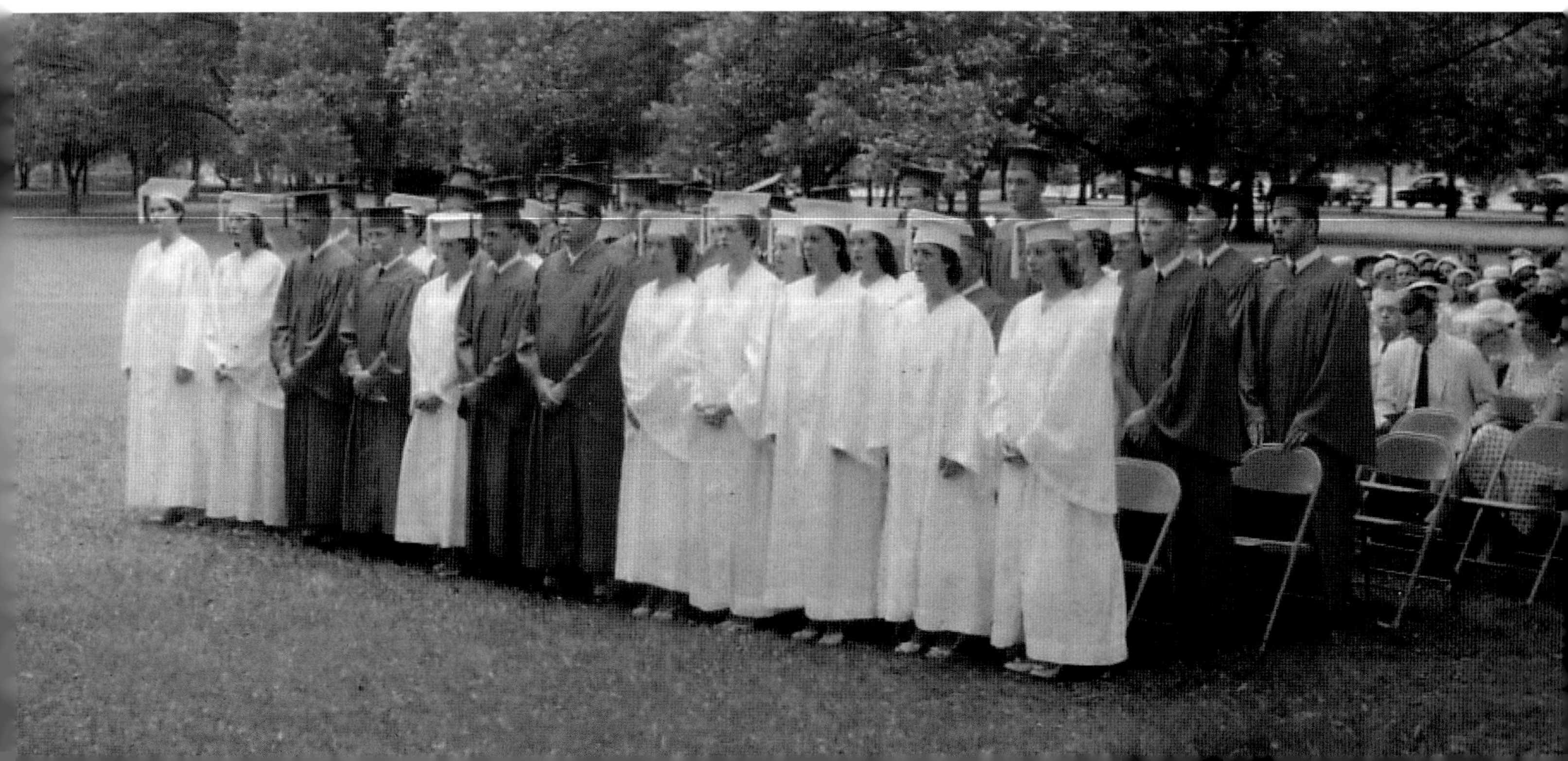

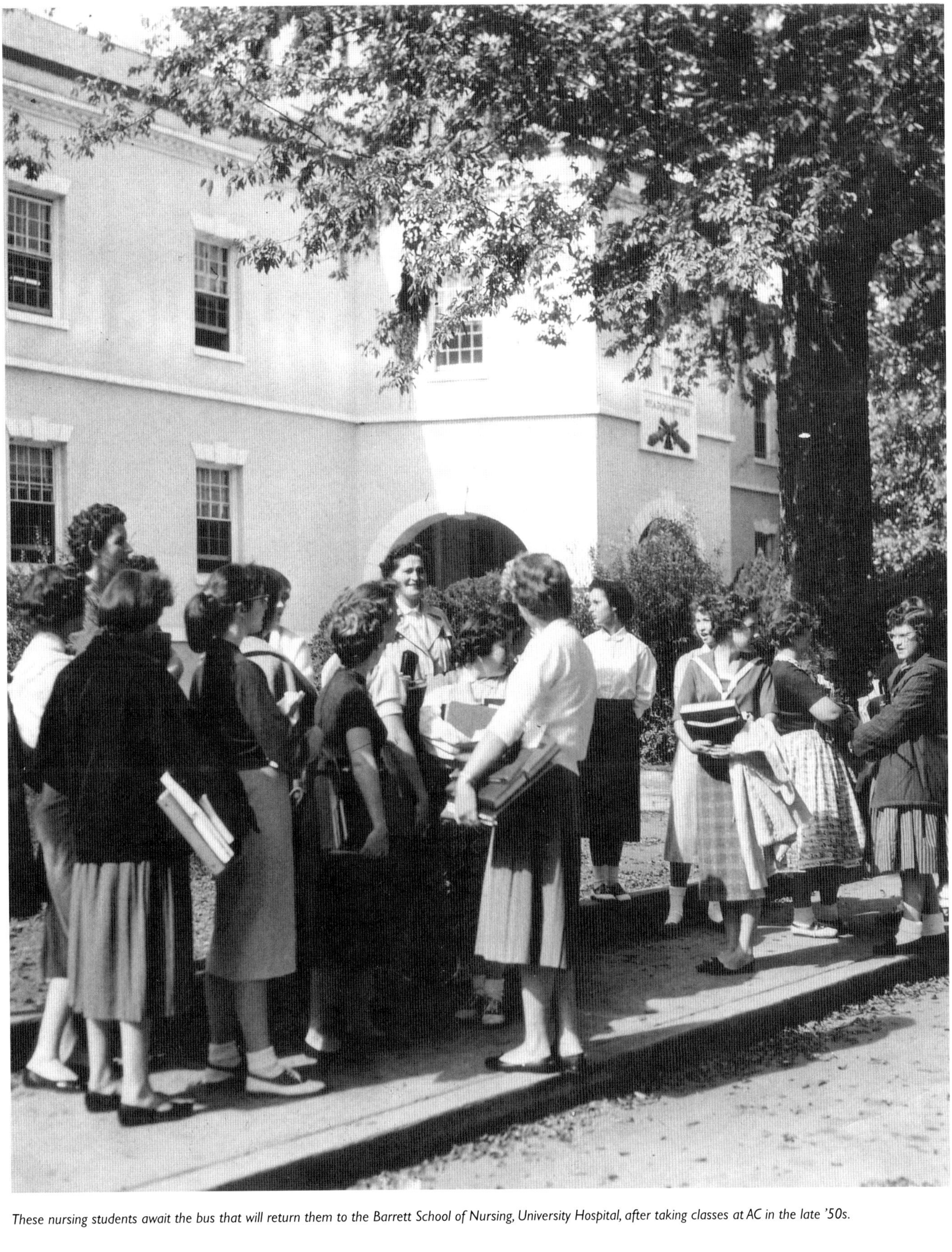

*These nursing students await the bus that will return them to the Barrett School of Nursing, University Hospital, after taking classes at AC in the late '50s.*

Hiring of new faculty began in earnest, the numbers more than doubling to eighty-seven, with 34 percent holding doctorates in 1967. (Only six of the thirty-five faculty had doctorates in 1964.) Also in 1967, the college received SACS accreditation, opened a center at Fort Gordon, and added an associate in nursing degree. AC's 2,500 students took courses in twelve departments: Behavioral Science, History and Political Science, Business Administration, Chemistry, English, Biological Science, Mathematics, Modern Languages, Physics-Earth Science, Fine Arts, Physical Education, and Nursing Education. AC's first four-year class of 181 students graduated in 1967.

The 1970s saw steady growth. Enrollment grew from 2,500 in 1970 to 3,739 in 1978. The academic program grew with new undergraduate degrees and majors—bachelor's degrees in music and computer science and associate's degrees in applied science, criminal justice, secretarial studies, and general studies—as well as the first master's degrees in business administration, education, and psychology. ROTC began. The college also responded to needs in the surrounding community, establishing the Center for the Study of Private Enterprise, the Augusta Institute of Aging, and the Small Business Development Center.

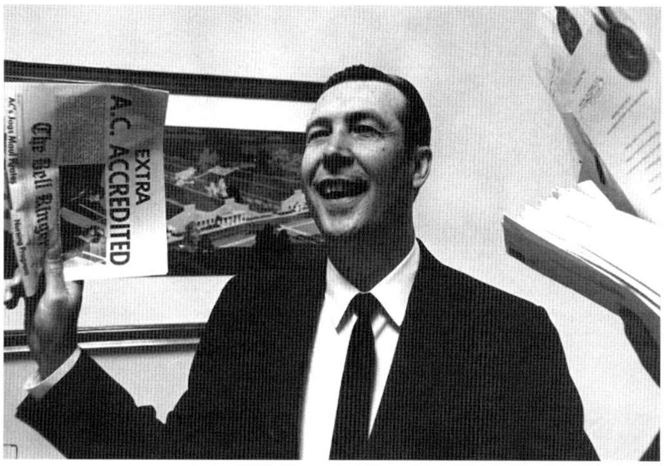


*Left: AC President Gerald Robins holds up a* Bell Ringer *student newspaper announcing accreditation.*

*Below: Art Professor Janice Williams Whiting worked with students in one of her classes in painting.*

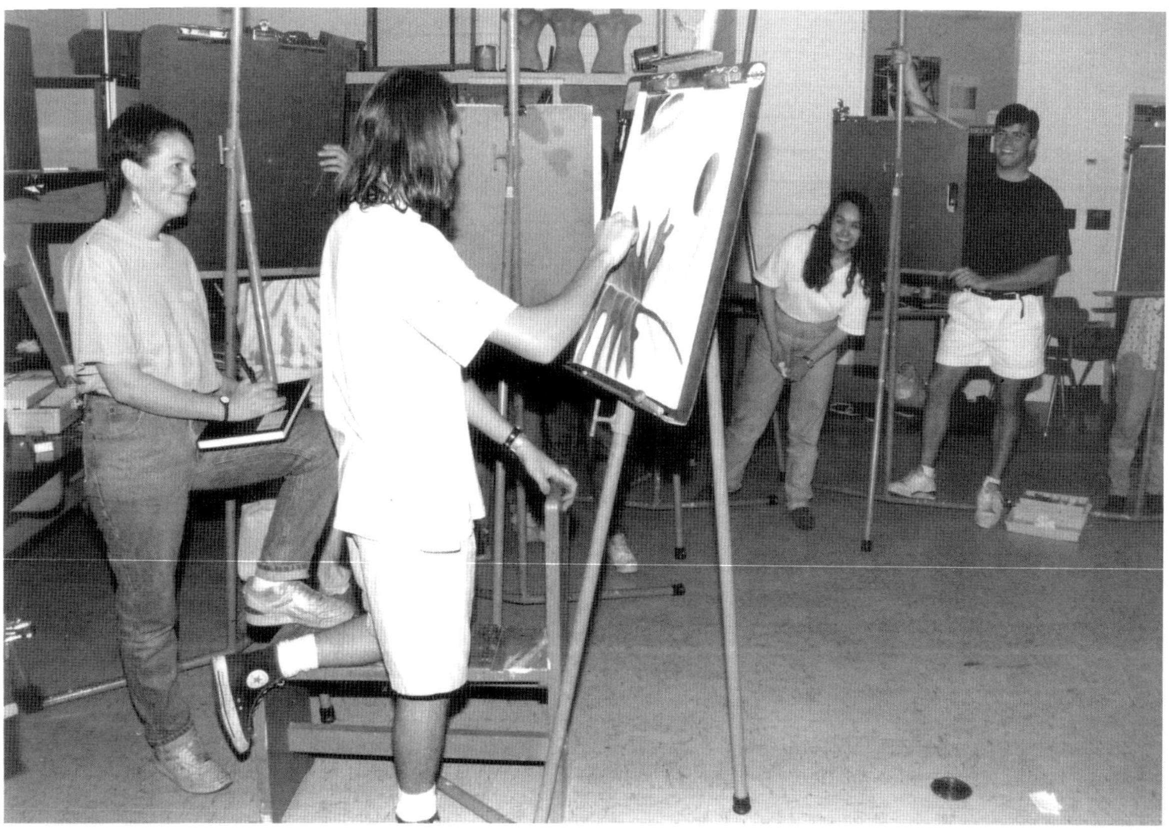

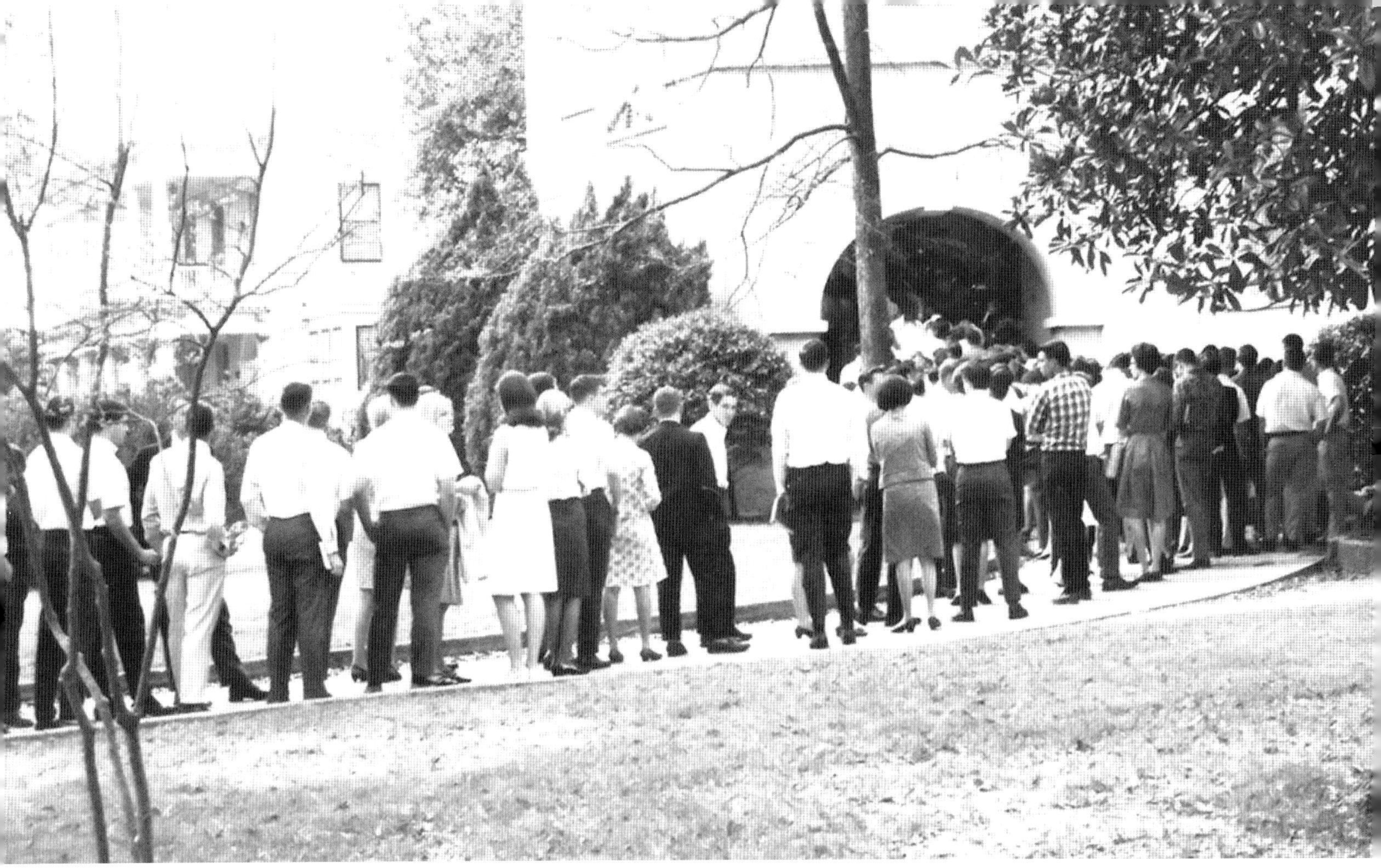

*Before computers, registration was a long process. These students wait in the registration line to enter Payne Hall, hoping the classes they need will still be open.*

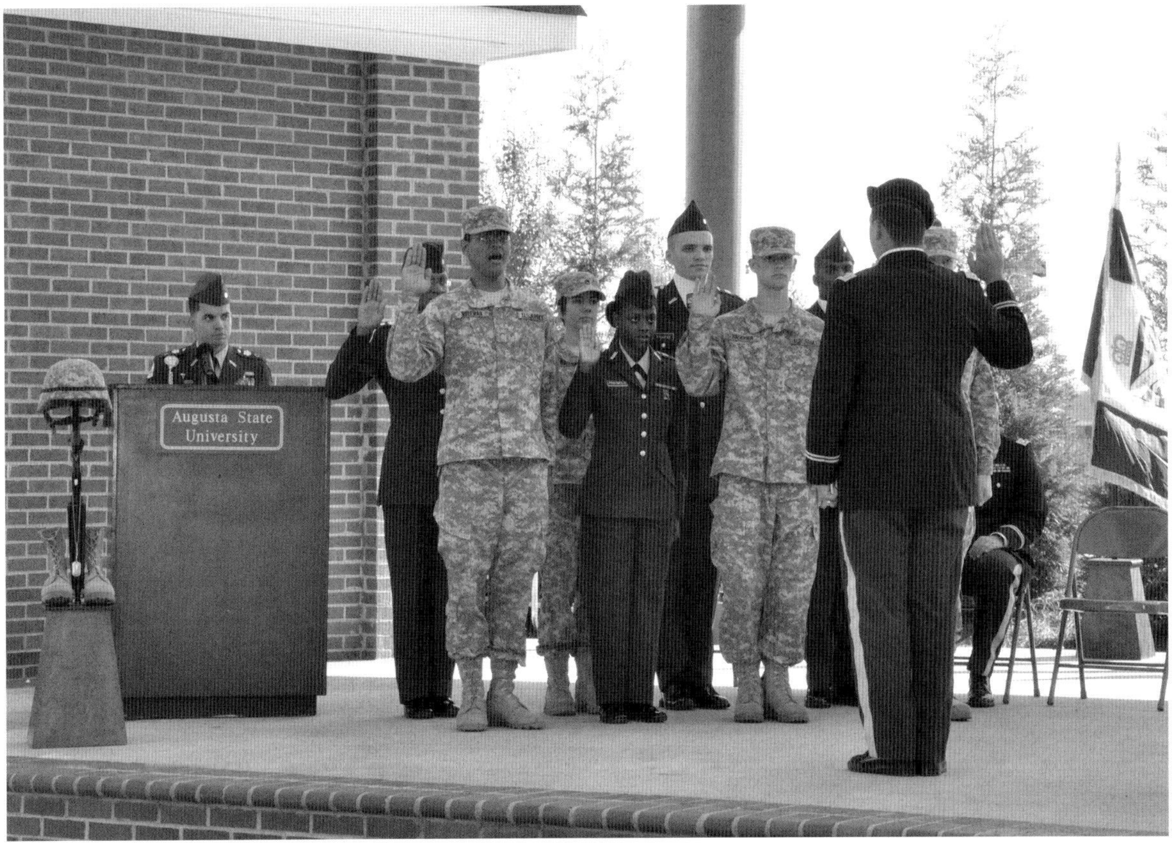


*With the raising of their right hands, ROTC cadets take the U.S. Army contracting oath. This 2010 photo shows the oath being giving prior to the annual Veterans Day observance.*

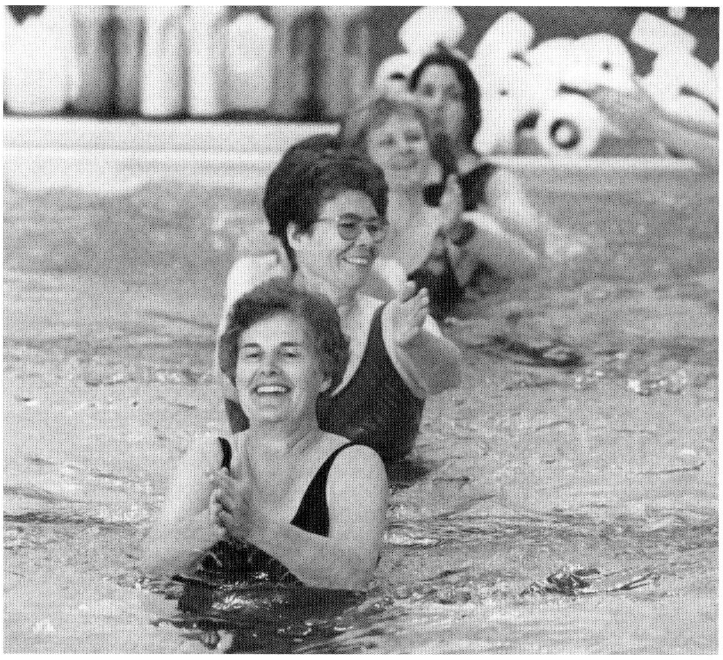

*Above: The ability to swim was a requirement for graduation from ASU until 2007. Students could demonstrate proficiency, have an exemption, or enroll in a swimming class. The pool also provided recreational and fitness activities.*

*Below: ASU students enjoyed classes that were occasionally held outdoors. Dr. Robert Bledsoe (pictured) instructs a German class.*

The 1980s saw new majors in communications and health and physical education, a new specialist in education degree, and several cooperative graduate degree programs in education with the University of Georgia and Georgia State University. Two more centers were established: the Research Center and the Center for the Creative Arts. The University System's first eminent chair was created at AC, endowed by William S. Morris III, and the Cree-Walker Foundation endowed two other chairs.

In the 1990s, the mission of the institution became focused: "excellence in teaching, advancement of knowledge, and enrichment of the community in a climate which fosters humane values and a life-long love of learning." This formulation remained the core of the institution's mission right up to the point of consolidation twenty years later. In the '90s, the School of Education boomed in enrollment. After years of preparation, the School of Business won accreditation by the Association to Advance Collegiate Schools of Business in 1999. That same year, the

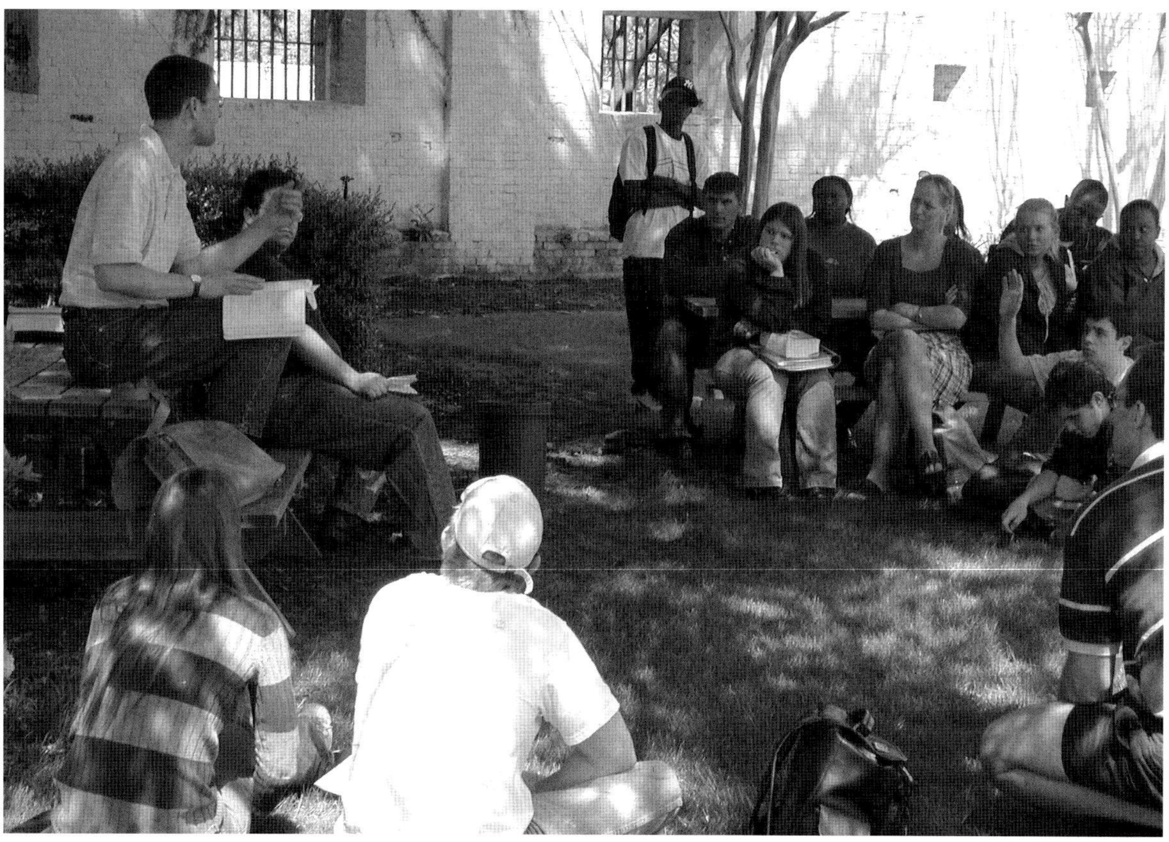

School of Arts and Sciences was named in honor of alumna and benefactor Katherine Reese Pamplin. In 1996, historian Edward J. Cashin founded the Center for the Study of Georgia History.

In 1996, the regents renamed many university system institutions, and Augusta College became Augusta State University. Each of the three schools at ASU became colleges. That same year the institution inaugurated its honors program. Two years later, along with MCG and other state institutions, ASU converted from quarters to semesters. Tougher admissions standards, also mandated by the regents, resulted in the creation of University College within ASU, creating the equivalent of a junior college within the university as a point of entry for students not meeting the new requirements.

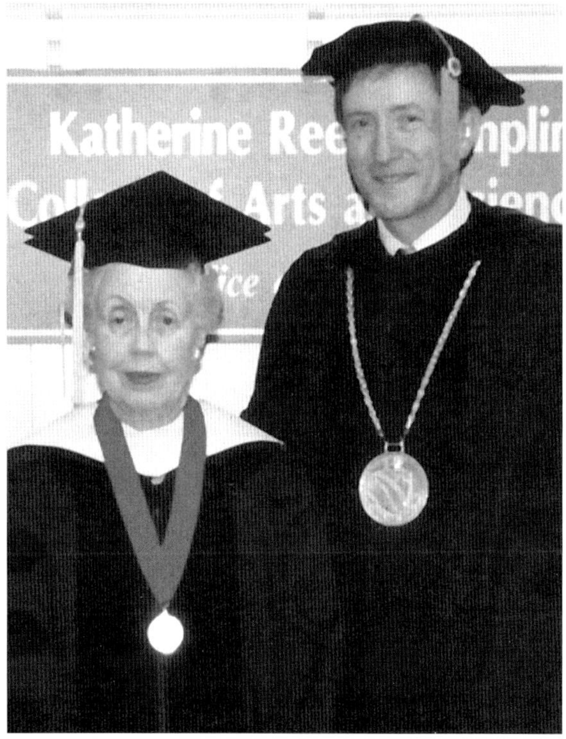


*Above: Alumna Katherine Reese Pamplin received the institution's first honorary doctorate in 1996. The following year, in recognition of her endowment to the university, the College of Arts and Sciences was named in her honor. (She is shown with President William A. Bloodworth Jr.)*

*Below: In 1996, Augusta College became Augusta State University. At graduation, students received tee shirts inscribed, "Our College Days are Over."*

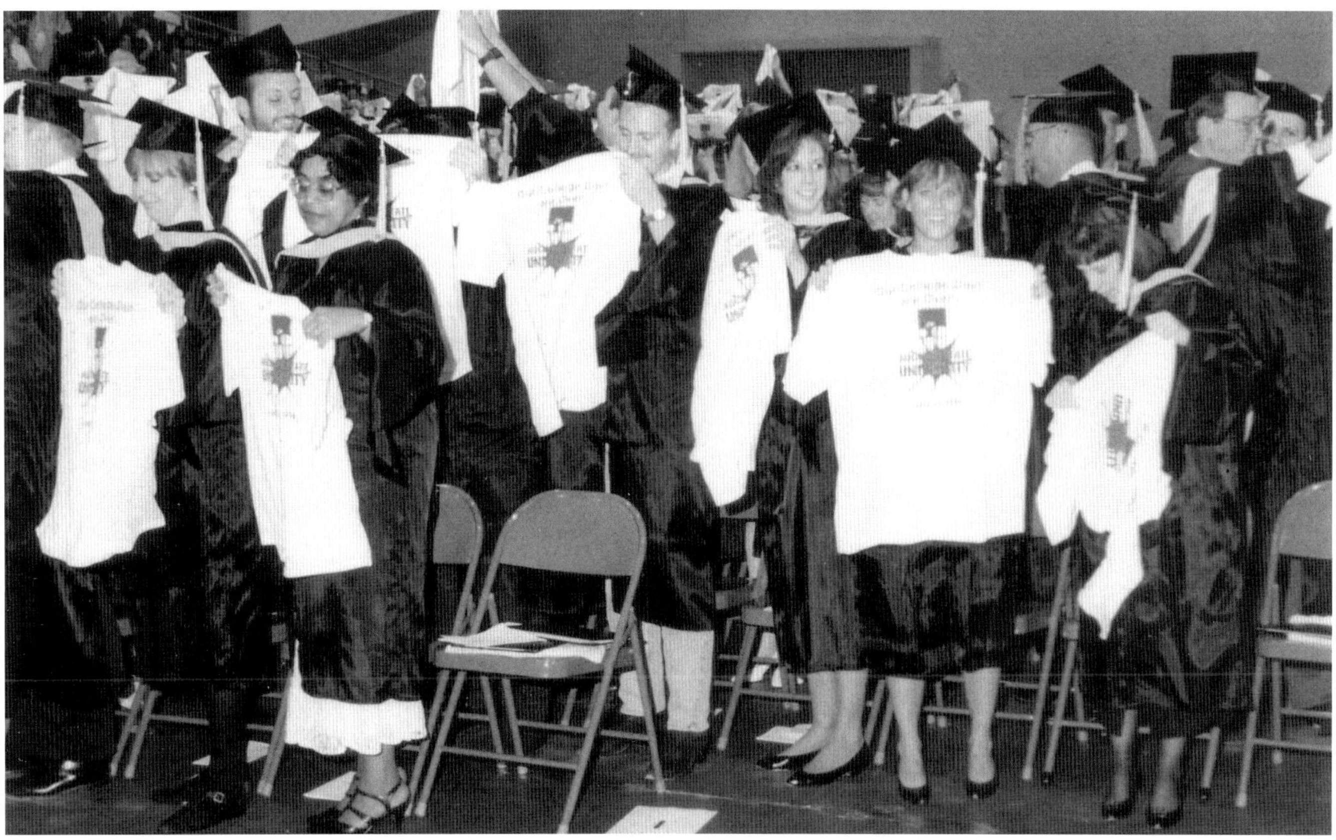

As the world shrank through digital communication, improved transportation, and international agreements in business, global awareness became increasingly important. Exchange programs with Mid-Sweden University in Sundsvall and the Dosso Dossi Art Institute in Ferrara, Italy, had been established in 1991. Ten years later, a certificate in European studies collaborative program began with Germany's University of Munich. A new exchange program began with Senegal in 2007. The study abroad program became increasingly popular, offering learning opportunities on almost every continent.

Collaborative programs proliferated. A cooperative doctoral program in education leadership with Georgia Southern University was added in 2000. A program with the University of West Georgia allowed new web-based courses in electronic commerce. ASU's Department of Nursing partnered with Doctors, St. Joseph, and University Hospitals to provide LPNs with a fast track to an associate in nursing degree. A memorandum of understanding (MOU) with Georgia Tech established a cooperative pre-engineering degree program.

In virtually every discipline, many courses included "service learning" components, part of the institution's mission to serve the community. Renovations to campus also enhanced the way courses were taught, with state-of-the-art electronic media in every classroom and multiple computer labs.

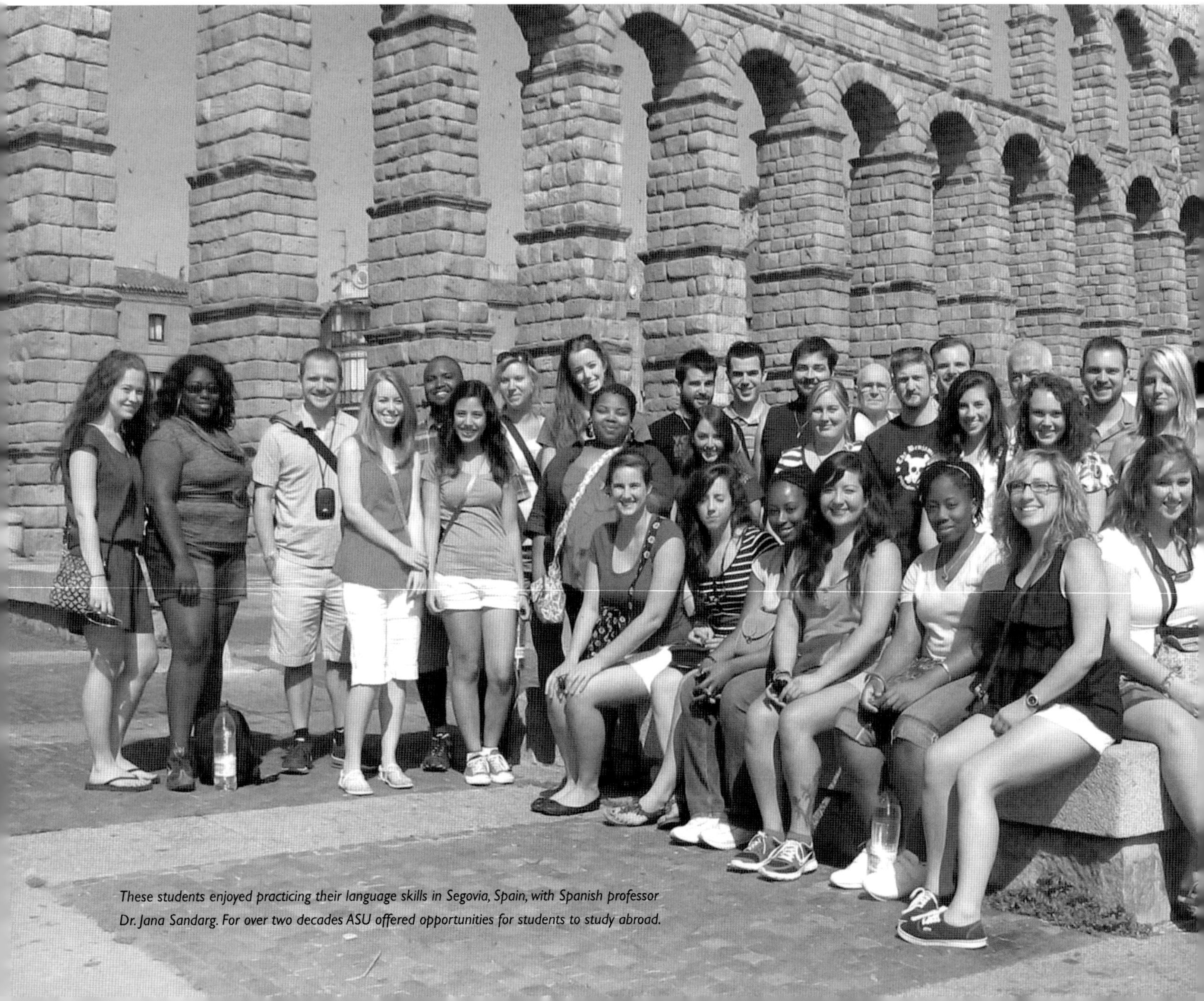

*These students enjoyed practicing their language skills in Segovia, Spain, with Spanish professor Dr. Jana Sandarg. For over two decades ASU offered opportunities for students to study abroad.*

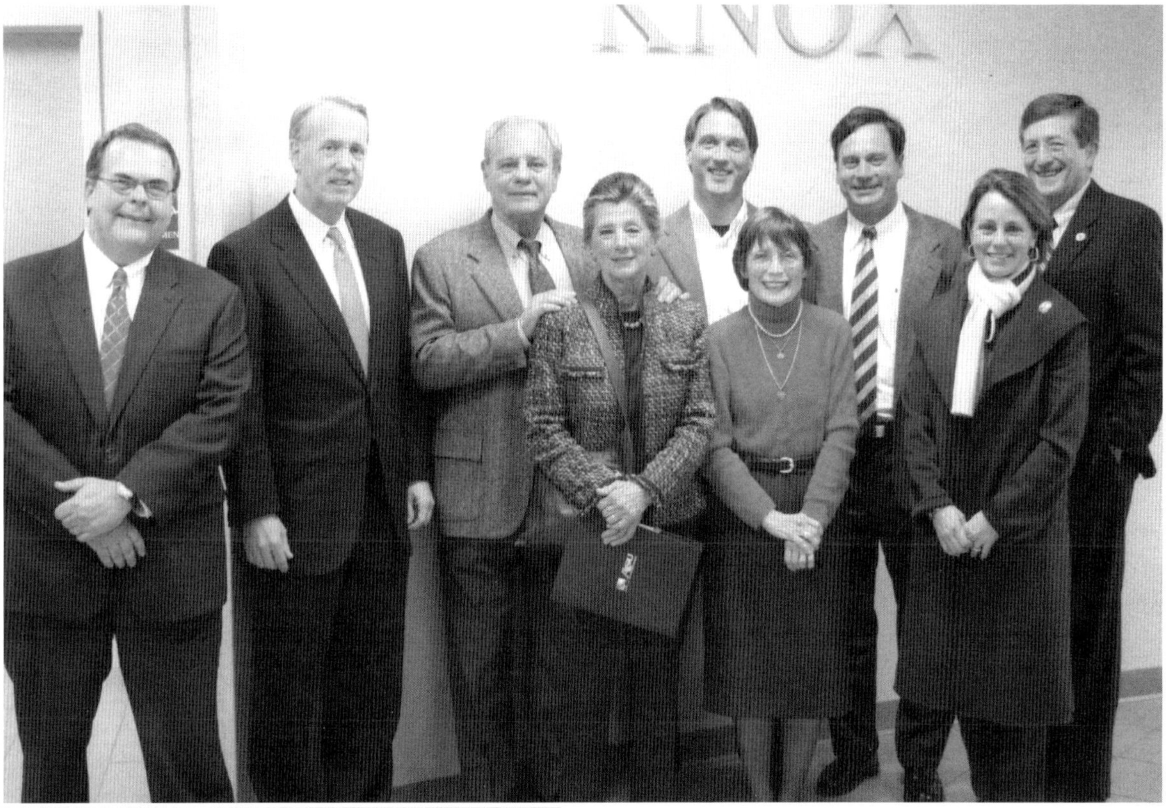

Members of the Knox family and Hull College benefactor James Hull Jr. posed with university officials after the opening of the Knox School of Accountancy in the Hull College, made possible by the family's philanthropy.

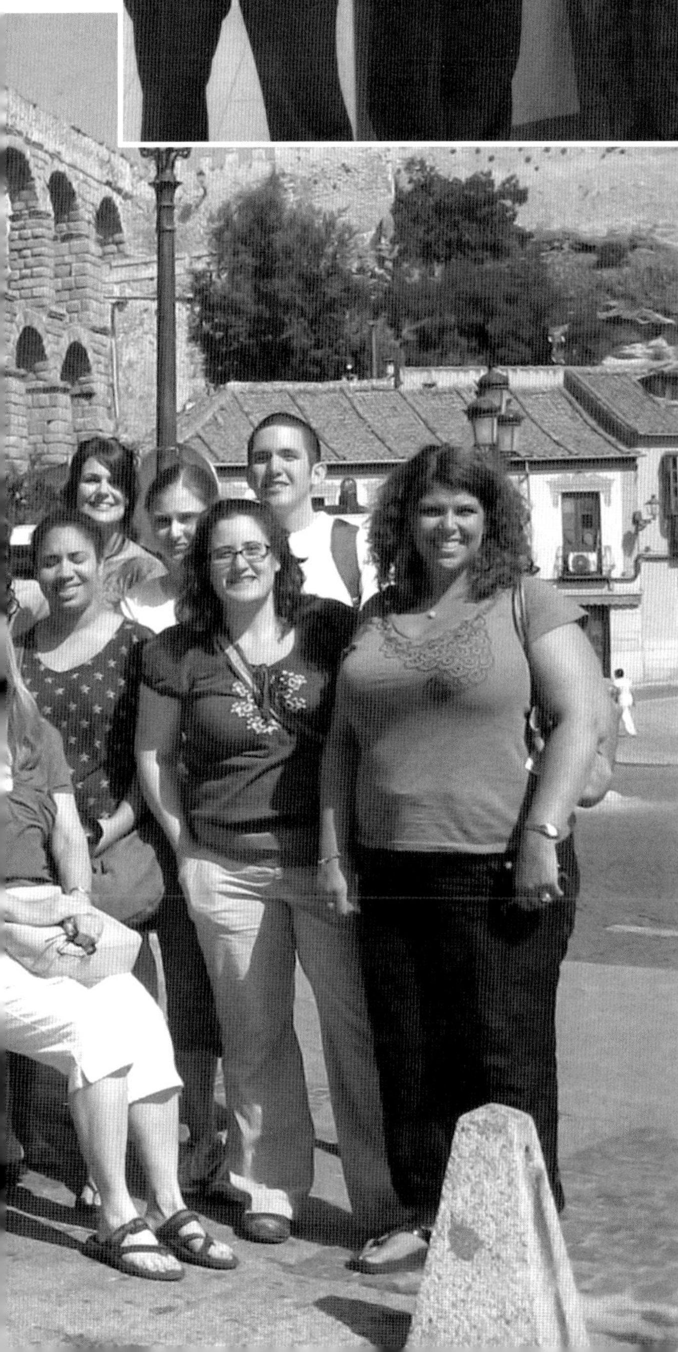

All three of ASU's colleges went through enormous changes in the 2000s. Major gifts to the College of Business Administration resulted in renaming the college the James M. Hull College of Business in 2006 and creating the Knox School of Accountancy within it in 2008 with a Peter S. Knox III Distinguished Chair of Accounting. For four consecutive years, *Princeton Review* named the Hull College one of the nation's top business schools.

The College of Education had its accreditation from the National Council for Accreditation of Teacher Education reaffirmed with no areas needing improvement. It also won accreditation for its counselor education program and began offering master of arts in teaching and master of education in teacher leadership degrees. A major National Science Foundation PRESTIGE grant made a five-year

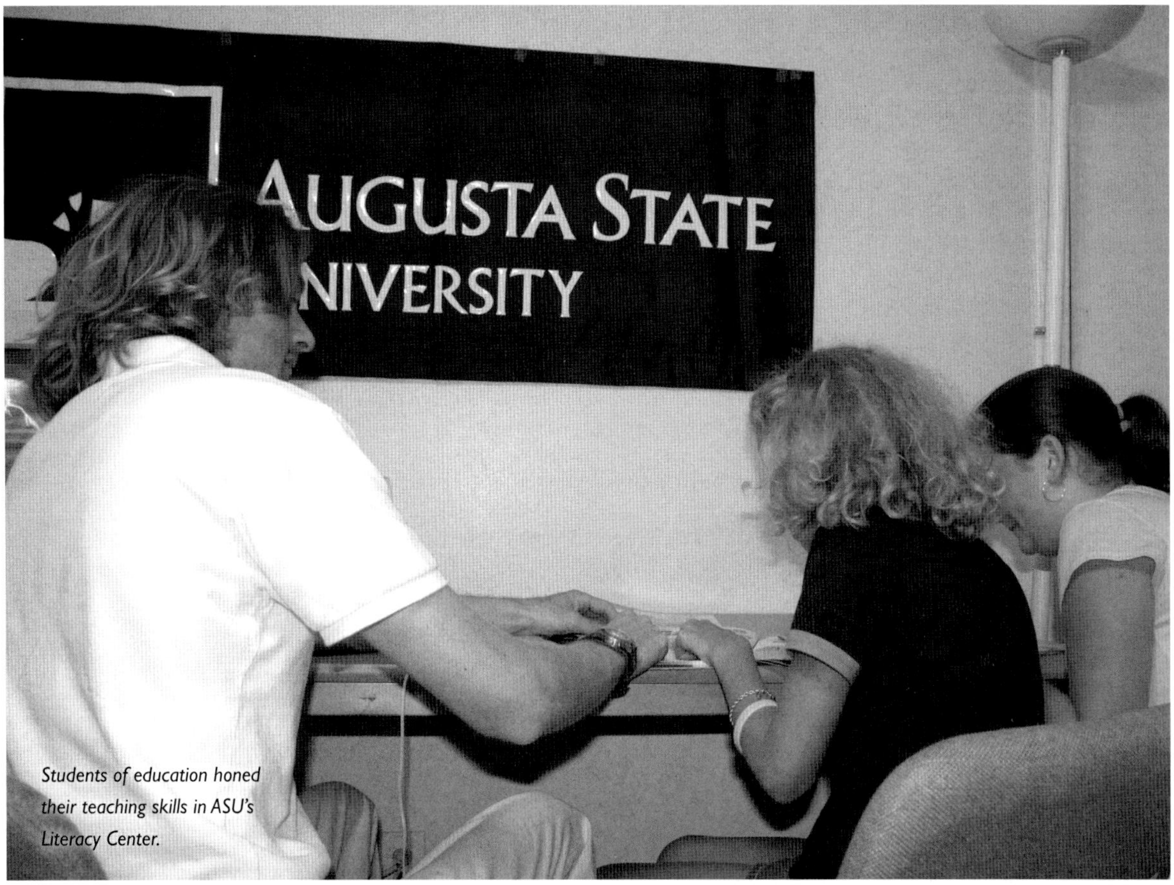

Students of education honed their teaching skills in ASU's Literacy Center.

program integrating the bachelor and master of science in education degrees possible.

The Pamplin College of Arts and Sciences won accreditation for a program in social work, added bachelor's degrees in social work and nursing, and accreditations for the master's of public administration degree and the nursing program. New tracks were added in forensic science and nuclear science. In 2012, the Pamplin College itself was split into two colleges: the Pamplin College of Arts, Humanities, and Social Sciences and the College of Science and Mathematics.

By the second decade of the new millennium the academic programs of Georgia Health Sciences University and Augusta State University had come a long way since their humble beginnings, but both still reflected what their respective founders had sought—institutions of higher learning that imparted knowledge and prepared students for their futures through excellent teaching.

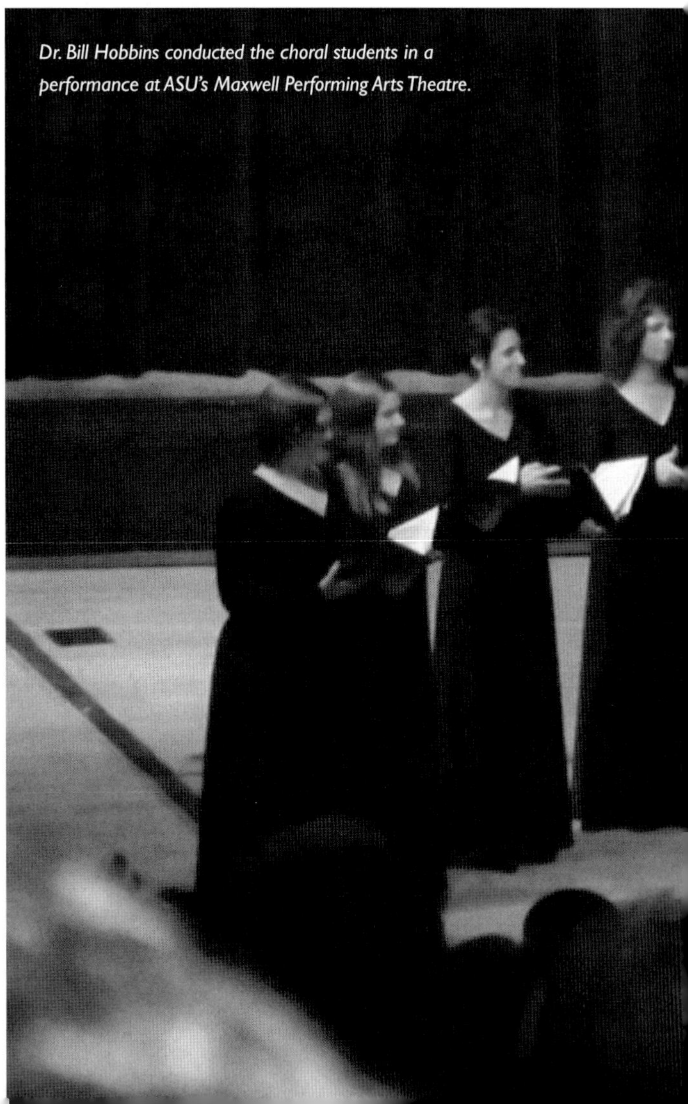
Dr. Bill Hobbins conducted the choral students in a performance at ASU's Maxwell Performing Arts Theatre.

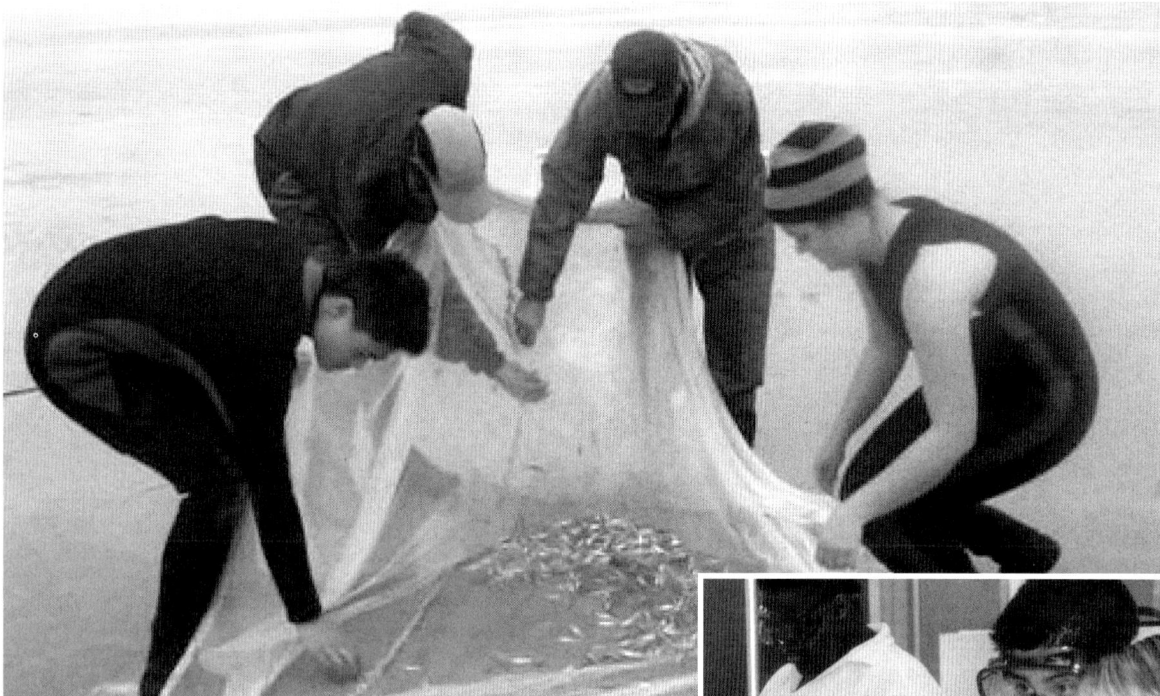

*Above: Biology students and graduates experienced marine research at St. Catherines Island as part of a long-term study of its fish population.*

*Right: Wearing protective goggles, ASU students perform chemistry experiments in their laboratory class.*

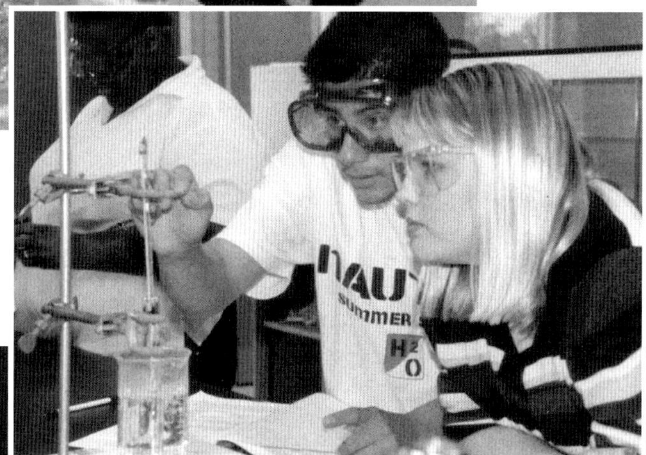


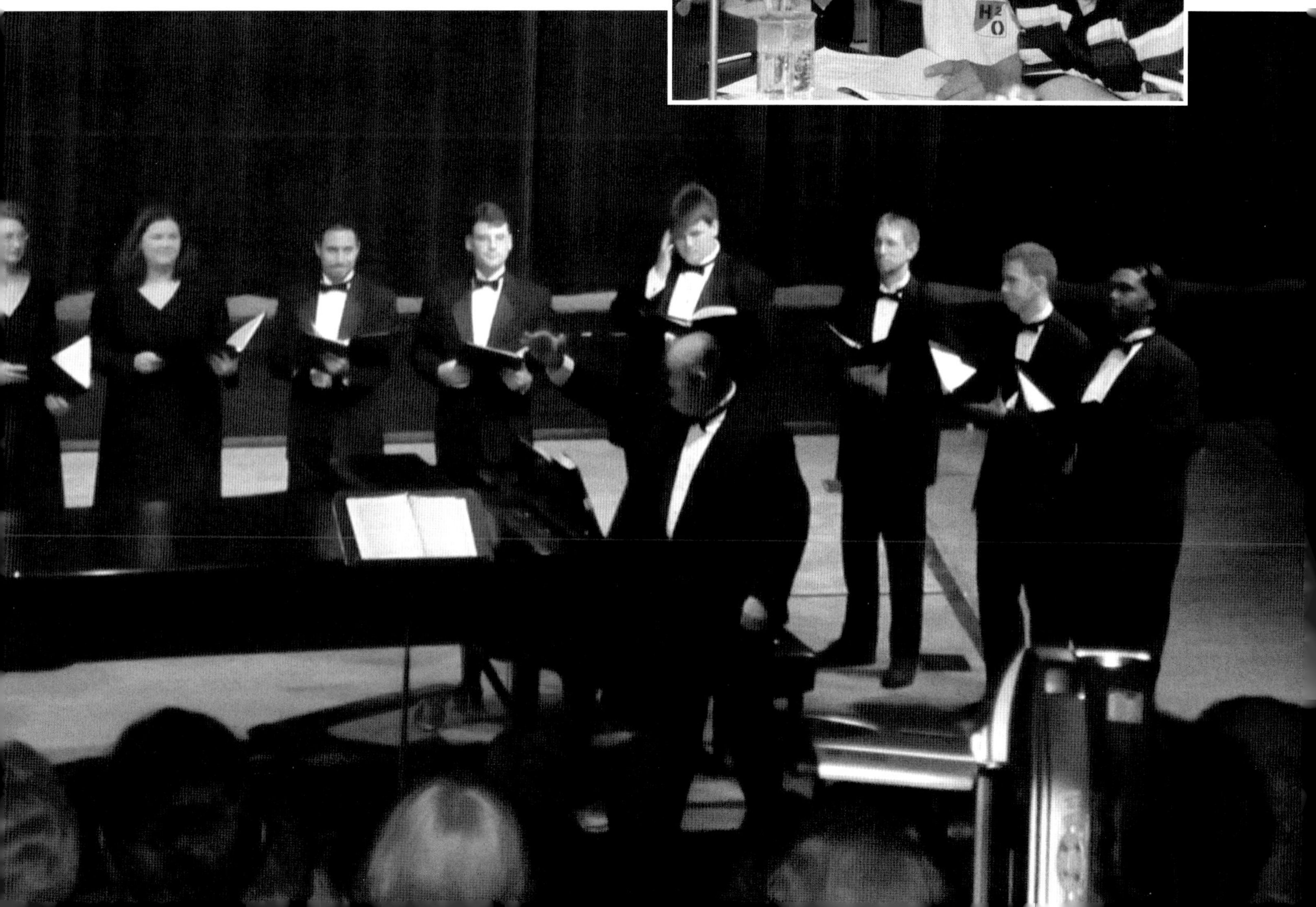

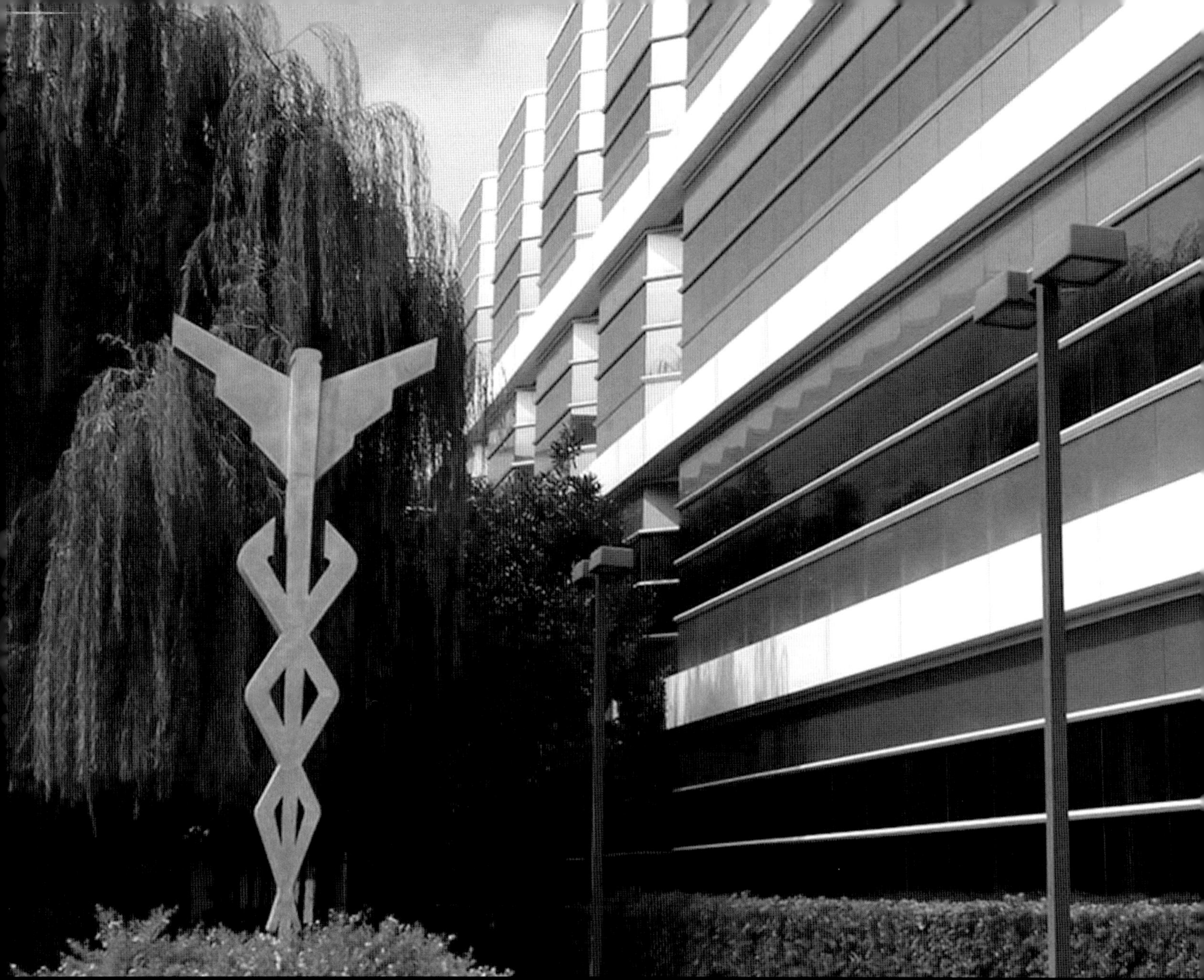

# RESEARCH:

## *Contributions of Discovery and Creation*

From its earliest years the Medical College of Georgia (MCG) created a culture that encouraged research and set a standard for medical treatment that continues to the present day. Even before founding the institution, Dr. Milton Antony was performing cutting-edge surgery, including the first lung surgery in the United States in 1821. He began publishing the *Southern Medical and Surgical Journal* in 1836 to report medical advances made by MCG faculty and other physicians.

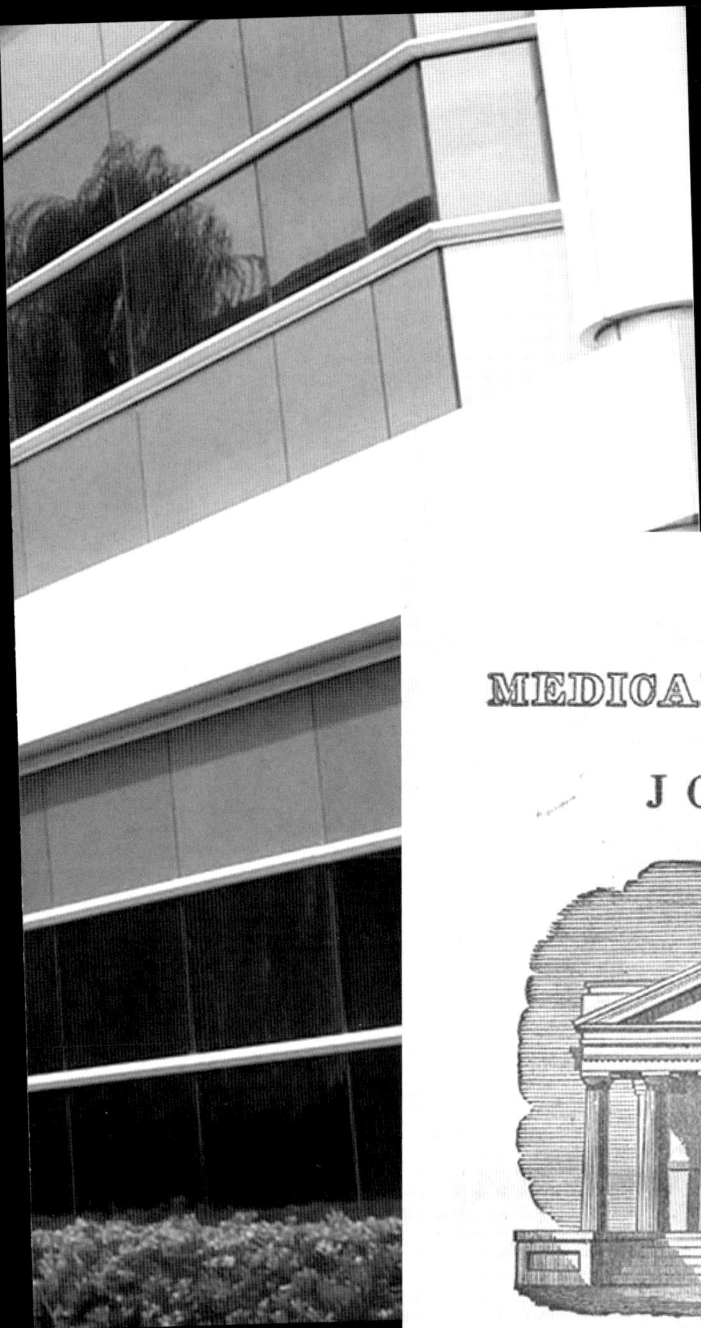

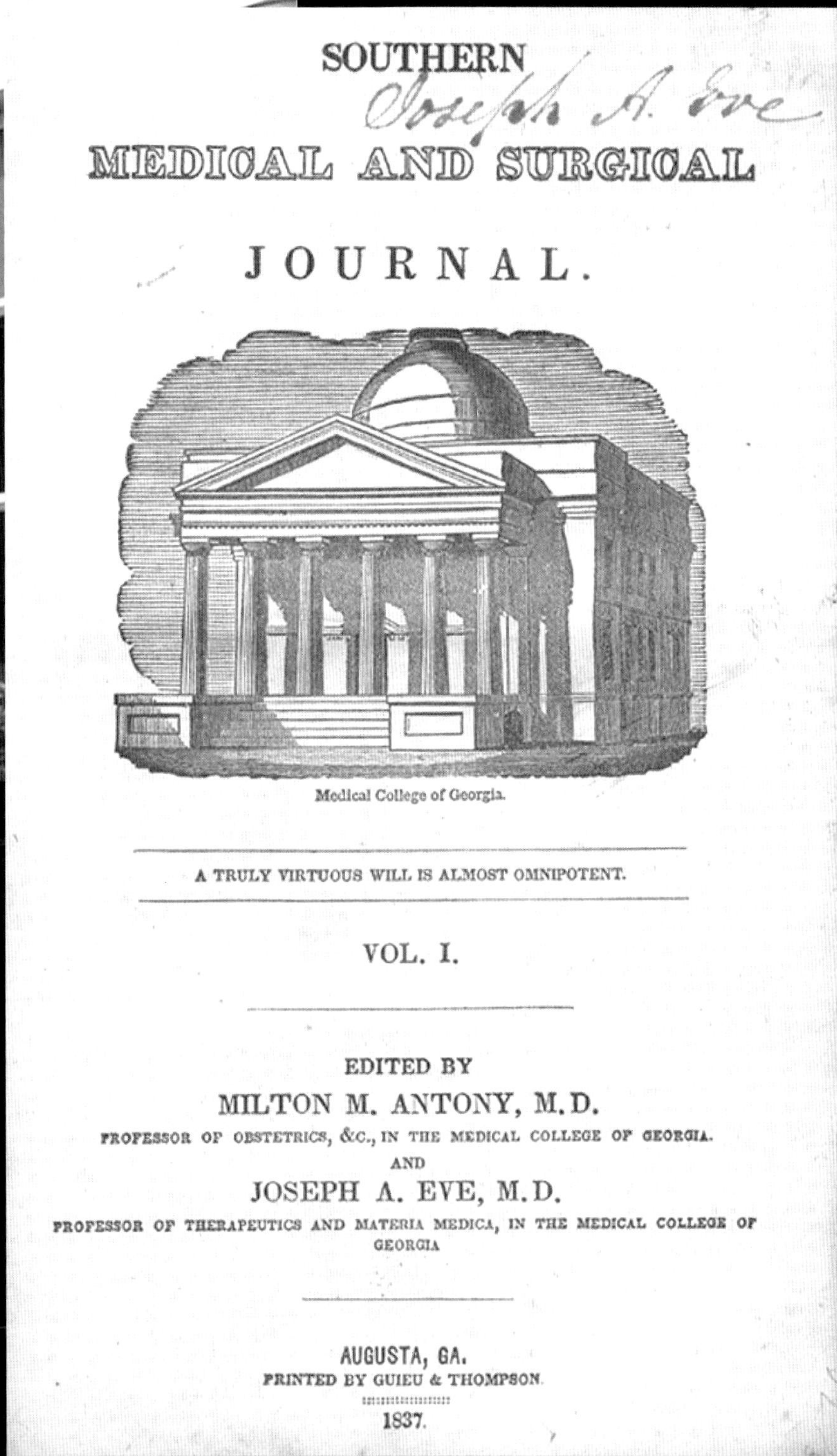

SOUTHERN

Joseph A. Eve

MEDICAL AND SURGICAL

JOURNAL.

Medical College of Georgia.

A TRULY VIRTUOUS WILL IS ALMOST OMNIPOTENT.

VOL. I.

EDITED BY

MILTON M. ANTONY, M.D.

PROFESSOR OF OBSTETRICS, &C., IN THE MEDICAL COLLEGE OF GEORGIA.

AND

JOSEPH A. EVE, M.D.

PROFESSOR OF THERAPEUTICS AND MATERIA MEDICA, IN THE MEDICAL COLLEGE OF GEORGIA

AUGUSTA, GA.

PRINTED BY GUIEU & THOMPSON.

1837.

*First published in 1836 by the faculty of the Medical College of Georgia, the* Southern Medical and Surgical Journal *brought recognition to the institution and kept physicians abreast of new practices in medicine.*

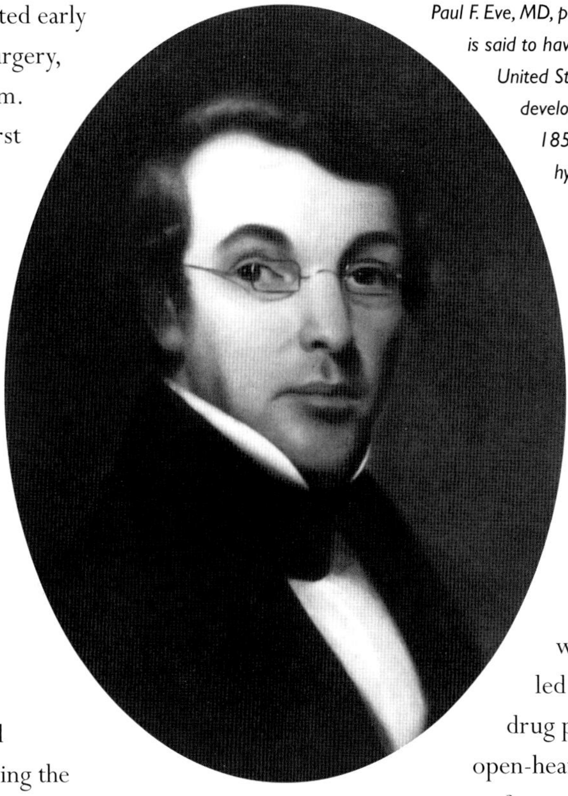

*Paul F. Eve, MD, professor of surgery and later dean, is said to have been the first surgeon in the United States to use chloroform, an anesthetic developed by a Scottish physician. In 1850, Eve performed the nation's first hysterectomy.*

Other faculty members adopted early efforts to eliminate pain in surgery, using hypnosis and chloroform. Medical firsts included the first hysterectomy in the country, performing ligature of the ischiatic artery for aneurysm, and developing the doctrine of reflex vasomotor reaction. The "Dugas Sign," a simple clinical test for diagnosis of a dislocated shoulder developed by Dr. Louis Dugas, is still used today. Technological advances included several instruments for use in gynecological operations and lithotomy and the surgical contribution during the Civil War of ligating large arteries of the extremities to arrest gangrene.

A multi-volume *Modern Medicine* (1906) contained a chapter on dengue fever contributed by MCG faculty member Thomas D. Coleman, the only Georgian and one of the few southern contributors. The chapter ushered in the twentieth century, which was an era of important discoveries and innovations by Medical College of Georgia faculty. Early to mid-twentieth century contributions included work on blood transfusion, sickle cell anemia, and wartime nutrition. The invention of the Hamilton Manometer in the mid-1940s paved the way for cardiac catheterization. MCG's first winner of the prestigious Lasker Award published research in 1948 that laid the groundwork for today's beta-blocking drugs used in heart surgery and control of high blood pressure, as well as made discoveries that led to the development of the drug propranolol. In 1956, the first open-heart bypass surgery in Georgia was performed at MCG.

MCG researchers over the years have contributed significantly to the treatment of reproductive system diseases and disorders including groundbreaking work on fertility, studies of gender-related disorders and sex determination, and treatment of a widely endemic venereal disease. Instruments were invented to make childbirth safer as well.

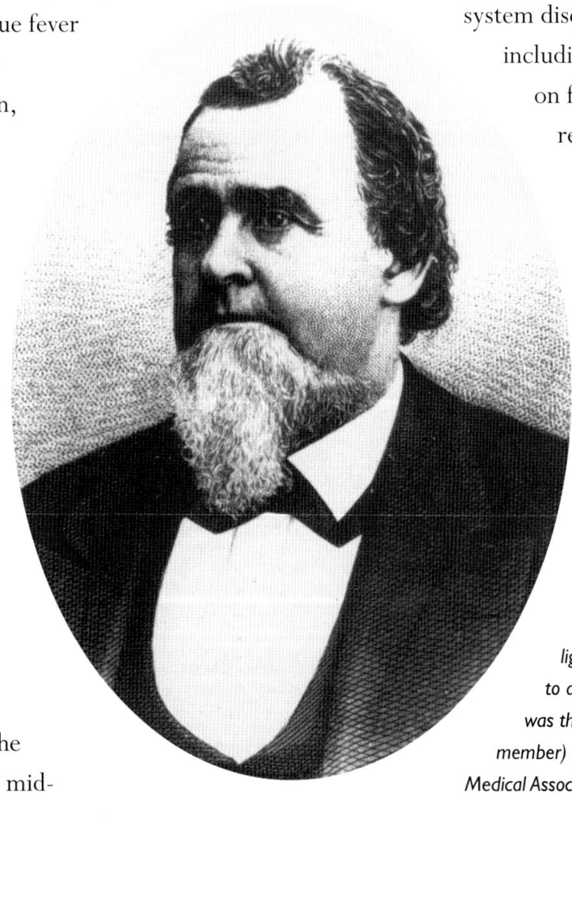

*Henry F. Campbell, an MCG graduate and professor, presented a doctrine of reflex and lithotomy, invented several instruments for use in gynecological operations and lithotomy, and began the practice of ligating large arteries of the extremities to arrest gangrene. In 1884, Campbell was the first alumnus (and second faculty member) to become president of the American Medical Association.*

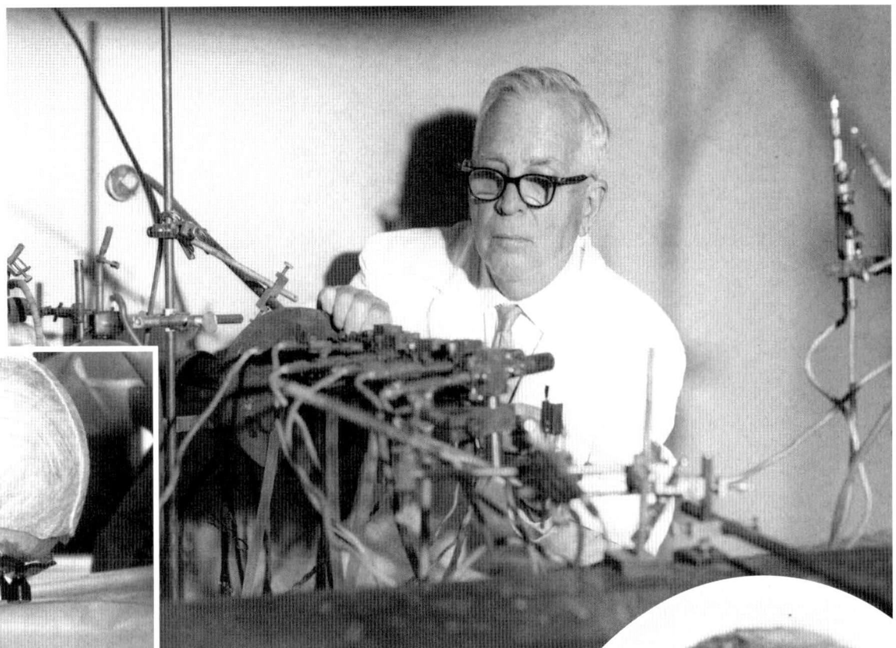

Right: William F. Hamilton, PhD, chairman of Physiology for almost twenty-five years and inventor of the Hamilton Manometer, distinguished himself in hemodynamic and cardiovascular research.

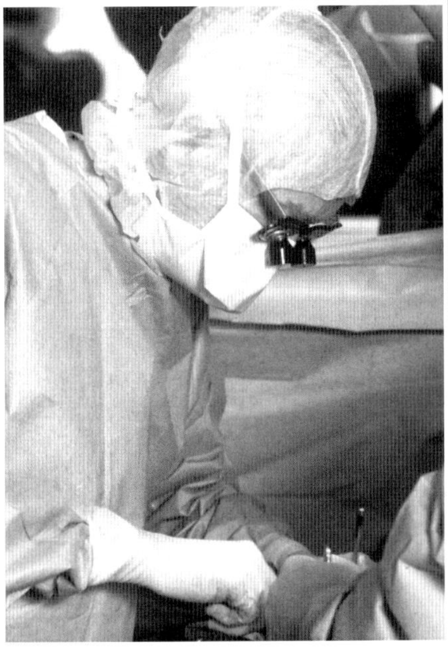

Left: Robert G. Ellison, MD, performed Georgia's first open-heart bypass surgery at MCG in 1956. He established the first cardiopulmonary laboratory in the state. He also improved techniques for cardiothoracic surgery and for treatment of esophageal and lung cancer.

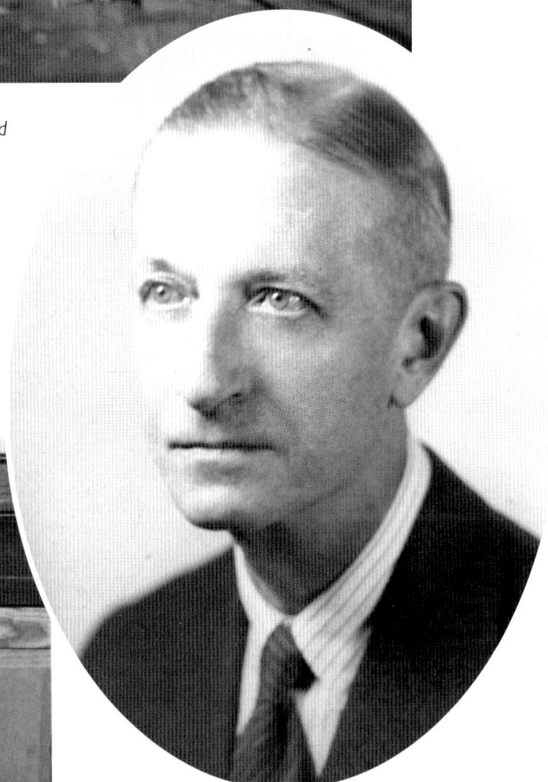

Virgil P. Sydenstricker, MD, chairman of the Department of Medicine from 1922 to 1957, was a medical student when he co-authored an article with Nobel Prize winner G. H. Whipple on a system of blood transfusion that became the basis for today's blood banking and transfusion practices. In 1923, he published the first case report of sickle cell anemia with autopsy findings. During World War II, he helped develop the K-ration and oversaw the medical and nutritional care of sixty thousand prisoners released from German prisons. He also demonstrated that pellagra resulted from a niacin deficiency, which earned him a nomination for the Nobel Prize.

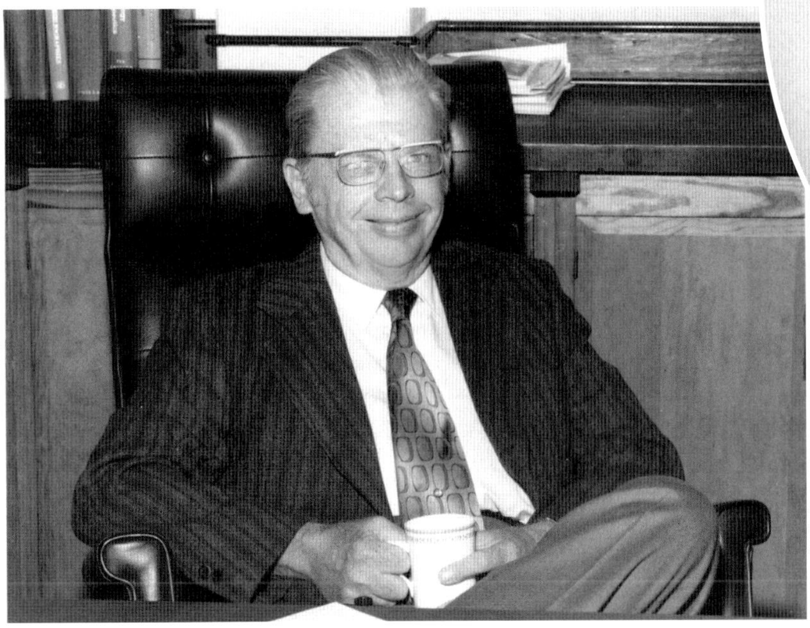

Raymond P. Ahlquist, PhD, chairman of Pharmacology and MCG's first Lasker Award winner, published research in 1948 that laid the groundwork for today's beta-blocking drugs used in heart surgery and in treatment of hypertension. His discoveries also led to the development of the drug propranolol.

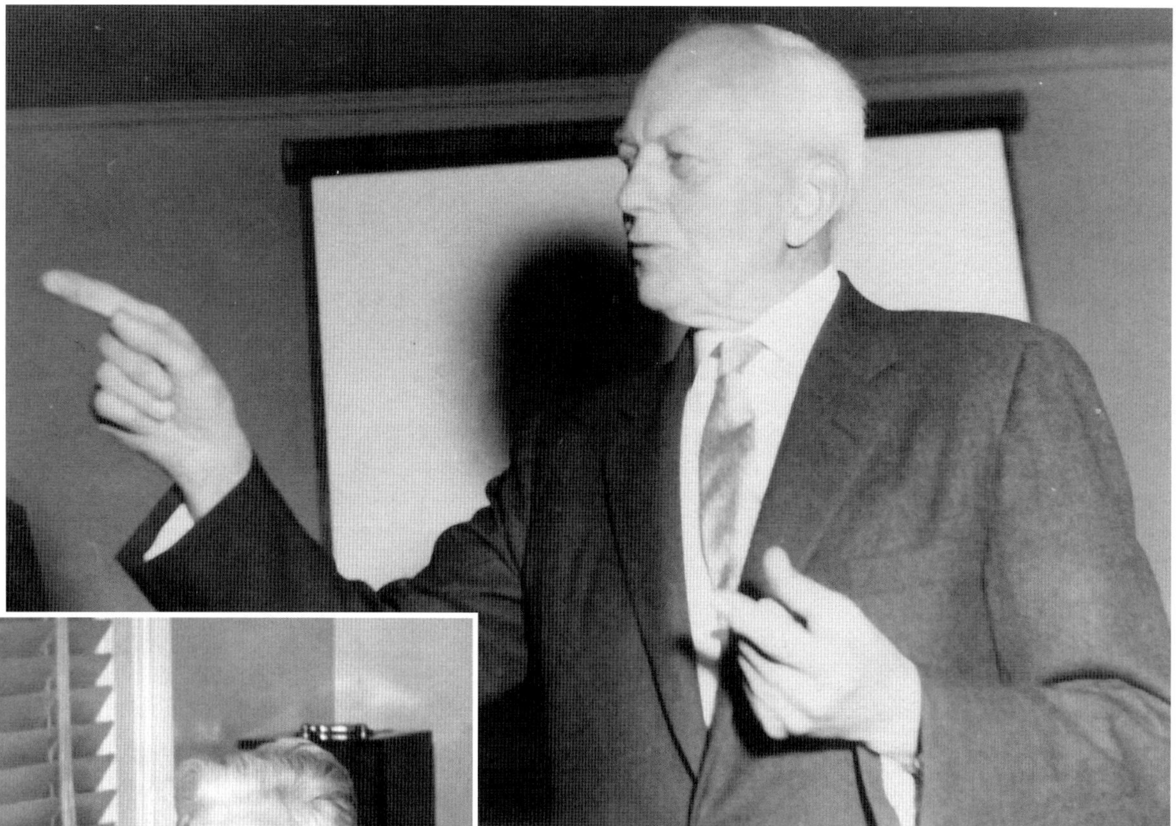

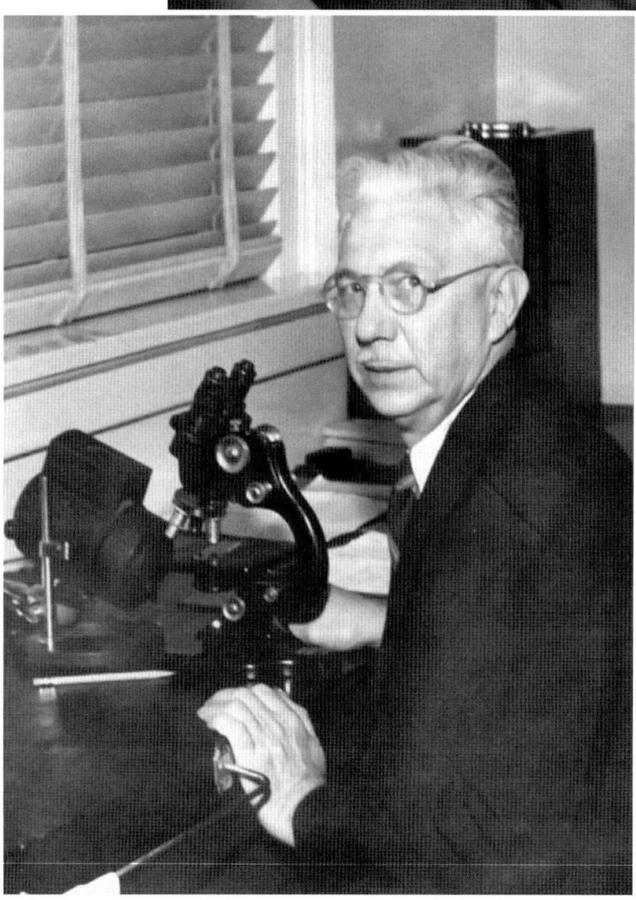

*Above: Richard Torpin, MD, chairman of Obstetrics and Gynecology, made significant contributions both through his writings and the invention of several surgical instruments that make childbirth safer including the Torpin Insufflator, the Torpin Uterine Packer, and other instruments.*

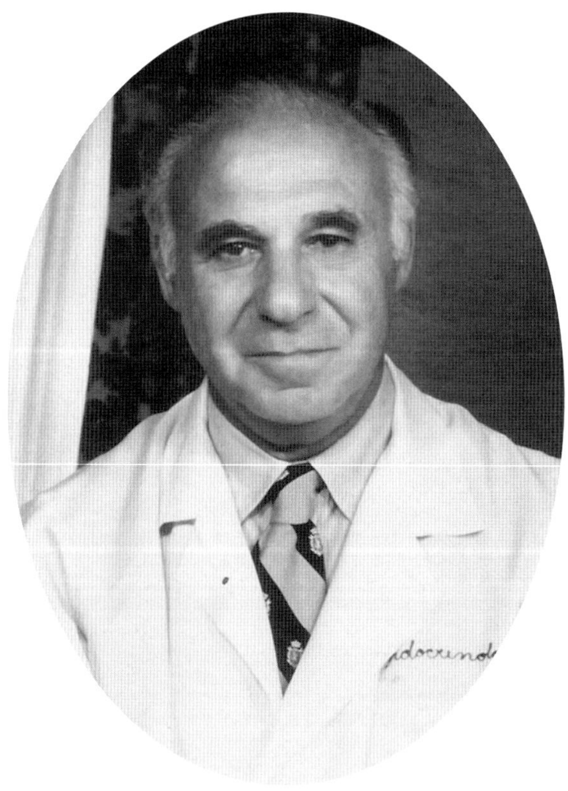

*Edgar Pund, MD, (above), a faculty member and later MCG president, and Robert Greenblatt, MD, (right) chairman of the Department of Endocrinology, described the pathonomic cell in granuloma inguinale, a widely endemic venereal disease. Greenblatt's finding that mycin antibiotics could cure the disease was a major contribution to public health; his research also laid the groundwork for fertility and birth-control treatments.*

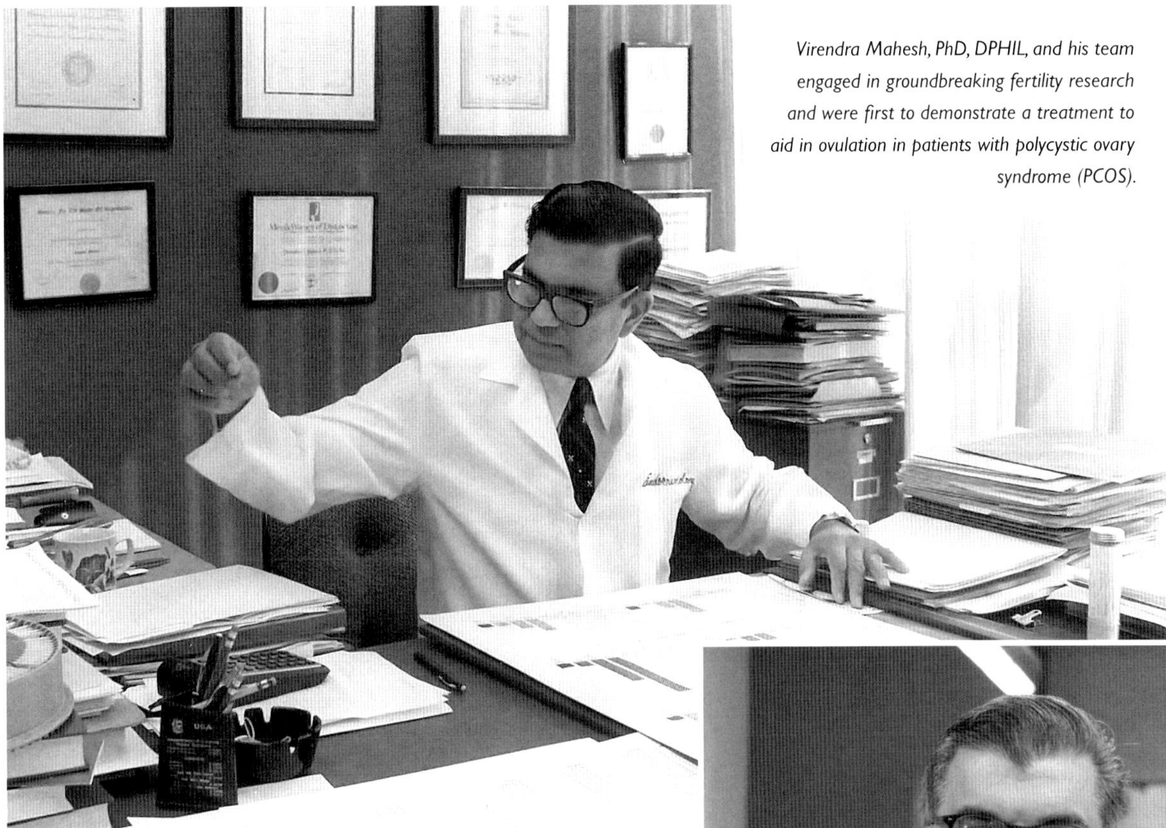

*Virendra Mahesh, PhD, DPHIL, and his team engaged in groundbreaking fertility research and were first to demonstrate a treatment to aid in ovulation in patients with polycystic ovary syndrome (PCOS).*

*Below: Reproductive endocrinologist Paul McDonough, MD, is known internationally for his contributions related to the molecular biology of mammalian sexual development. He performed the first prenatal diagnosis of congenital adrenal hyperplasia using a specific biochemical marker in amniotic fluid as well as the first DNA analysis in amniotic fluid for the same disorder.*

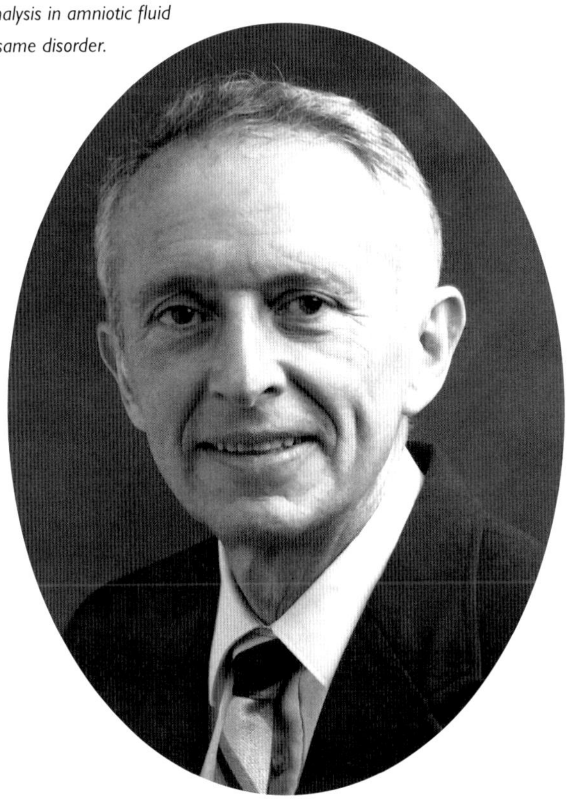

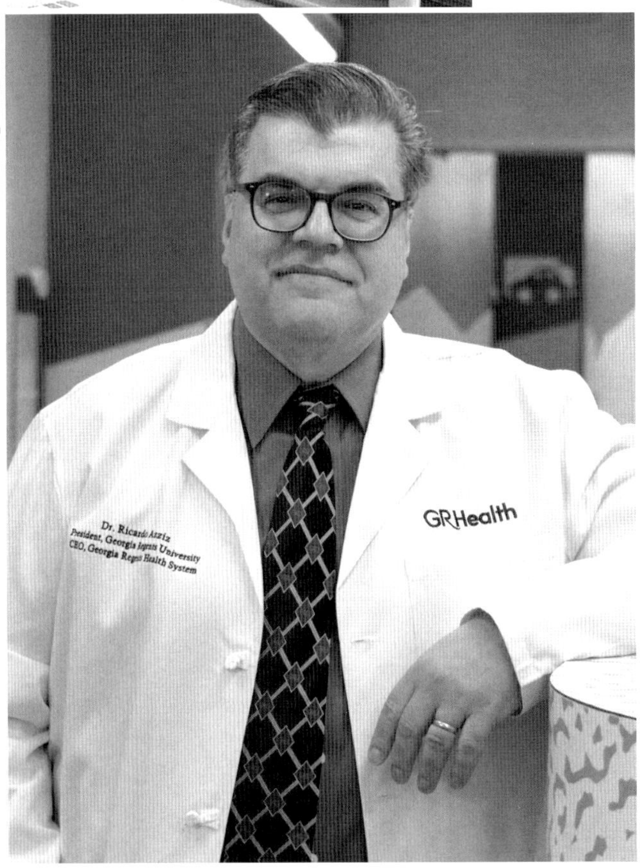


*Above: Ricardo Azziz, MD, MPH, MBA, professor of Obstetrics and Gynecology, has been recognized internationally for his research on hormonal abnormalities of women, focusing primarily on androgen excess disorders, adrenal hyperplasia, and polycystic ovarian syndrome. He has authored or edited seven textbooks, over four hundred articles, and numerous other publications.*

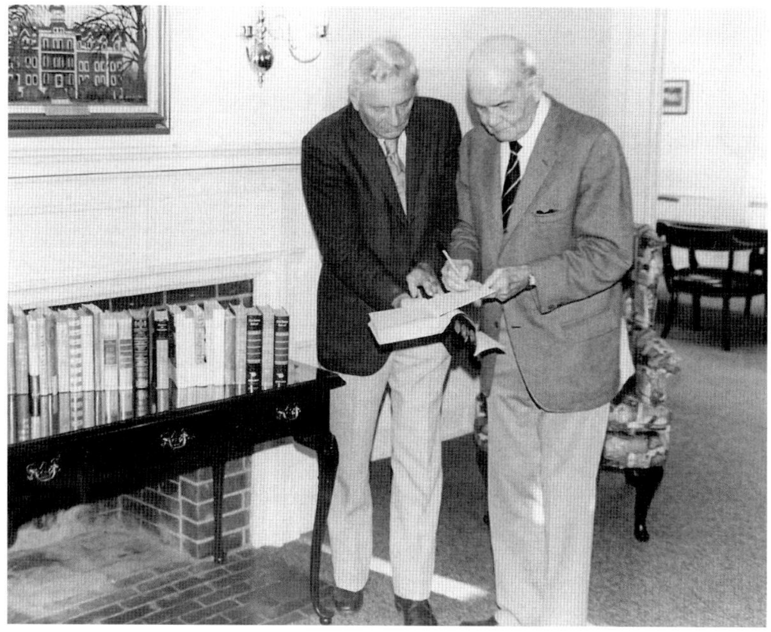

*Right: Psychiatrist Hervey M. Cleckley's 1941 book,* The Mask of Sanity, *considered a seminal work describing psychopathic personality, has been reissued multiple times, most recently in 2003. In 1957, Cleckley and Corbett H. Thigpen, MD, presented the first case study documenting a patient displaying more than two personalities. The resulting book,* The Three Faces of Eve, *was published in fourteen languages and made into a popular movie. Both Cleckley and Thigpen were MCG alumni and faculty members.*

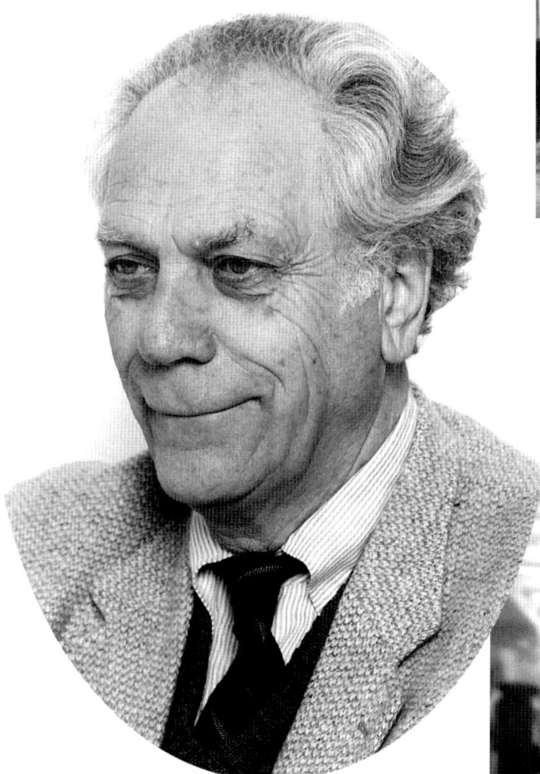

*Left: Titus H. J. Huisman, PhD, DSc, professor in the Department of Hematology and Oncology from 1959 to 1995 and author of over one thousand papers, identified thalassemia and many other hemoglobin variants that, among other things, led to nationwide newborn screenings for hemoglobin-related disorders. By the time of his death in 1999, his labs had discovered over half of the seven hundred known hemoglobin variants.*

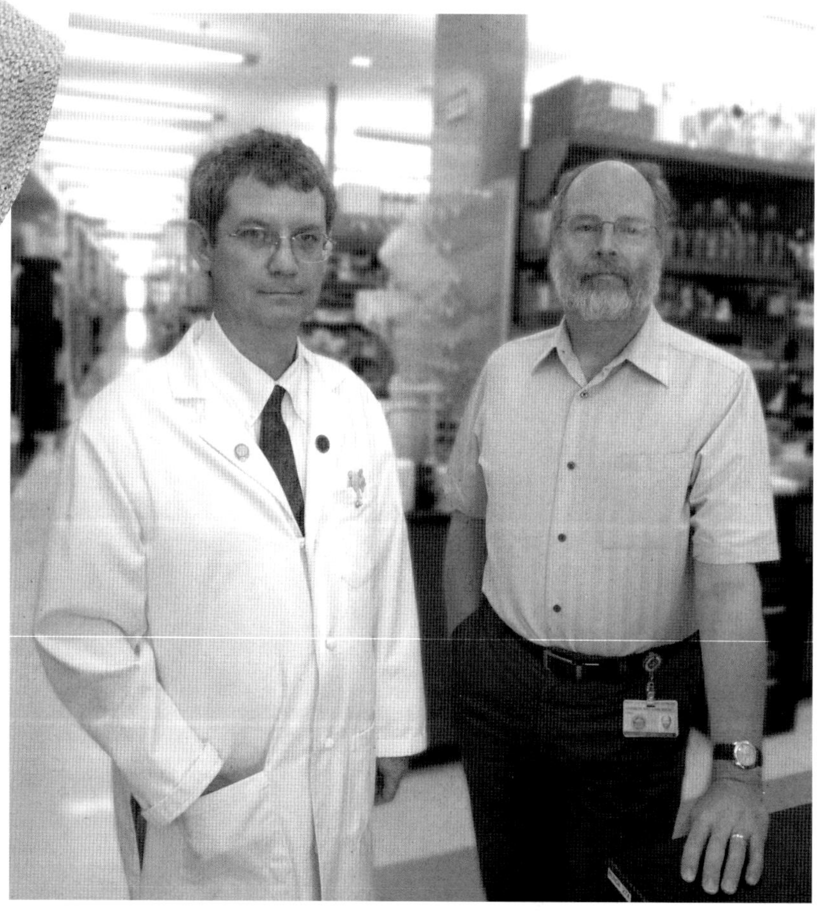

*Right: Pediatric oncologist David Munn, MD, (left) and immunologist Andrew Mellor, PhD, (right) identified the enzyme IDO's role in preventing a mother's immune system from rejecting a fetus and showed that immune cells can produce this enzyme. Both studies appeared in* Science *in 1998. Their subsequent findings showed tumors use IDO to protect themselves from the immune response. The university patented technologies to inhibit IDO as a way to battle cancer. Conversely, IDO's ability to selectively inhibit the immune response is being explored for its potential in treating autoimmune diseases such as arthritis.*

In the second half of the twentieth century significant contributions came in a variety of fields including hematology, immunology, drug abuse, hypertension, stroke, Gulf War Syndrome, emergency medicine, and Alzheimer's disease. Recently, research on the regeneration of bone tissue and the prevention of bone necrosis has been underway at the university. In dentistry, patients are seeing the result of bioengineering and regenerative treatments and therapies as researchers continue to develop and evaluate new materials, implants, and products. Children have benefited from MCG research on sickle cell anemia and juvenile diabetes, early pet exposure and allergies, health promotion and disease prevention, and childhood obesity.

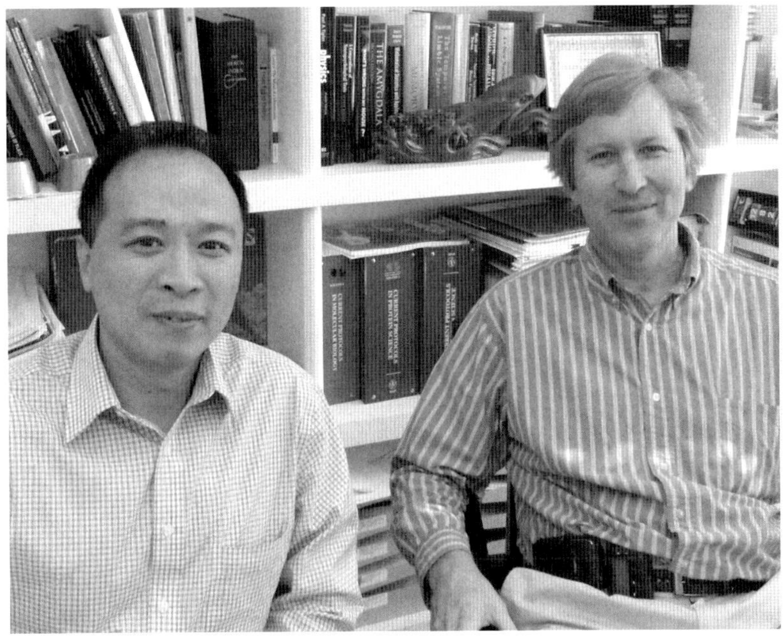

*Neuroscientist Joseph Tsien, PhD, (left) and vascular neurologist David H. Hess, MD, (right) co-direct the Brain and Behavior Discovery Institute. Hess, an innovator in stroke treatment, found stroke victims could be effectively diagnosed and treated through the emerging capabilities of the Internet. This led to the development of a telestroke network system now used at more than one hundred hospitals in several states. Tsien's groundbreaking research into the genetic factors affecting memory led to the identification of the NR2B subunit of the NMDA receptor, which has prompted the discovery by other researchers of over two dozen other genes that affect memory.*

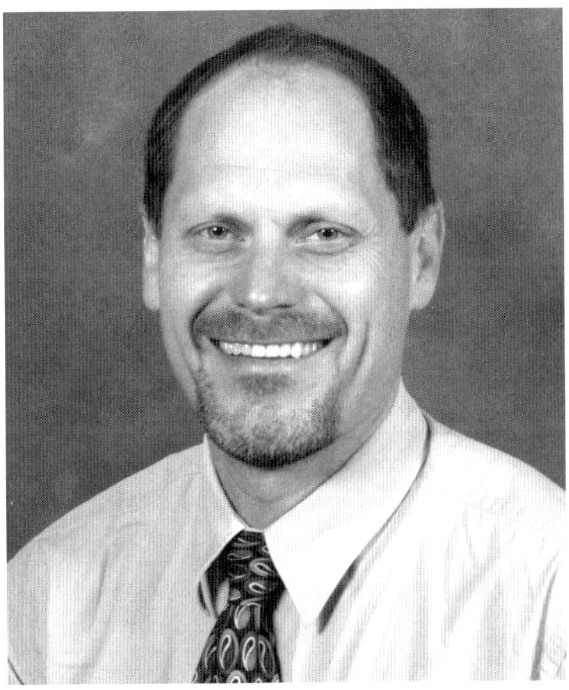

*Above: Richard Schwartz, MD, emergency medicine physician, worked with Birmingham ER physician John Croushorn, MD, to develop an abdominal aortic tourniquet that can prevent bleeding to death for soldiers in the field and other trauma patients. The device, used in war zones and stateside, earned a 2012 Popular Science Invention Award.*

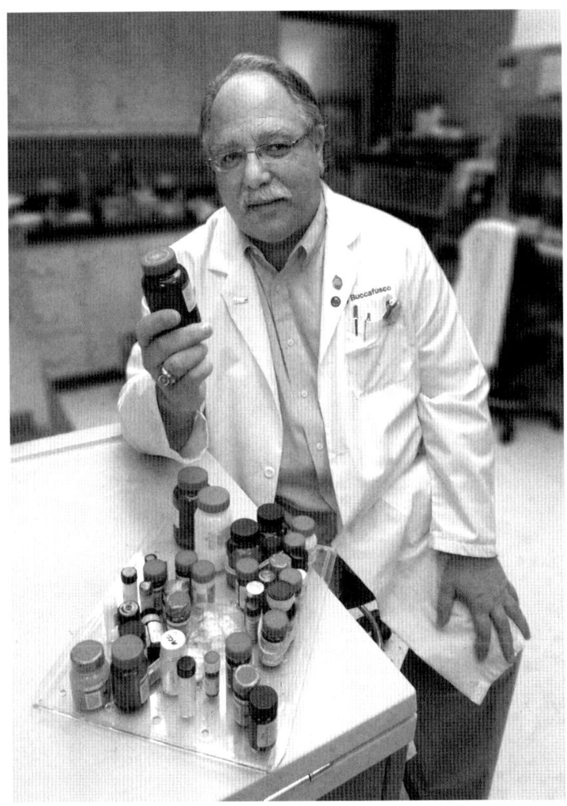

*Right: Internationally renowned pharmacologist Jerry Buccafusco, PhD, published over two hundred articles and four edited books that made contributions to the study of drug abuse, hypertension, Gulf War Syndrome, and Alzheimer's disease. He was the founding director of the Alzheimer's Research Center, where he developed biomarkers for early detection as well as novel therapies for the disease.*

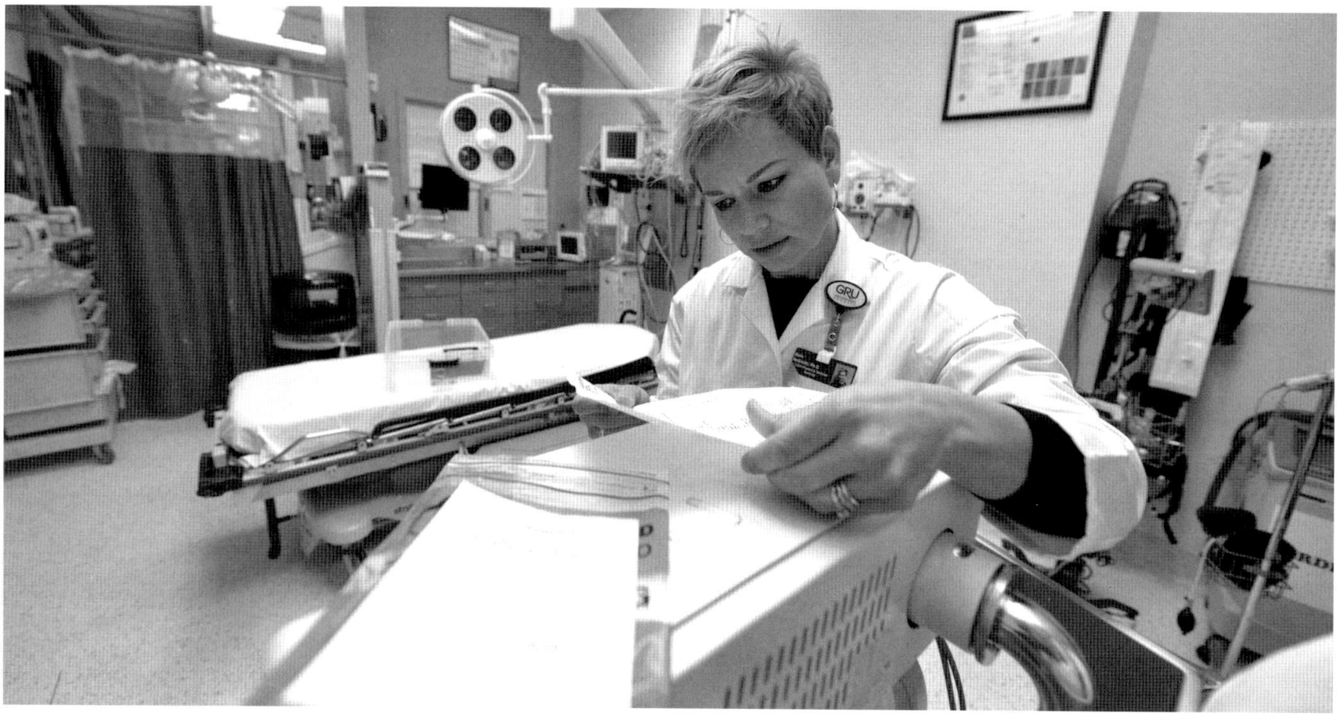

*Elizabeth G. NeSmith, RN, PhD, has been researching the treatment and prevention of sepsis and organ failure following trauma as well as the influence of stress on inflammatory response.*

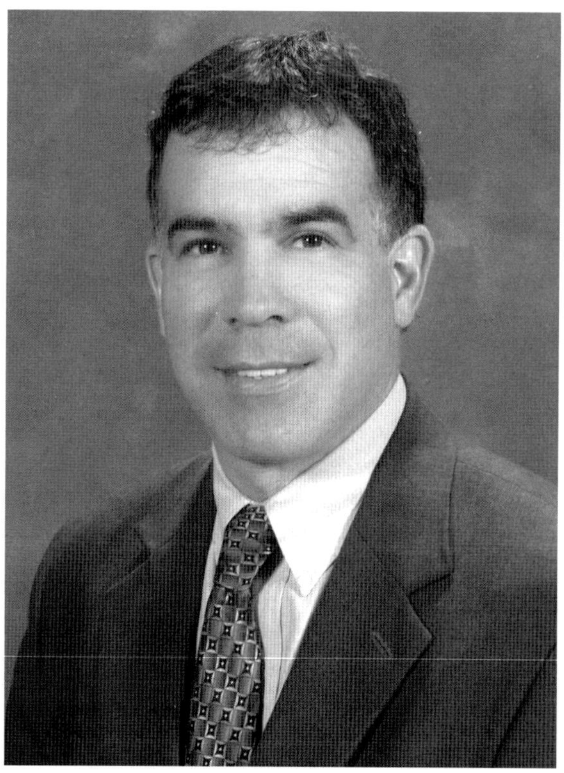

*David Terris, MD, otolaryngologist, pioneered robotic and minimally invasive thyroid surgery. He developed a new Robotic facelift thyroidectomy that results in a scarless surgery.*

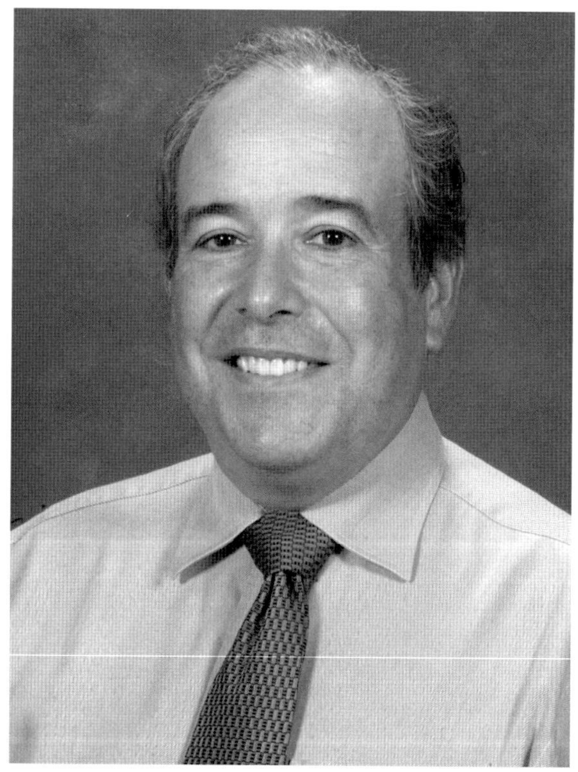

*Carlos Isales, MD, director of the Institute of Regenerative and Reparative Medicine, has published over 110 articles and sixteen book chapters related to the regeneration of bone tissue and the prevention of bone necrosis.*

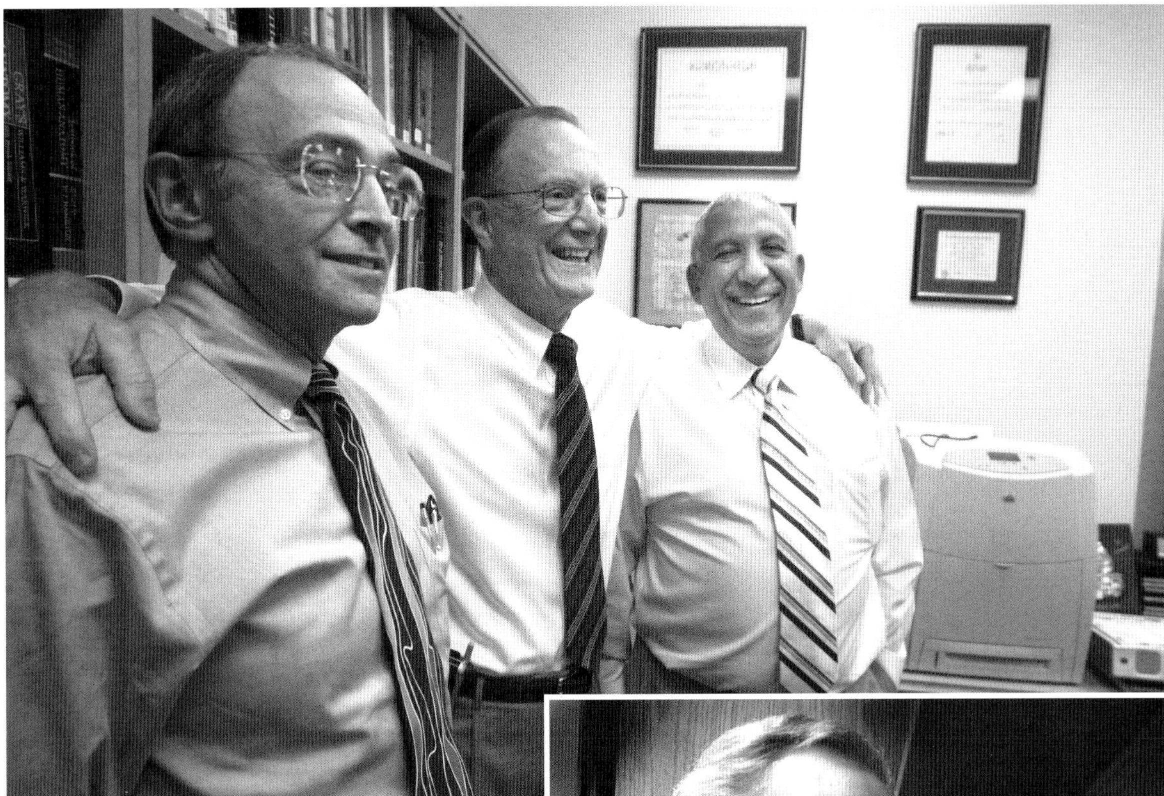

*Above: George S. Schuster, DDS, PhD, (left) conducted important research on the effects of dental materials on cell membranes. He holds several patents relating to green tea polyphenol compositions and methods for treating immune disorders. David H. Pashley, PMD, PhD, (center) studied the structure and function of dentin, particularly resin-dentin bond longevity. His discovery that oxalic acid was extremely effective in reducing dentin sensitivity led to his formulation of a topical dental desensitizing gel. Mohamed Sharawy, PhD, (right) has an interest primarily in applied research related to bone regeneration, implants, and bioengineering using bone cells. The three have published more than one thousand papers, articles, and books in their fields.*

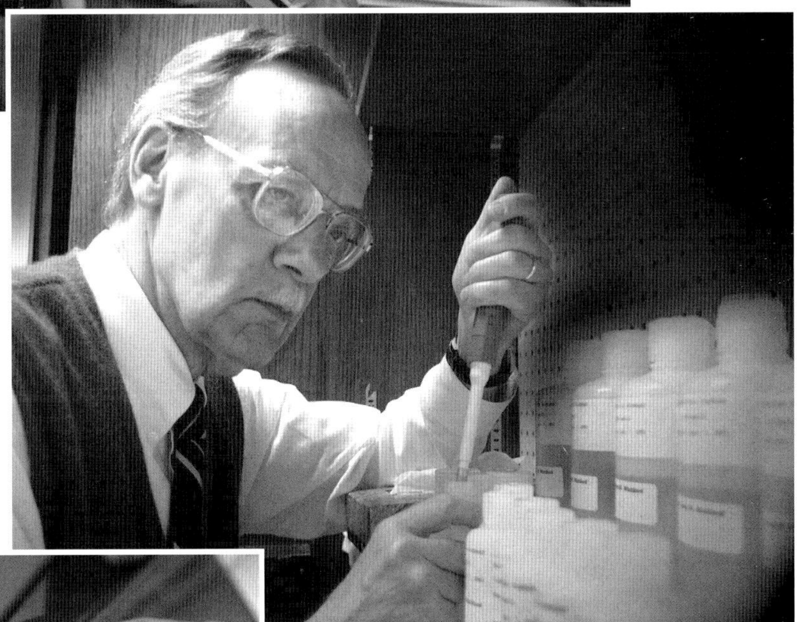

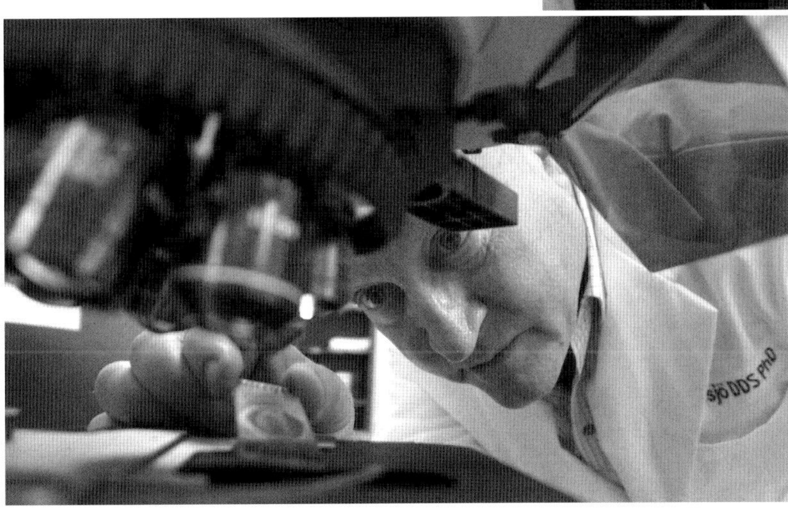

*Above: Gary Whitford, DMD, PhD, is a world-renowned fluoride scientist. He has consulted on fluoride metabolism in several countries as well as to the American Dental Association, World Health Organization, and Centers for Disease Control and Prevention.*

*Left: Ulf M.E. Wikesjo, DMD, DDS, PhD, has authored or co-authored more than 150 abstracts and 230 articles, reviews, and chapters on craniofacial tissue engineering and implant/bone interface, leading to greater understanding and breakthrough treatments in the field of periodontal regenerative therapies.*

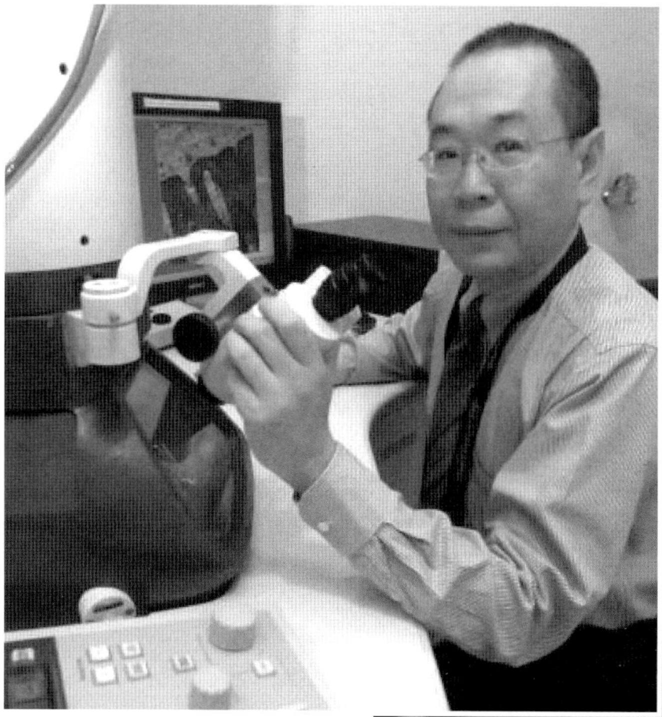

*Left: Franklin Chi Meng Tay, PhD, chairman of the Department of Endodontics, has published more than four hundred peer-reviewed papers in international journals. He is studying a new nanotechnology technique to extend the longevity of tooth-colored fillings.*

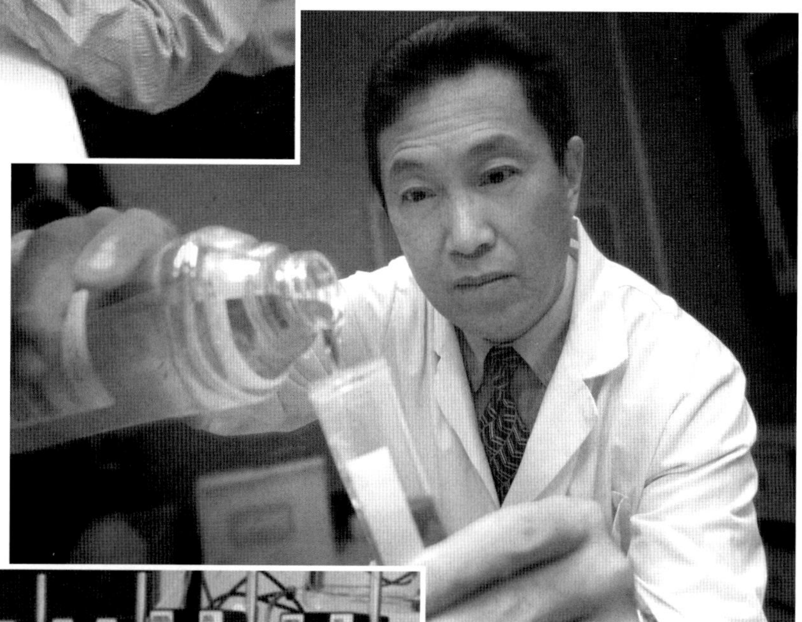

*Right: Stephen Hsu, PhD, College of Dental Medicine, has researched for more than a decade the effects of green tea as UV protection, antioxidant, anti-carcinogen, anti-ager, anti-inflammatory, and accelerator of keratinocyte differentiation and wound treatment as well as a variety of other disorders and diseases. He holds a number of patents including ones for commercial products developed for dry mouth and for skin disorders.*

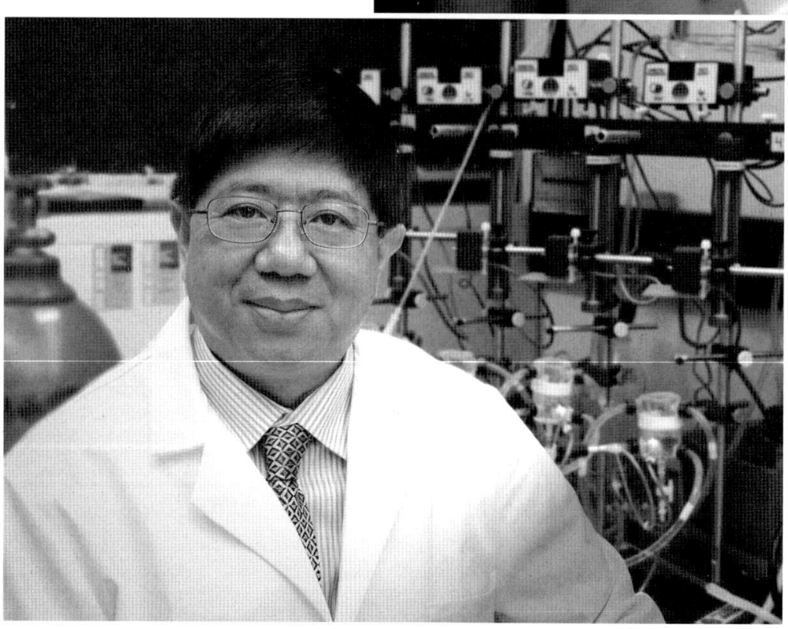

*Geneticist Jin-Xiong She, PhD, is helping lead an international initiative to uncover the interaction of environment and genetics in causing type 1 diabetes in children. Internationally the TEDDY study is following nine thousand children from birth to age fifteen, tracking variables including infections, vaccines, and diet among others. This unprecedented study should lead to earlier identification of susceptibility, possible preventative treatment, and more effective treatment.*

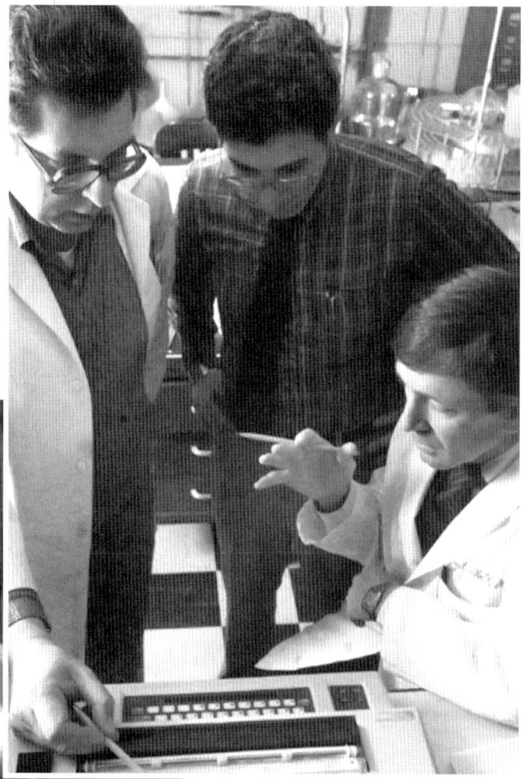

*Right and below: Robert Adams, MD, neurologist, (below) and Virgil C. McKie, MD, (seated right) pediatric hematologist/oncologist, published in the* New England Journal of Medicine *their use of painless Transcranial Doppler as the first non-invasive method for identifying children with sickle cell disease who also are at risk for stroke. Their later studies showed regular blood transfusions could significantly reduce stroke risk.*

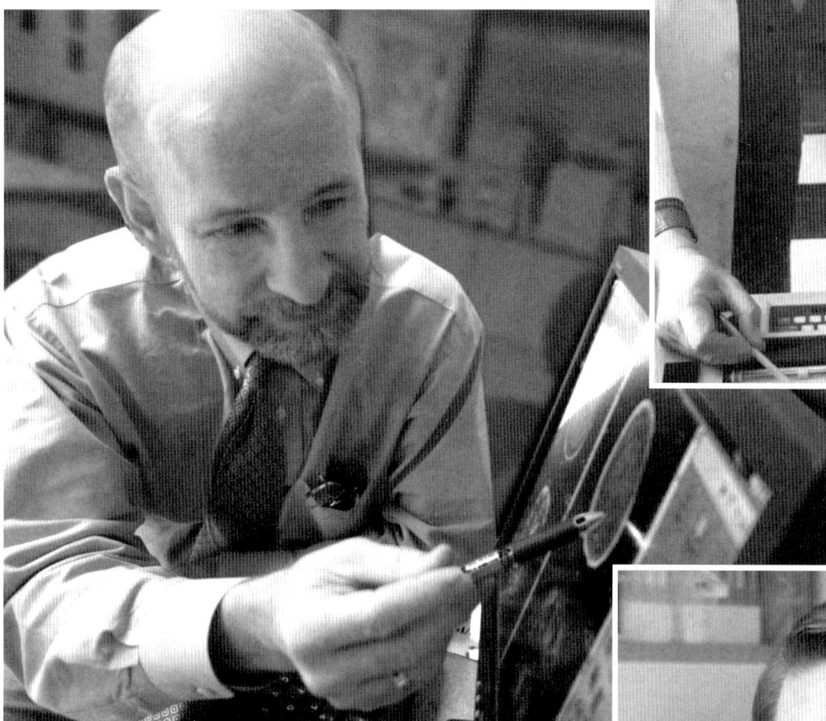

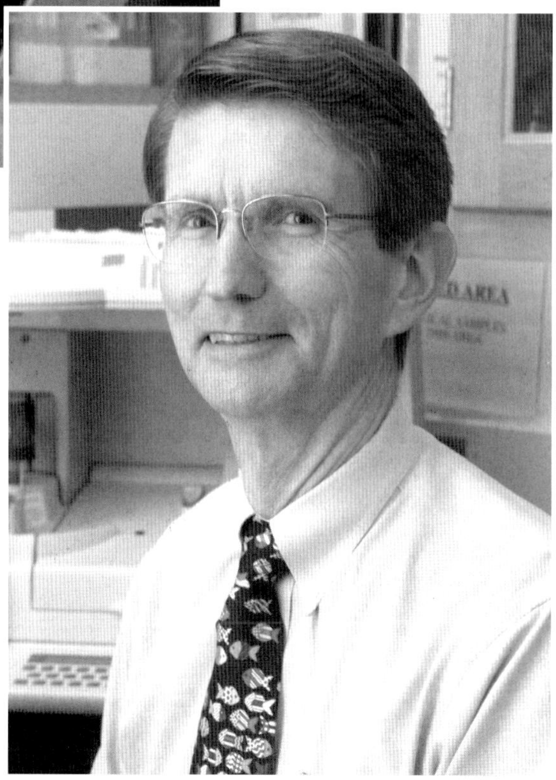

*A 2004 study, led by allergist/immunologist Dennis Ownby, MD, overturned the long-held belief that young children need to be kept away from animals to avoid developing allergies. His study, published in the* Journal of the American Medical Association, *showed children in homes with dogs and cats have significantly reduced risk of developing common allergies and asthma.*

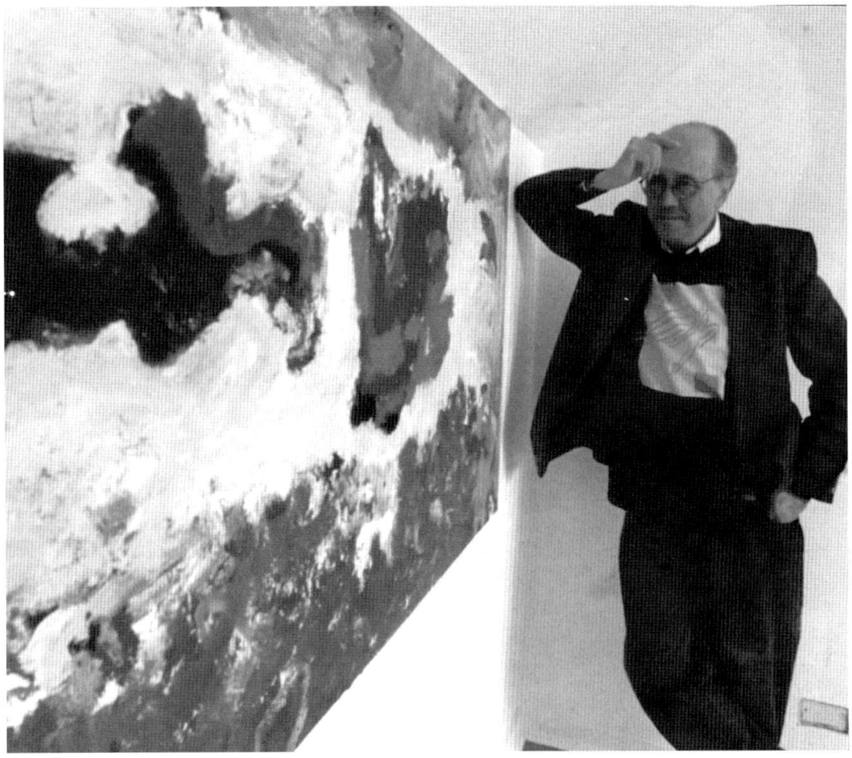

For the most part, research took a different form at Augusta State University (ASU) where education in the liberal arts and specialized professions were the core of its foundation. Even with teaching as the primary mission, faculty also made significant contributions to their disciplines. Art professors exhibited paintings, sculptures, ceramics, and other media at local, state, national, and international galleries and spaces; won awards at juried shows; and placed their works in important collections throughout the country and world. The William S. Morris Eminent Chair in Art, established in 1988, was the first eminent scholar chair at any University System of Georgia institution. To date, four artists with national and international acclaim have been named Morris Eminent Scholars.

*Above: Internationally known visual artists Jim Rosen, Philip Morsberger (pictured), Tom Nakashima, and William Willis have the distinction of being Morris Eminent Scholars in Art.*

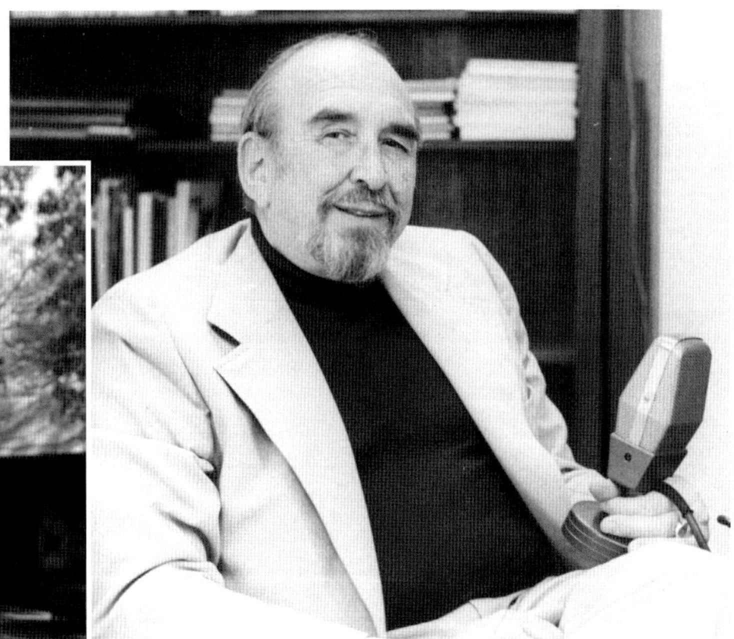

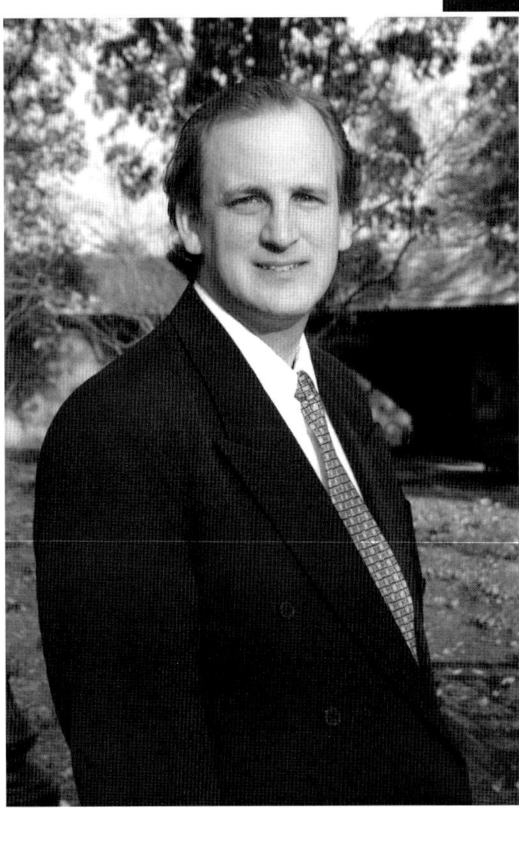

*Above: Harry Jacobs was the first chairman of the AC music department and founder of the university radio station (WACG). He also founded and conducted the Augusta Symphony, the Harry Jacobs Chamber Music Society, and the Etherridge Center Chamber Orchestra in Aiken.*

*Left: Pianist and university orchestra director/conductor Martin David Jones, DMA, who performs with orchestras throughout the nation, has been featured at Lincoln and Kennedy Centers and in solo at the National Gallery of Art.*

Music faculty have performed with Symphony Orchestra Augusta and other symphonies, chamber music groups, jazz ensembles, concert bands, and solo in venues including major music centers such as the Kennedy and Lincoln Centers. In addition to performing, some professors have also composed and produced CDs of their music.

Historians, literary professors, and creative writers have been active in scholarship. Historians have published books and journal articles examining

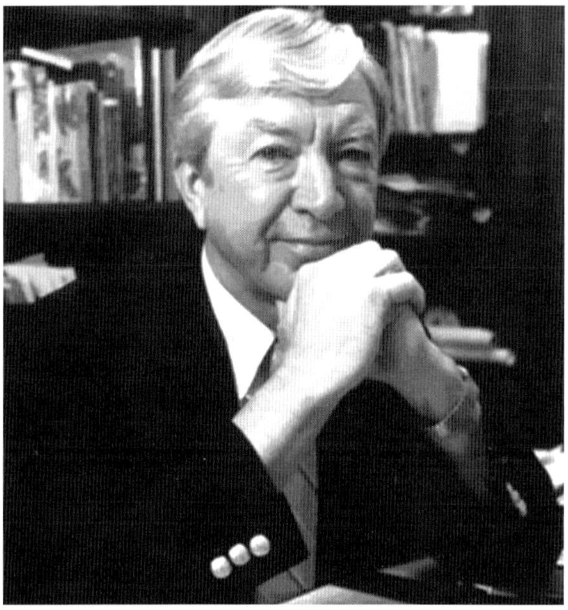

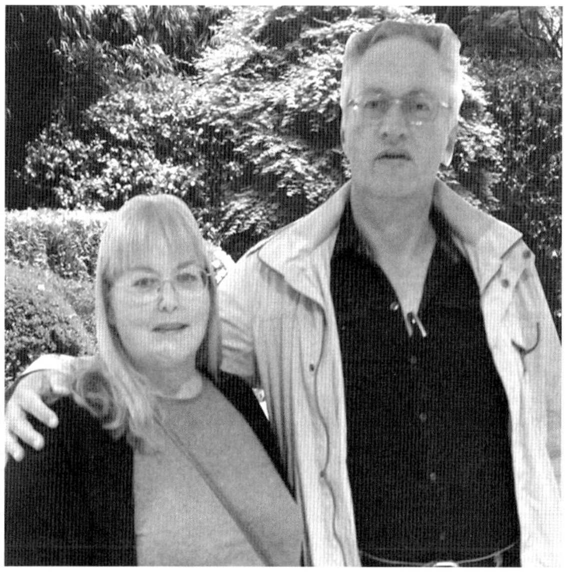

*Above: Debra and Hubert van Tuyll are both well-published scholars. Debra van Tuyll, PhD, Communications, published three books on the role of the press in the American Civil War and Hubert van Tuyll, PhD, History, authored five books on military and strategic history.*

*Left: Edward J. Cashin, PhD, authored many articles and more than twenty books, some award winning, focusing on histories of the community, state, and region. He founded the Center for the Study of Georgia History.*

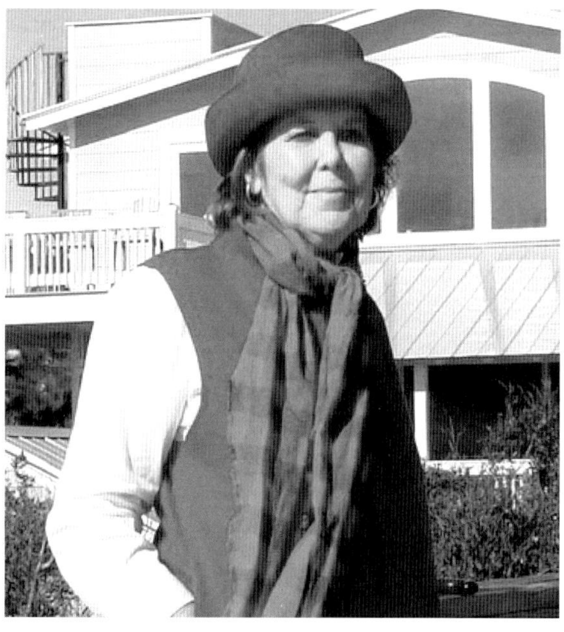

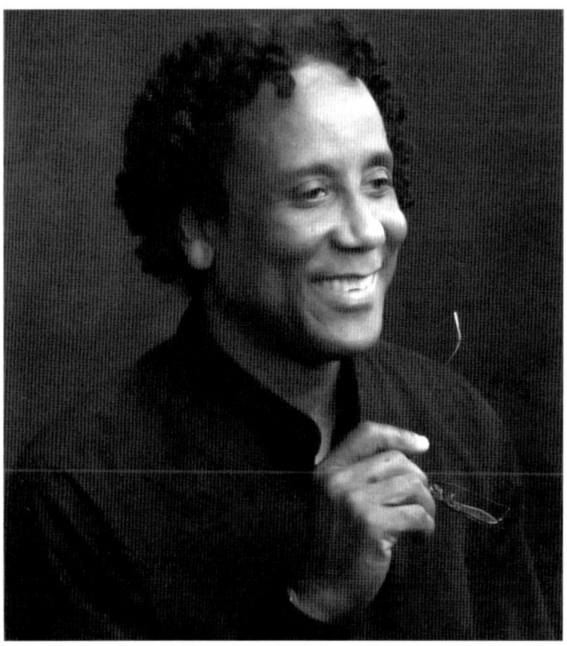

*Above: Writer-in-Residence Louise Shivers authored two acclaimed novels as well as her memoirs. Her novel* Here to Get My Baby out of Jail *was made into a Hollywood film.*

*Left: Professor Antony Kellman, MFA, has published five books of poetry and two novels. His work appears in anthologies and literary periodicals.*

various areas and historical eras of the United States, Britain and Europe, Latin America, and the Middle East. Faculty members have published novels, short stories, and books of poetry, as well as plays that have been performed throughout the country. They have also published books, DVDs, and CDs for teaching children literature and foreign language. Scholars in the humanities and social sciences have published articles in professional journals and chapters in books, reviewed books and manuscripts for presses and journals, and presented research at state, regional, national, and international conferences.

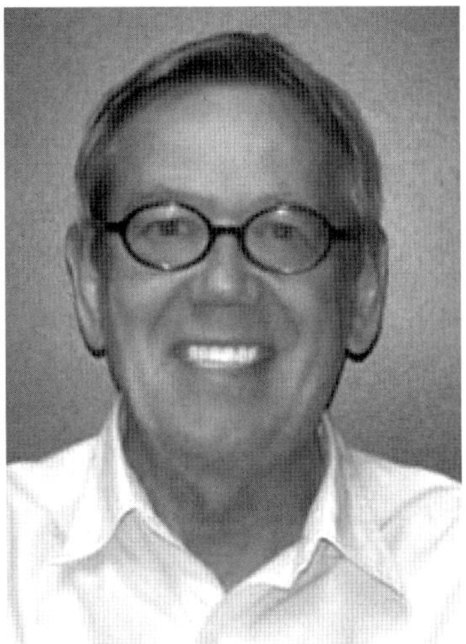

*Richard Davis Jr., MA, winner of thirteen literary and playwriting competitions from 1998 to 2012, has written over forty plays and musicals that have been produced off Broadway and in theaters across the nation. He has performed in or directed over thirty plays.*

Research and publication in the natural sciences began early. Chemists and physicists have published articles on topics including atomic and molecular physics and geological research with seismic clusters and waves, including a study of factors that affect the accuracy and uncertainty of measurement seismic wave gradients. Collaborating with Purdue University, an ASU faculty member set up a computer server at the institution that provides access for researchers from all over the world to perform multi-channel quantum defect theory calculations. Another ASU faculty member, in collaboration with Purdue, has participated in the analysis of data taken from experimentation in high-energy physics, which is published in several articles in national/international research journals.

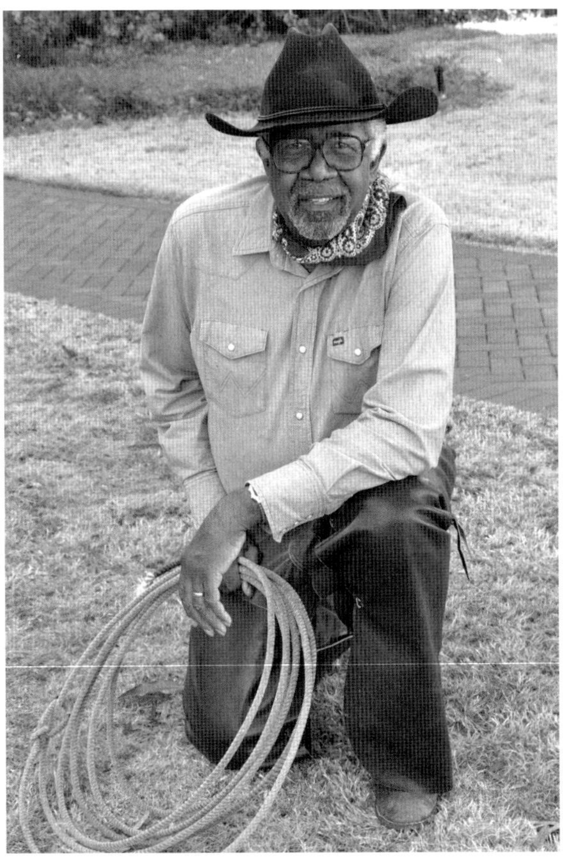

*History professor Michael Searles (Cowboy Mike) publishes and lectures extensively on the history of African Americans in the American West.*

*Kavel Scholar Trinanjan Datta, PhD, specializes in the areas of quantum and classical magnetism, using theoretical and computational tools to investigate magnetic properties of frustrated quantum magnets.*

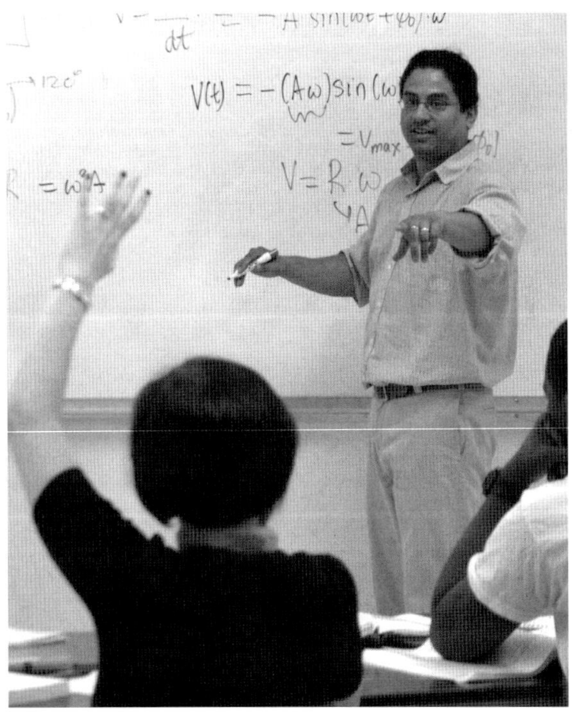

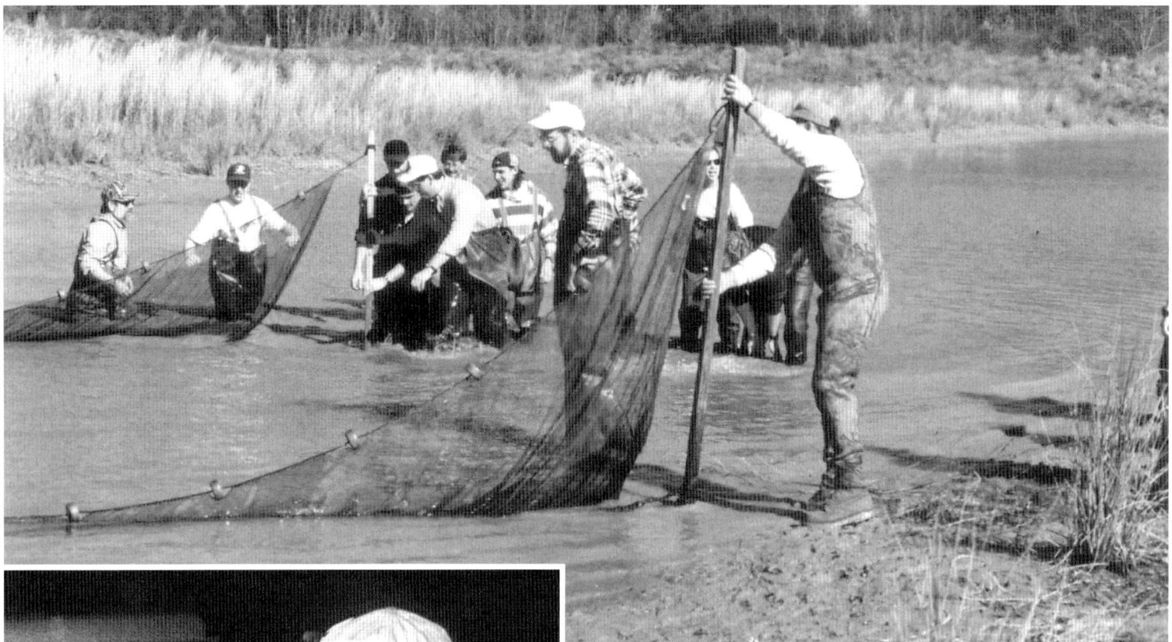

*Above: Monitoring the state's rivers and streams provided valuable data for environmental and ecological research studies.*

Biologists have made important contributions in life science that include, for example, a collaboration to develop a potential treatment for Trypanosoma cruzi, an often fatal parasite found in Latin America with no known vaccines, and to develop a potential new vaccine for several viruses, including herpes. ASU was also the academic home of one of the world's authorities on the birds of Africa.

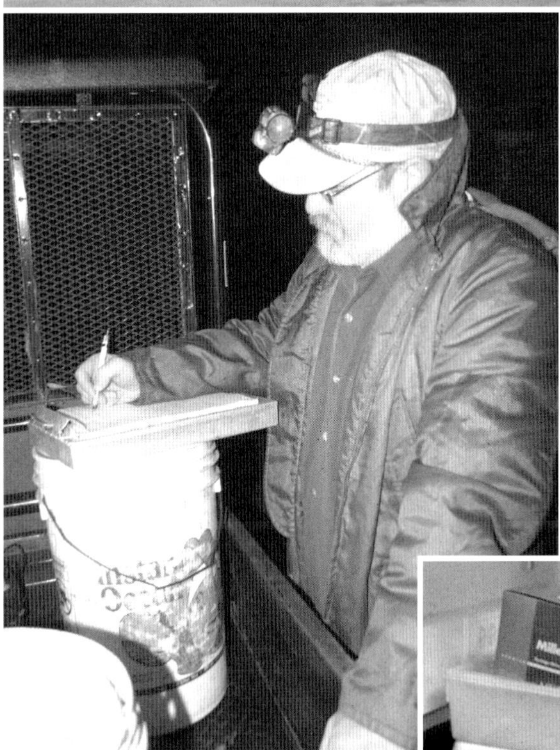

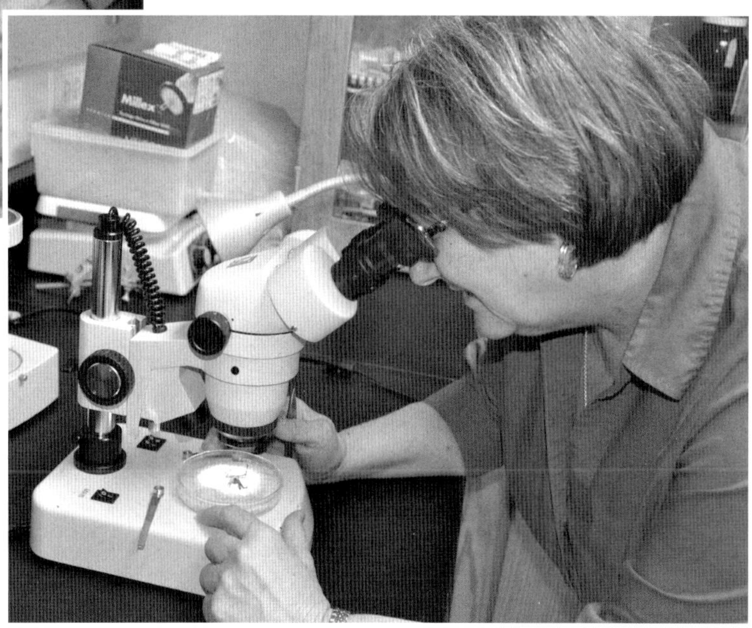

*Above: Since 1996, biology professor Bruce Saul, PhD, has been identifying and monitoring the diversity of fish species in local streams and at St. Catherines Island, Georgia. He has consulted internationally, and his data is used by other researchers studying migration patterns and environmental factors such as ocean salinity, weather, and water temperature.*

*Right: Biologist Cathy Tugmon, PhD, has been researching bacterial diversity on spiders, determining their resistance to antibiotics.*

Business research includes books of finance, textbooks, and many book chapters and journal articles in the fields of business management, accounting, and marketing. ASU economists include one of the world's foremost-published authorities on the economy of Thailand, as well as a well-published professor who consults with national and international agencies.

The research performed by faculty in the College of Education and published in books and educational journals has provided sound principles and practice for current and future educators. Notable also are the efforts to address literacy, including the creation of

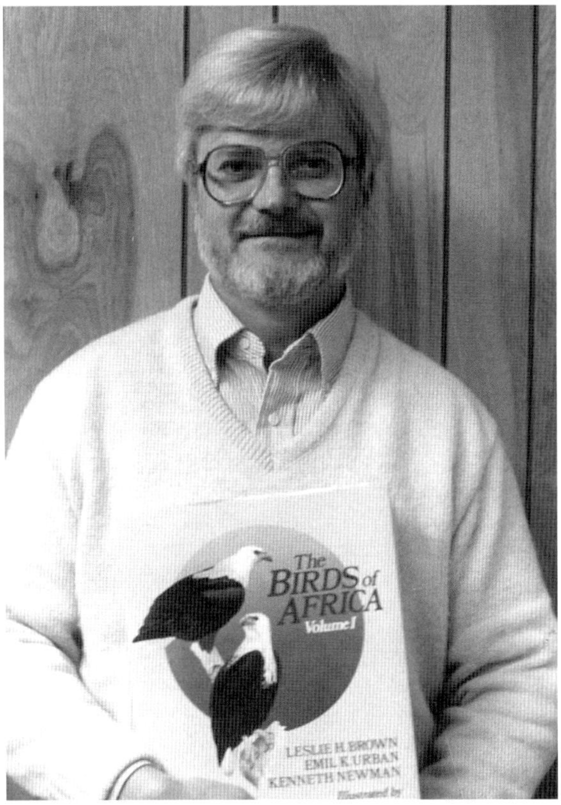


*Above: Emil Urban, PhD, former chairman of Biology and Calloway Professor of Biology, was an internationally known authority on the birds of Africa, chronicling over two thousand in a seven-volume collection. He also published books on birds of South America and Mexico.*

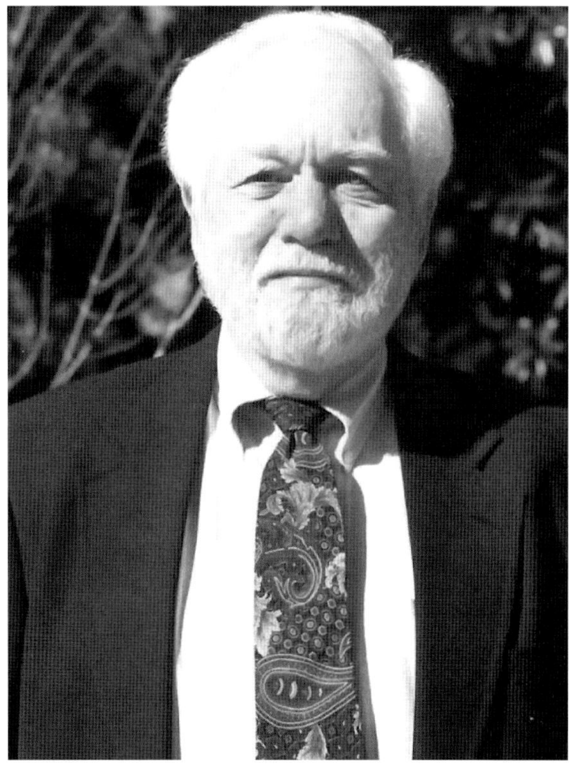

*Above: Political scientist Ralph Walker, PhD, drafted the charter for the consolidation of Augusta-Richmond County and served as a political analyst, strategist, media expert, and political commentator for over three decades. He was the founder of the ASU Research Center.*

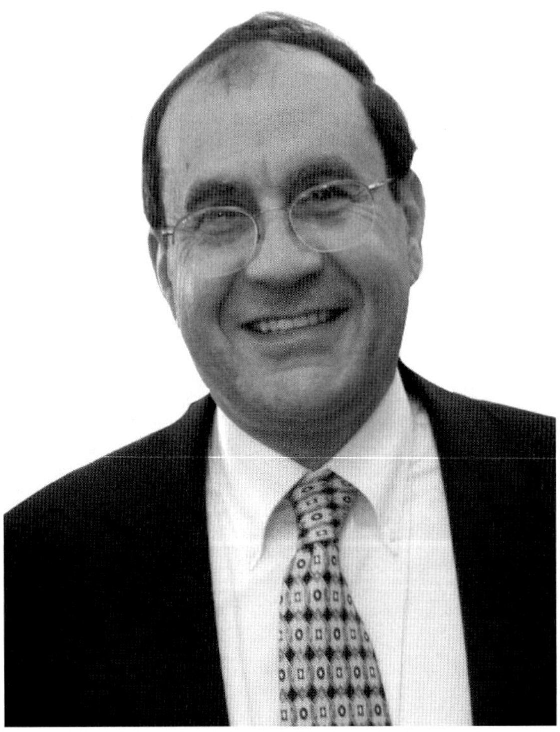

*Left: Nabil Ibrahim, PhD, former Grover C. Maxwell Distinguished Professor of Business, made significant contributions in the field of business management with two textbooks, thirteen book chapters, and many articles.*

a Georgia Regents University Literacy Center and its satellites.

These are but a few examples of the research that has been done over time at these two parent institutions. With such a history of research in every discipline, Georgia Regents University stands ready to become a great American research university. From lifesaving discoveries and technological advances to new perspectives on historical knowledge, from musical and artistic creations to better practices in education and business, GRU's wide range of interests—and research—will continue to add to knowledge and progress in all fields of endeavor.

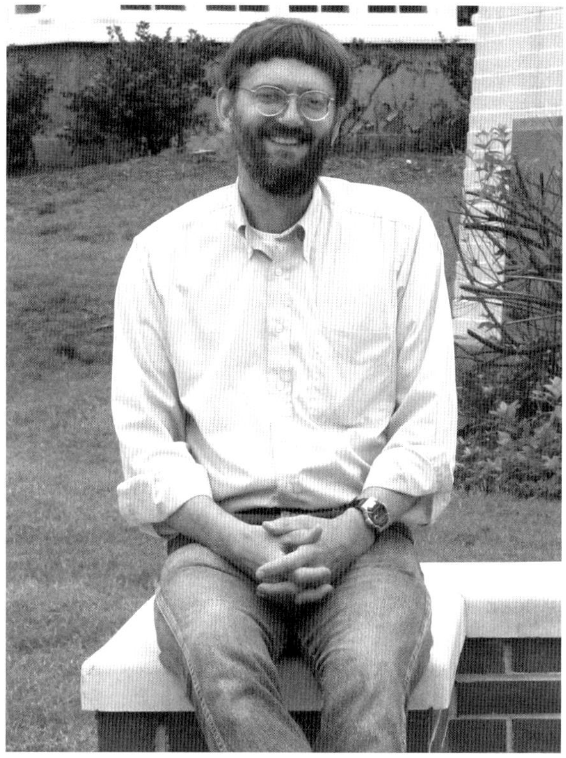

*Above: The work of Jurgen Brauer, PhD, professor of Economics, has been published in eight languages in a wide array of research journals. He has authored or co-authored nine books dealing with the economics of security, war, and peace; held fellowships at many universities throughout the world; and served as a consultant to the World Bank, United Nations, NATO, and other organizations and agencies.*

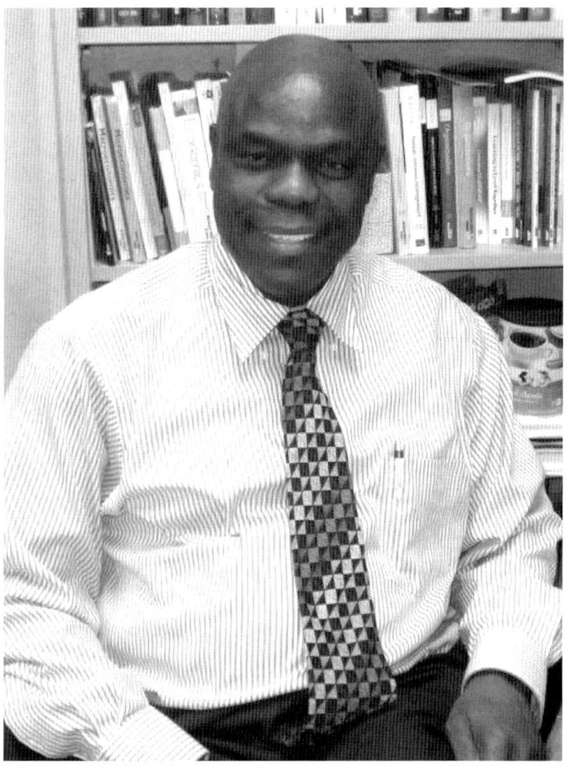

*Above: Olajide Agunloye, PhD, College of Education, served as a Fulbright Senior Specialist to Nigeria where he implemented a program to improve educational processes for disadvantaged and disenfranchised populations. He authored two books on inclusive education and has published numerous articles in professional journals.*

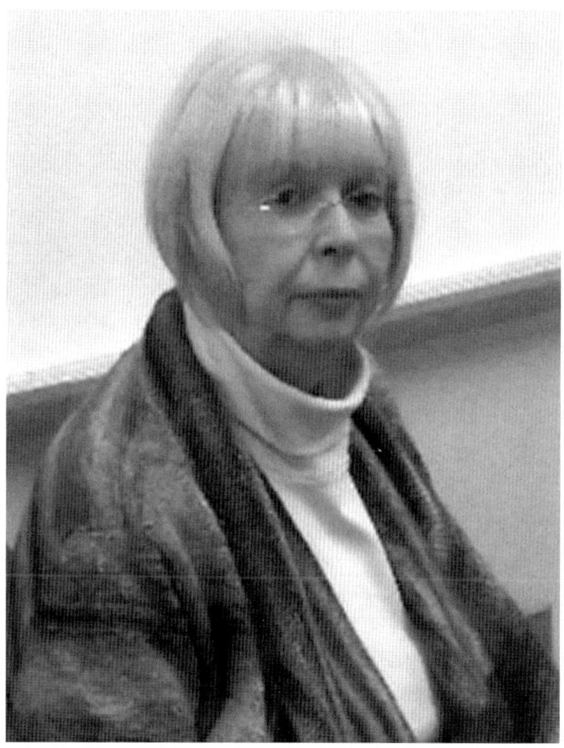

*Right: Paulette Harris, EdD, Cree Walker Professor of Education, has directly impacted thousands of teachers and hundreds of thousands of children through her literacy activities and publications. Since establishing the university's Literacy Center in 1990, she has worked with others to open a number of satellite centers in three counties.*

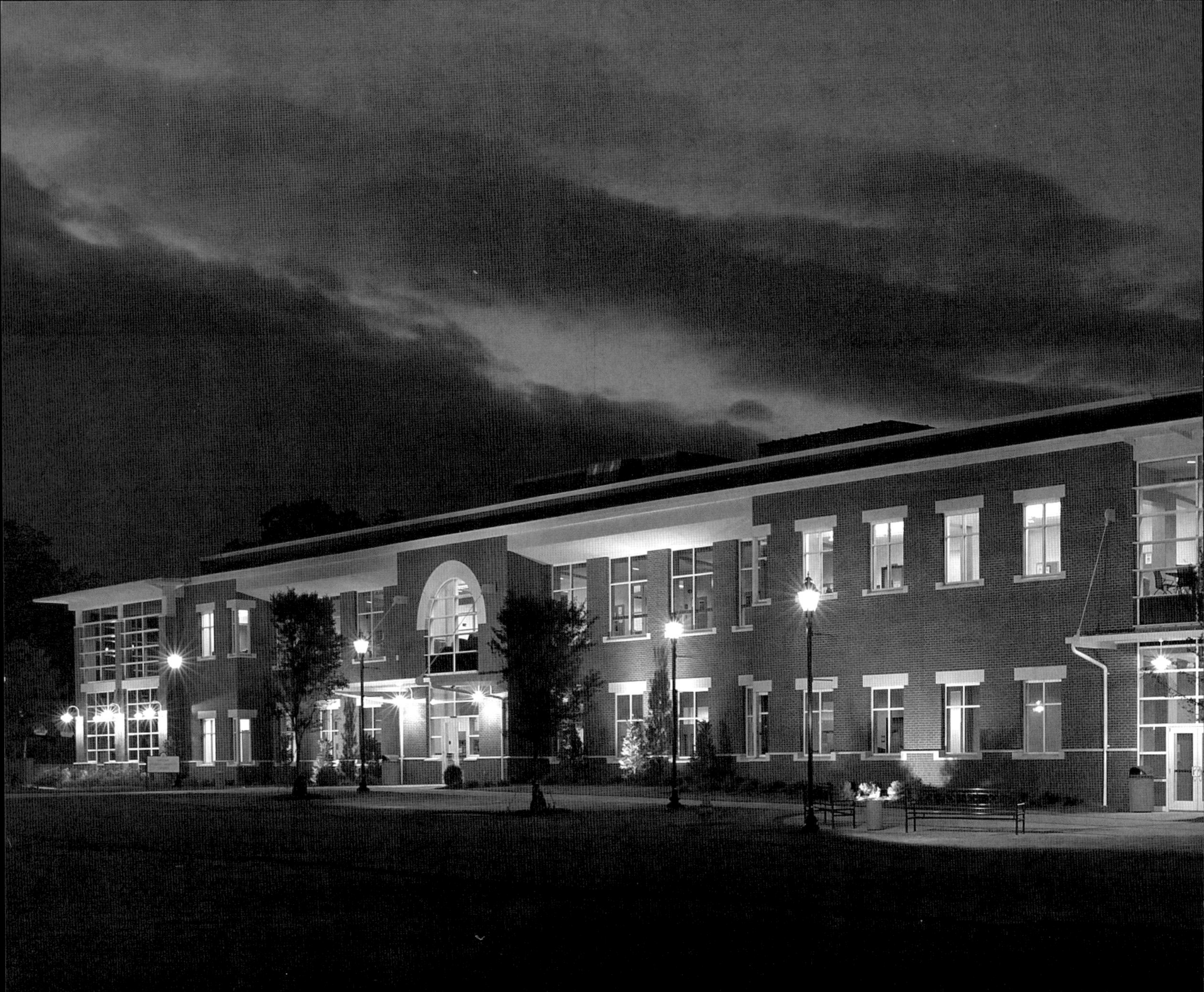

# Campus Life:

## *Experiences and Traditions Beyond the Classroom*

Campus life was practically nonexistent for students in the early days of Medical College of Georgia (MCG) as a daily regimen of medical lectures and studies left little leisure time for the aspiring physicians. The first student group, an outlet for the discussion of medical topics, did not organize until 1887. The following year the Society of Medicine formed so students could provide mutual instruction.

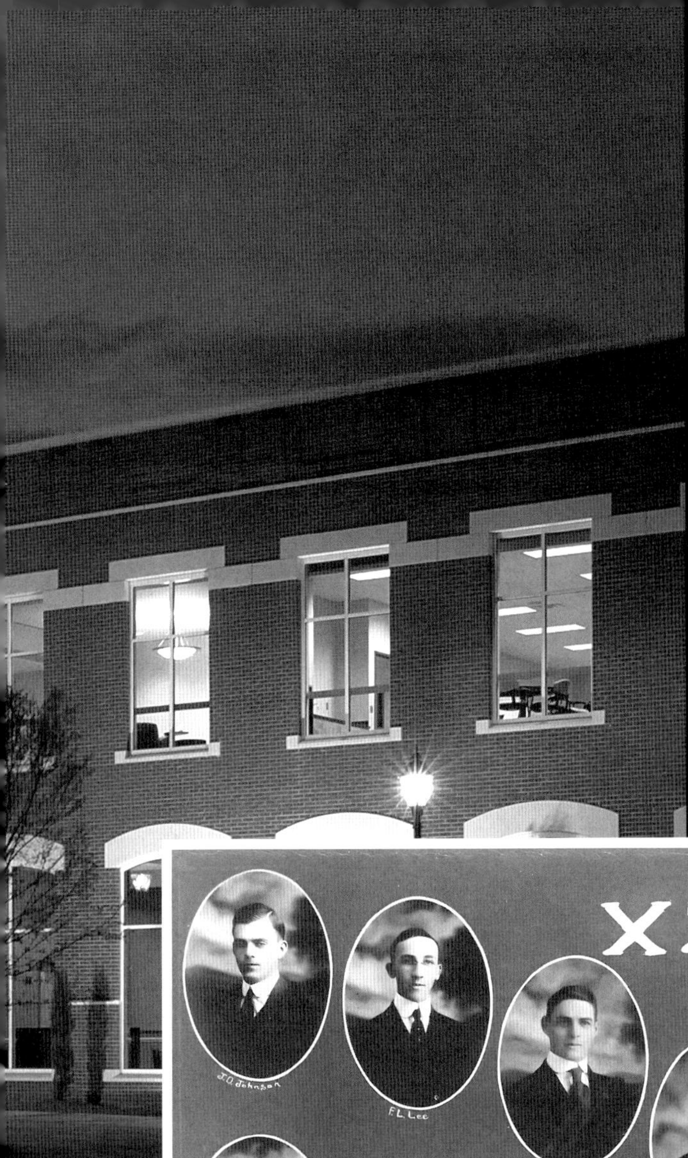

In the early 1900s, as the Medical Department of the University of Georgia, medical students performed in a Glee Club and the first fraternities were founded. Other clubs with both faculty and student members appeared as early as 1907, followed a few years later by a shortly lived Athletic Association and a "Mysterious Seven" group.

Student life expanded even further during the Roaring Twenties, with about twenty-six clubs and other offerings available, ranging from a Mandolin Club to the Demosthenian Literary Society. A national scholastic medical fraternity, Alpha Omega

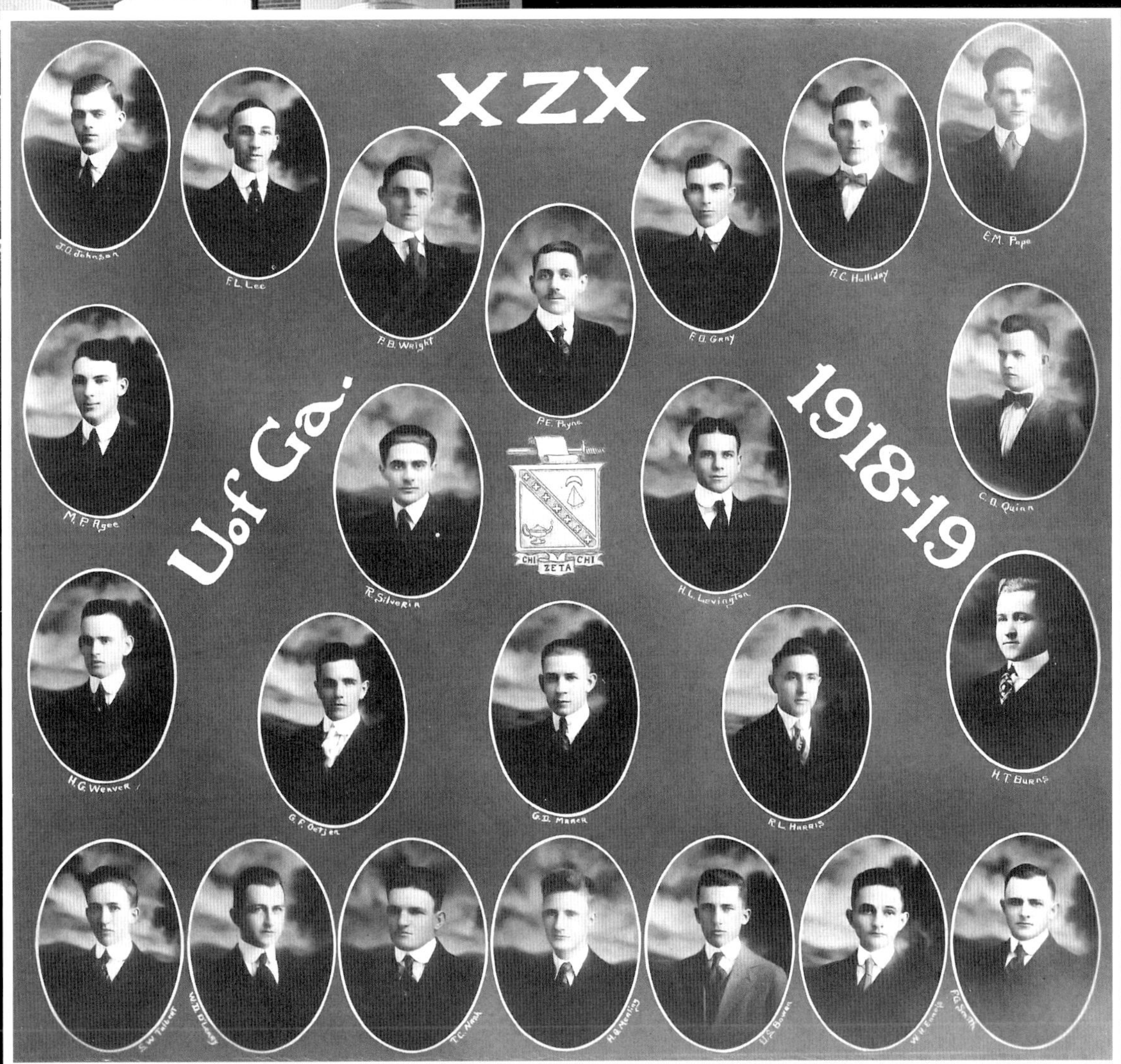


*The Alpha Chapter of Chi Zeta Chi chartered in 1903, becoming the first fraternity at MCG. The Alpha Gamma Chapter of Alpha Kappa Kappa followed in 1904.*

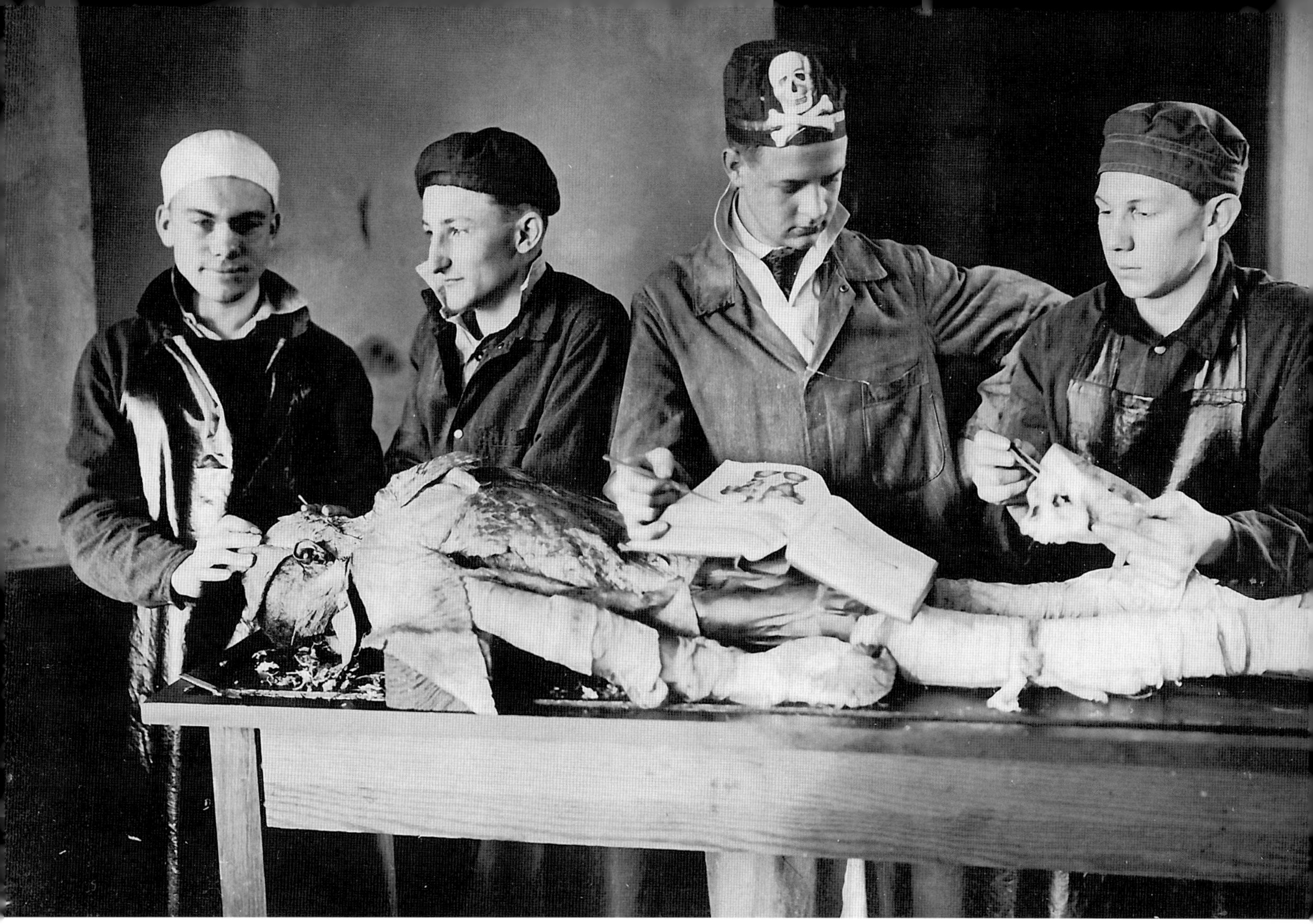

*Among the early clubs offered to MCG students were the No-Name, Coffin, and Skull and Cross Bones (shown).*

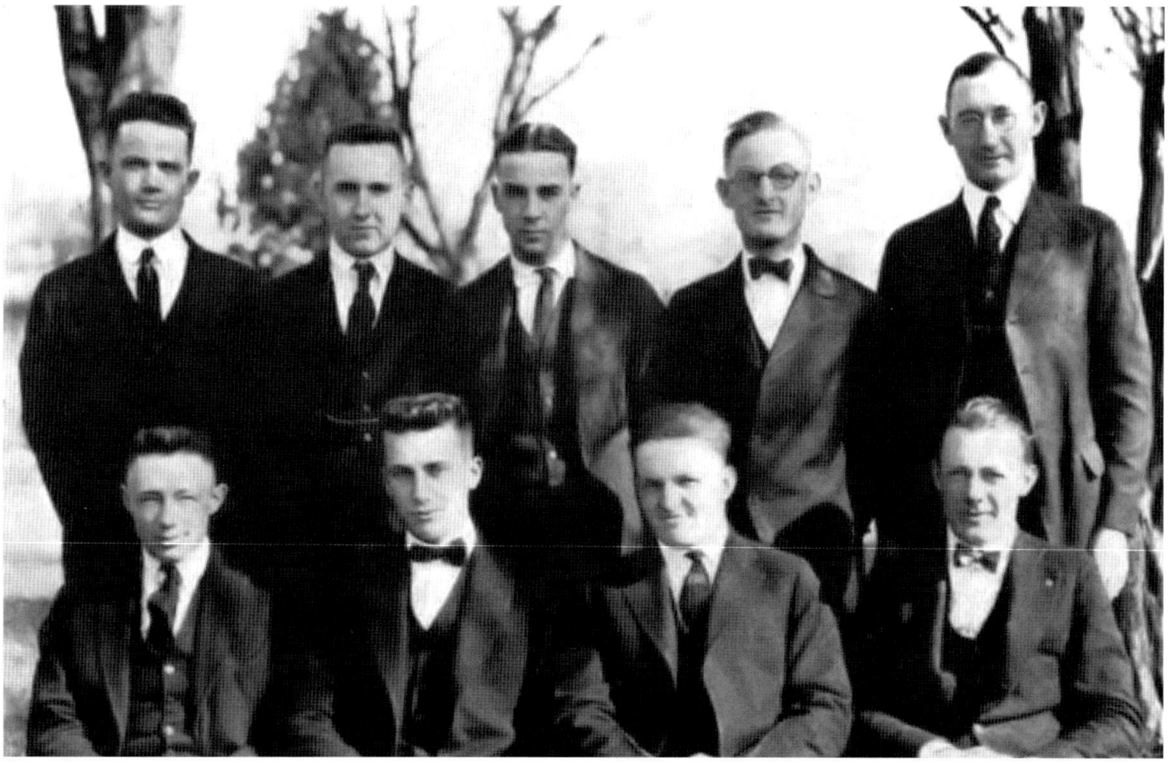

*The Student Council represented students' interests and concerns. (1922)*

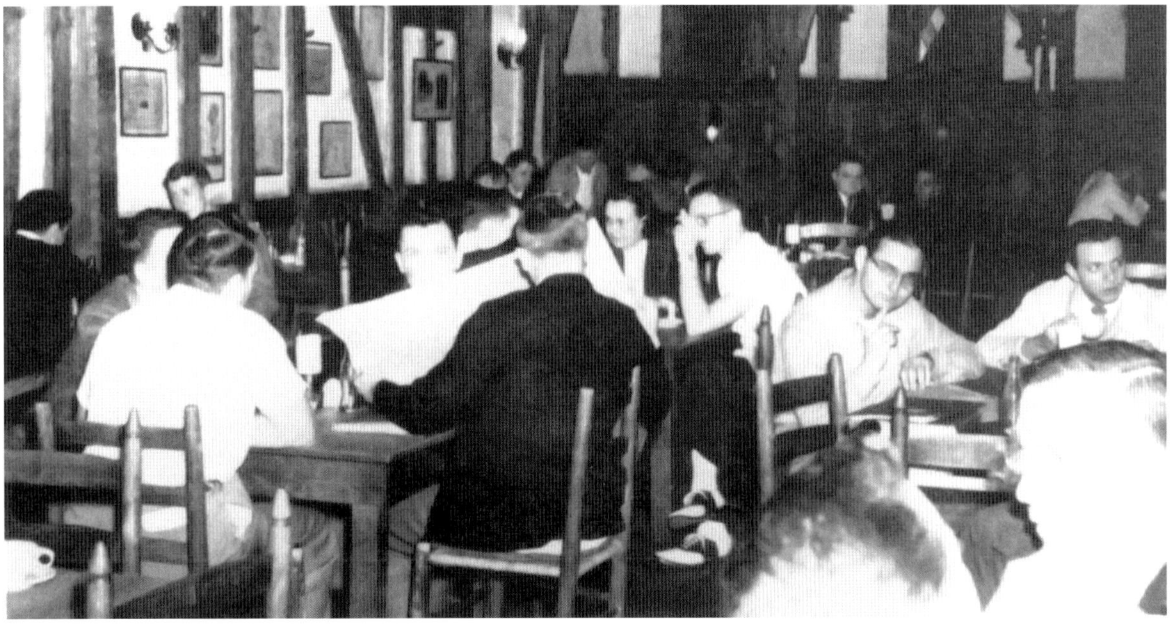

*The old pharmacy and surgery quarters of the Newton Building gave way in 1936 to the creation of the pub-style Alumni Tavern.*

Alpha, was granted a charter in 1926, and the 1930s saw the addition of more fraternities. Annual student-faculty get-togethers where students presented skits and impressions of faculty and vice-versa became the start of a new tradition.

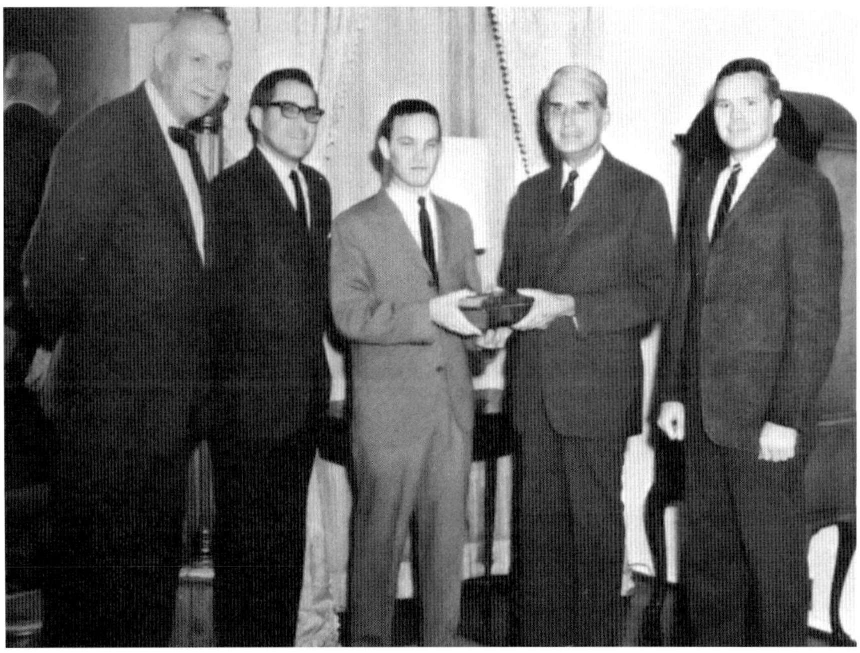

*Named in honor of one of the college's founders, the Milton Antony Society was comprised of faculty and students and encouraged the study of the history of medicine. (1954)*

While the 1940s focused on training physicians and nurses for the war, the 1950s brought back extracurricular activities. The 1940s began with the formation of the Faculty-Student Council to discuss matters of mutual interest, with its five faculty members being elected by the student body. Post-war years once again combined both work and tomfoolery, reflecting a renewed sense of optimism. *The Cadaver* student publication began in 1946 and the following year, the *Aesculapian*, MCG's first yearbook, was published.

Amid dinner meetings, journal clubs, and the still-popular student-faculty skits, a new focus reflected the fact that many students were a few years older. A Student Wives Association was launched, photos of medical students' babies were featured in the yearbook, and local restaurants and clubs such as the Red Lion began advertising "For Couples Only" evenings out.

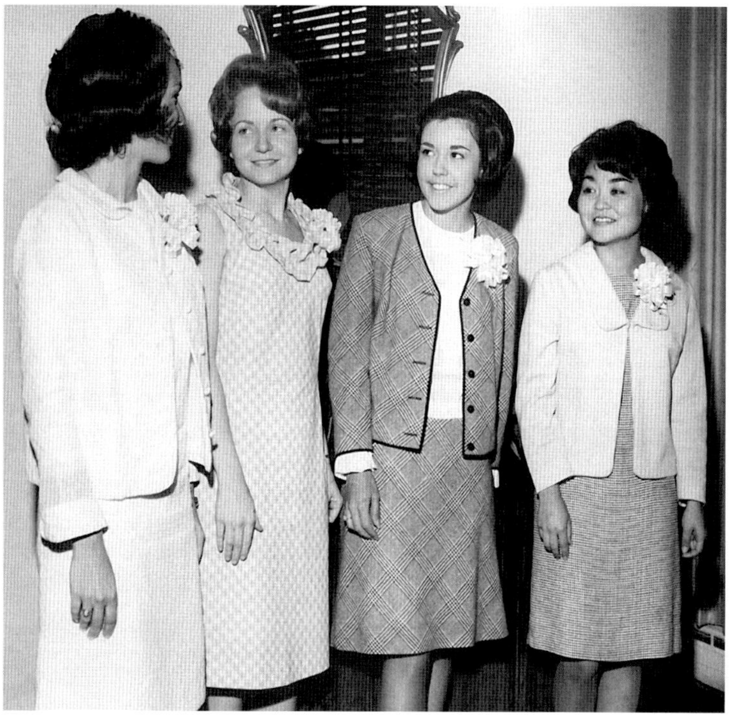

*Above: A Graduate Tea honored senior nursing students at MCG. (1966)*

*Below: Spouses of medical students formed the Medical Dames in 1947, which was known at various times as the Dames Club, the University Dames, or Student Medical Association Auxiliary. The '70s saw the emergence of Dames Married to Dental Students.*

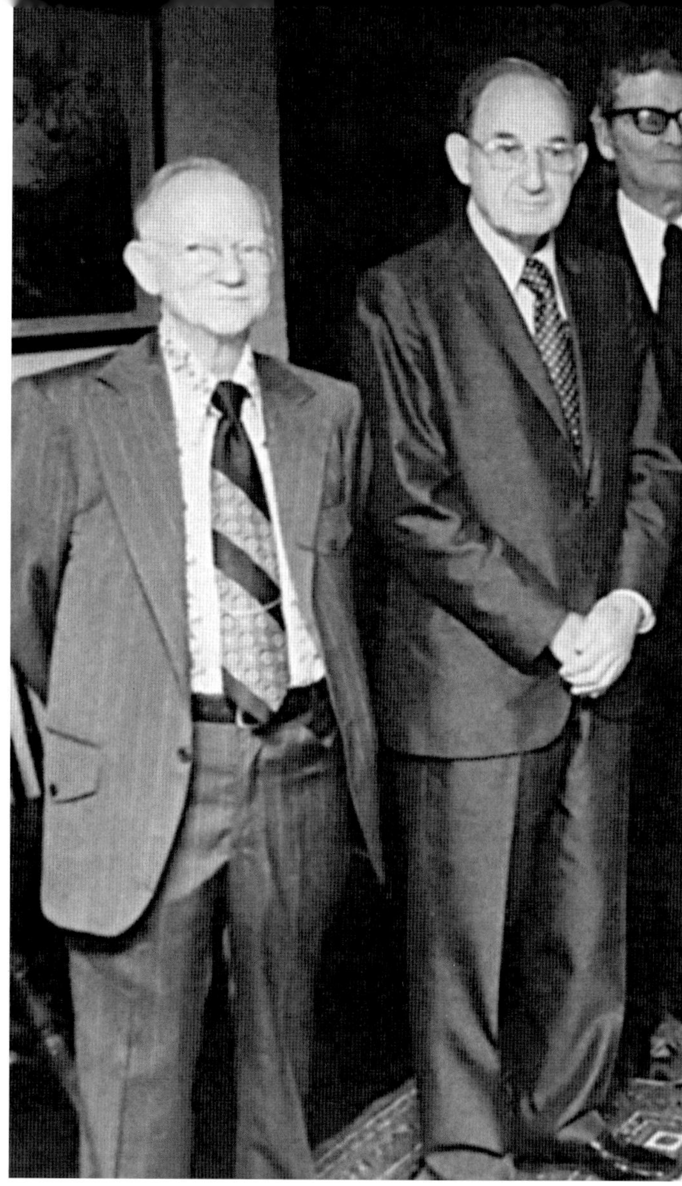

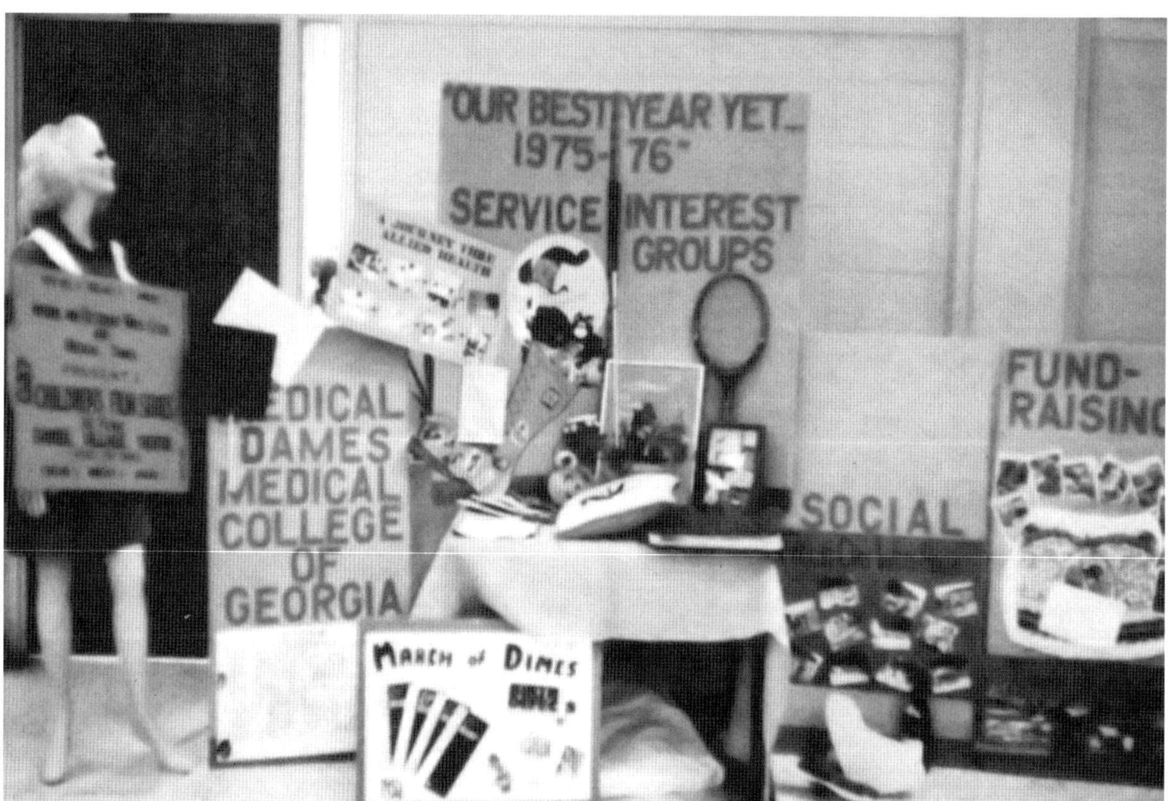

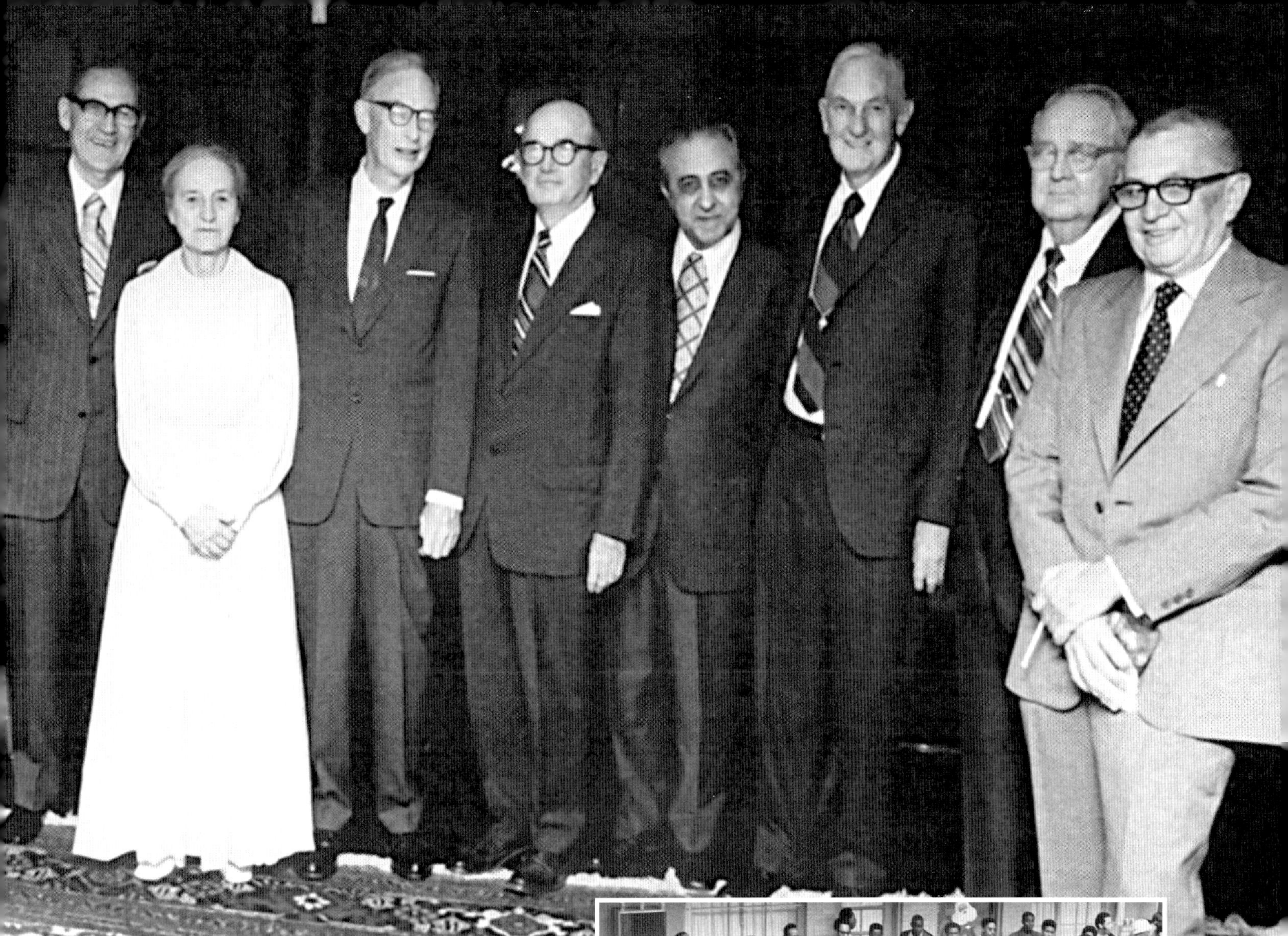

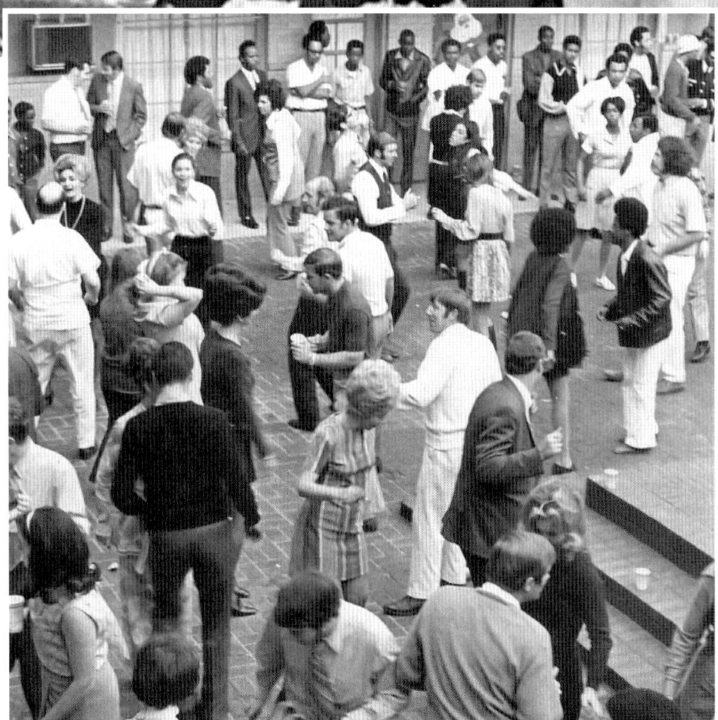

*Above: MCG's class of 1928 reconnected at a 1973 reunion.*

*Right: Dances and other get-togethers livened up MCG's Faculty Pavilion in the 1970s.*

Campus life became even more active in the 1960s and '70s. Influenced by the nation's civil rights movement, the demographics of the institution began to change and new organizations reflected it. MCG established a minority affairs program in 1969, and within a short time, a Black Student Medical Alliance was formed with Joseph Hobbs as president. Dance parties became the craze with events such as Greek Rush and the Freshman Brawl. Students dressed in sheets for fraternity toga parties. Intramural football and soccer; billiards and ping-pong tournaments; a film series; and arts, crafts, photography, and self-defense classes were all added. The classes joined activities such as Stunt Night and picnics. Squeaky's Tip-Top was a favorite place to hang out, and when Augusta College's Recreation Area at Clark's Hill was opened to medical students, it became a gathering spot for students of both institutions.

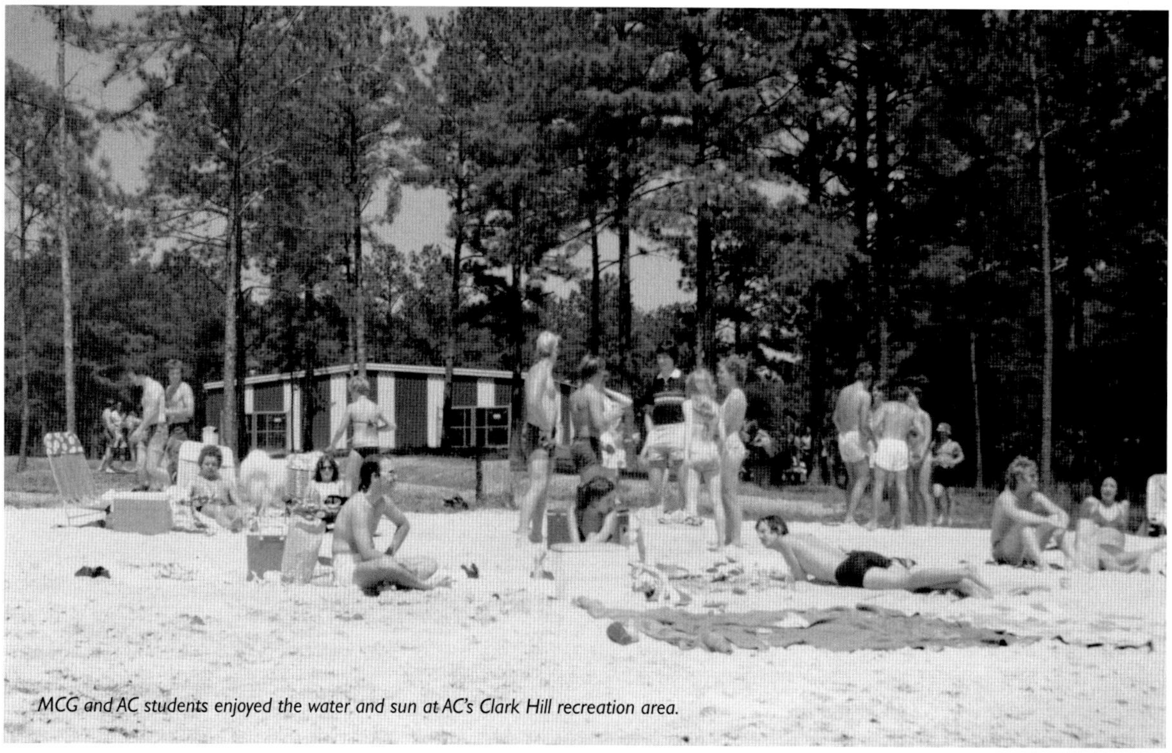

*MCG and AC students enjoyed the water and sun at AC's Clark Hill recreation area.*

*The Sophomore Parades brought students out to strut and stroll down Laney Walker Boulevard in outlandish costumes and riding on handcrafted floats.*

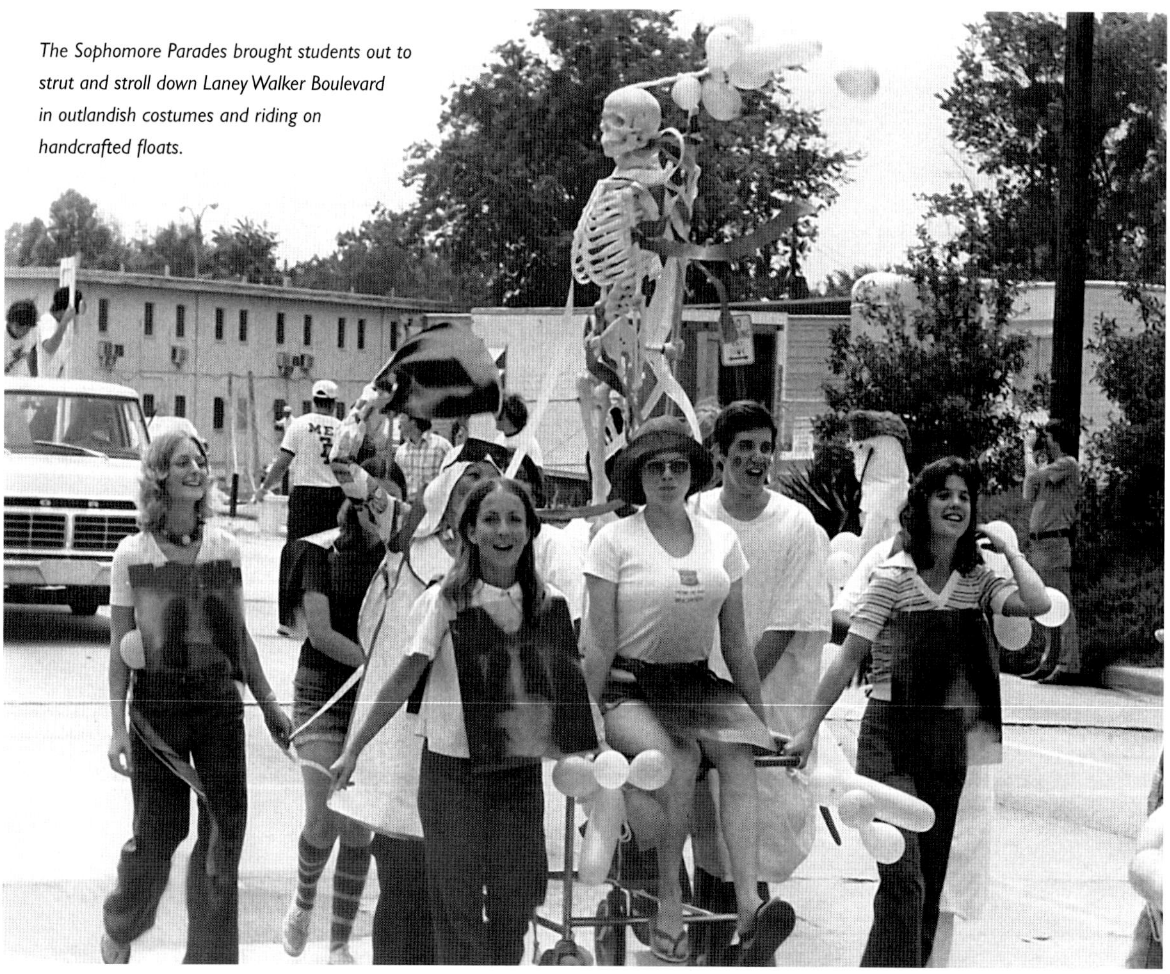

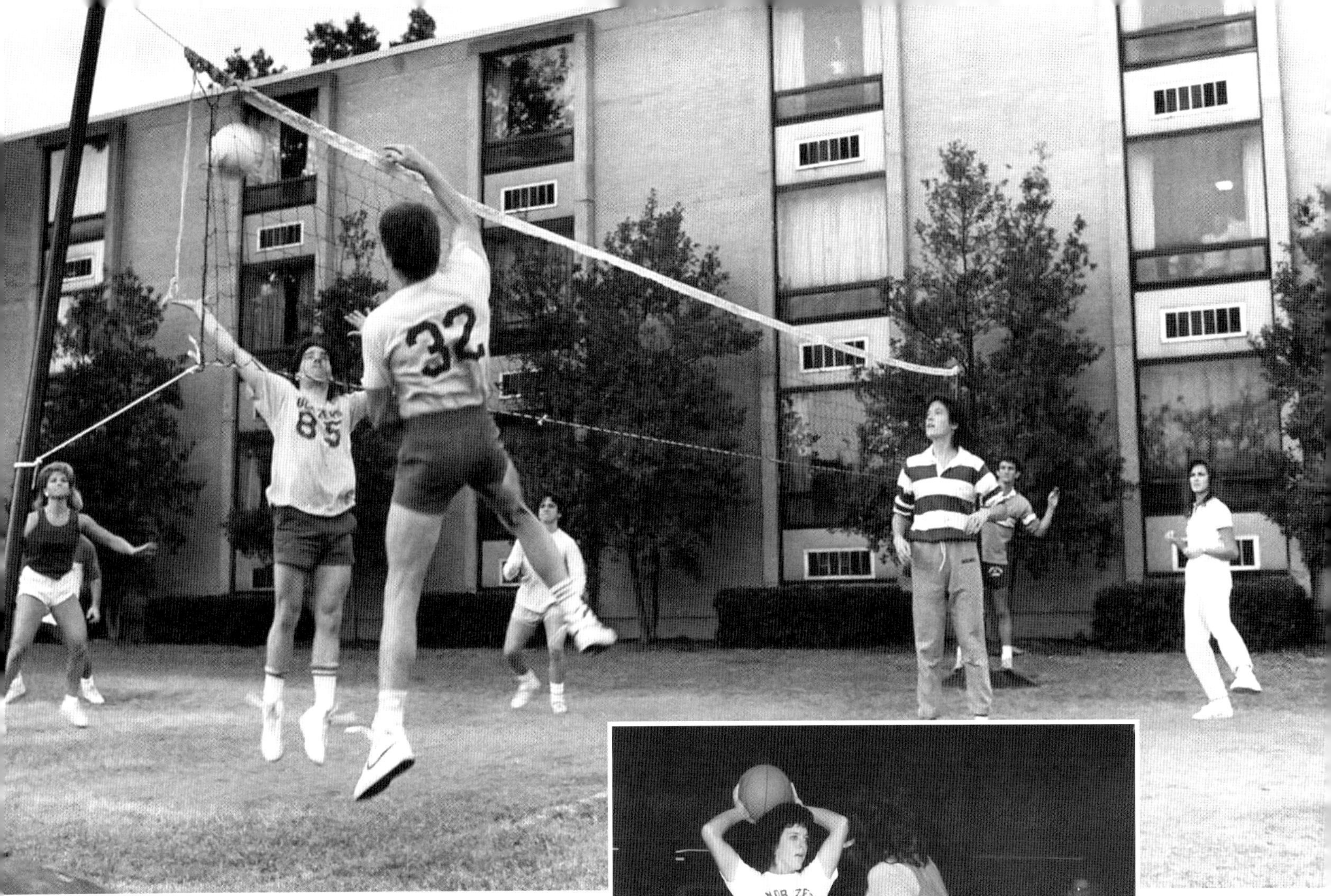


Above: Students in the physical therapy program took on challengers in a campus volleyball match.

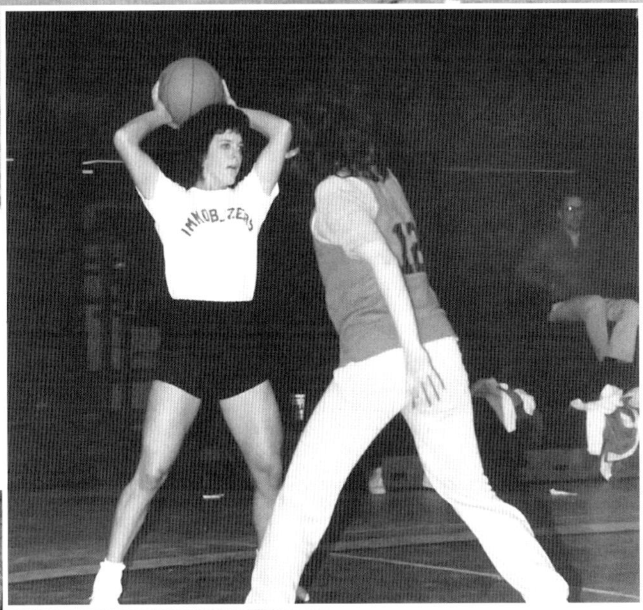

Right: The Immobolizers (physical therapy) took on the Shifting Dullness (senior medical students) in a campus match-up of women's basketball teams. A women's team competed in the city's recreation league, taking the championship in 1971.

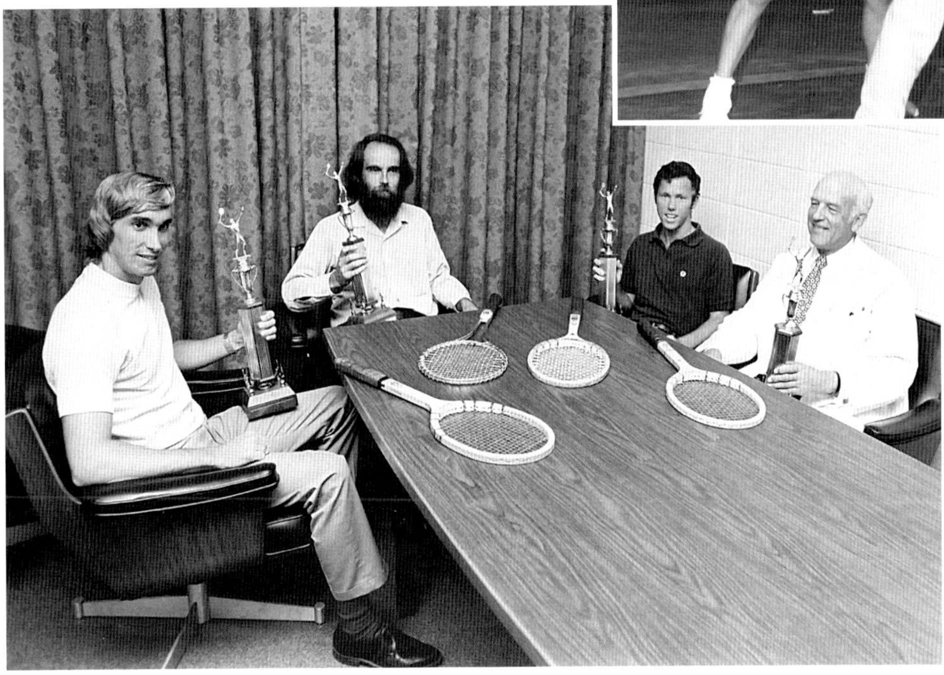

MCG students chose their own faculty partners to compete in an annual tennis tournament. On the right is Dr. William Moretz who served as president of MCG from 1972 to 1983.

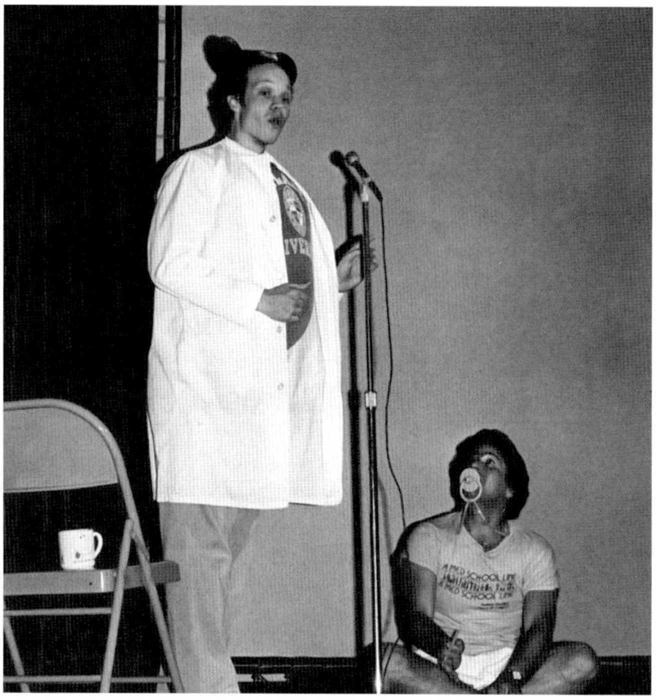

As the decade rolled over into the '80s and '90s, new activities at MCG included the Freshman Brunch and Pac-Man-it-is. Despite being part of what was dubbed the "Me" generation, students were becoming more aware of the world around them, taking opportunities to get even more involved in the local community. Doctors Ought to Care (DOC) launched in 1984, working with schools to talk to kids about better nutrition, tobacco and alcohol awareness, and more.

*Left: Seniors, and later the freshmen, organized the annual Stunt Night, sponsored by the Student-Faculty Council. Bert Berding and Steve Waronker clowned in this 1970s event.*

*Below: Anatomy faculty in the School of Medicine replicate the famous group pose shown in Rembrandt's* The Anatomy Lesson of Doctor Tulp *in this 1974 photograph.*

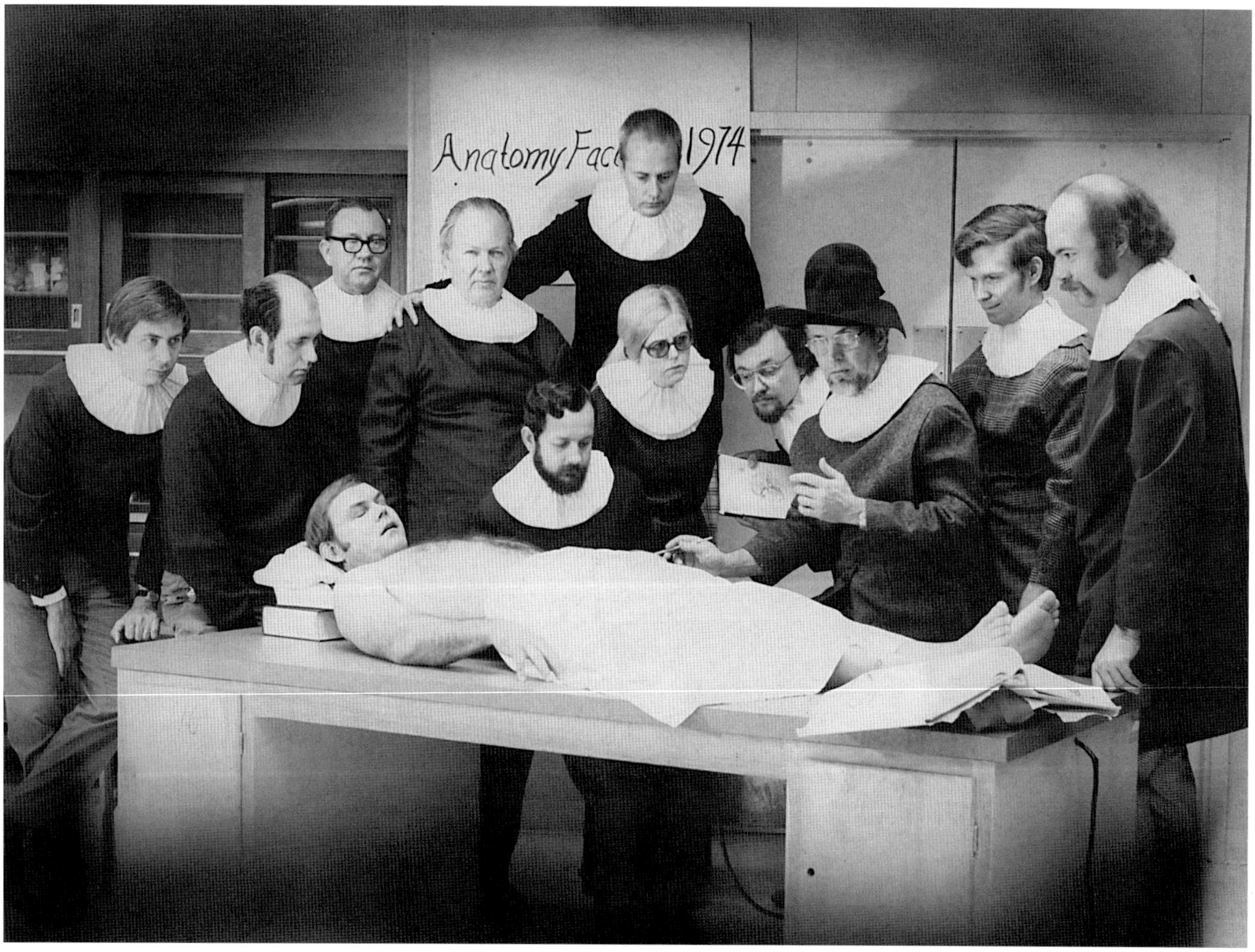

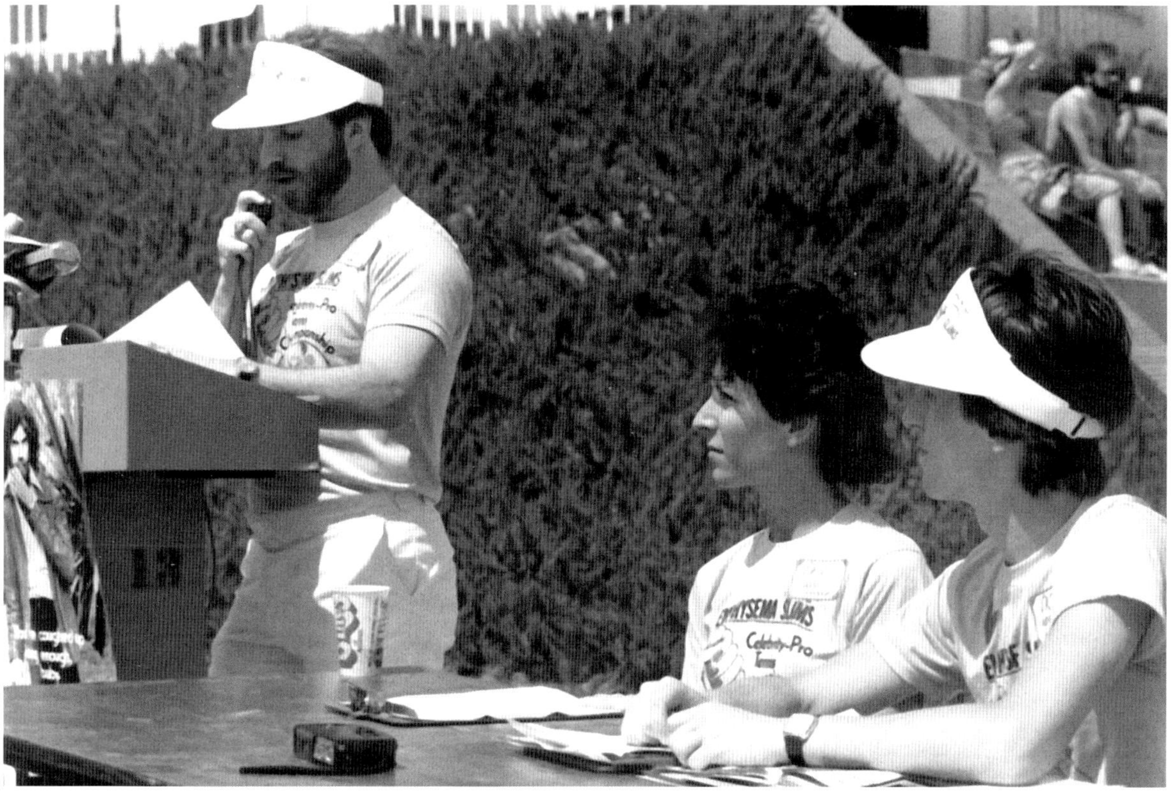


*Above: Doctors Ought to Care hosted the Emphysema Slims Tennis Tournament in 1985, a parody of the Virginia Slims Tourney, to highlight the dangers of smoking.*

*Right: MCG students embraced fitness in a 1980s aerobics class.*

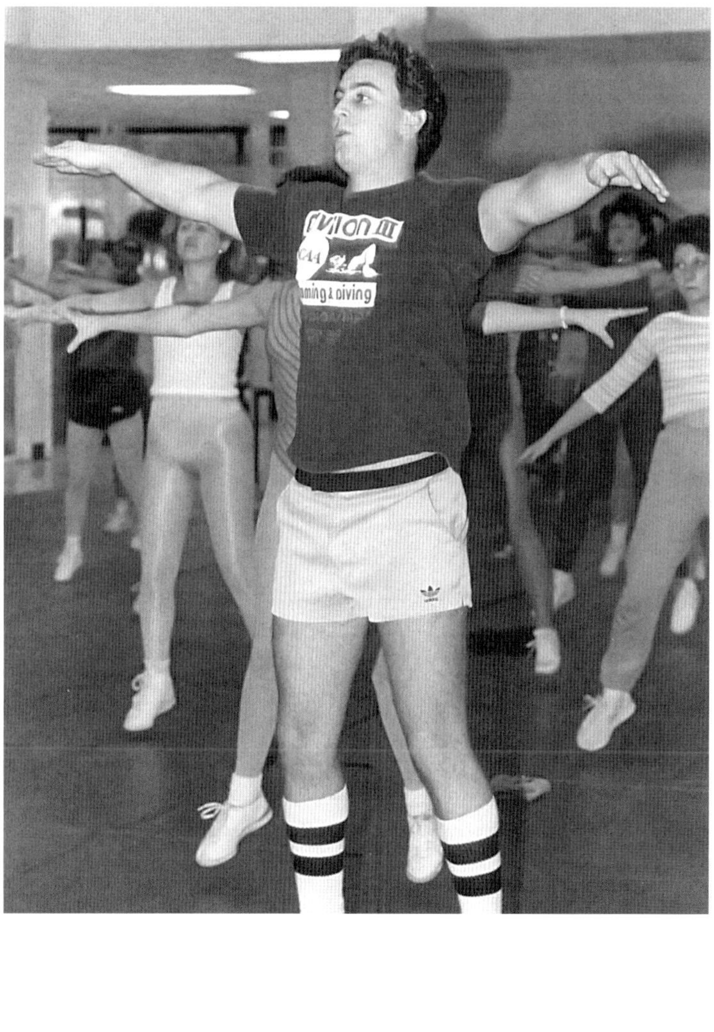

Students for Community Involvement worked with local sixth graders on how to live healthier lives. Campus wellness became important as well with the opening of a new student wellness facility and, beginning in 1986, an annual MCG 5K run.

Other activities provided opportunities for fun, fellowship, and relaxation. Greek life continued to be popular, and the student center became a prime location for annual dances. An important new tradition was born when senior medical students at MCG began dressing in wild costumes to celebrate annual Match Day festivities.

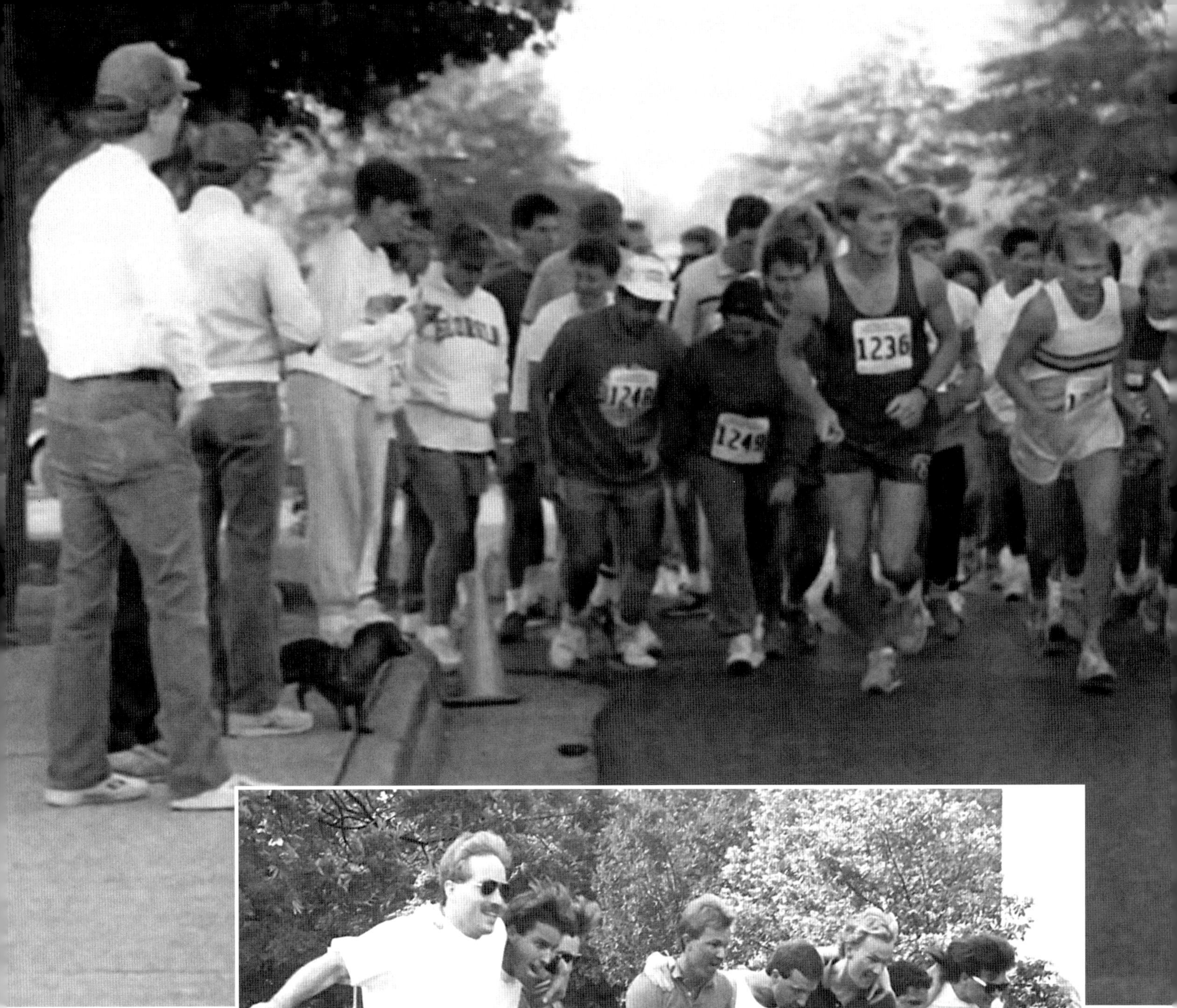


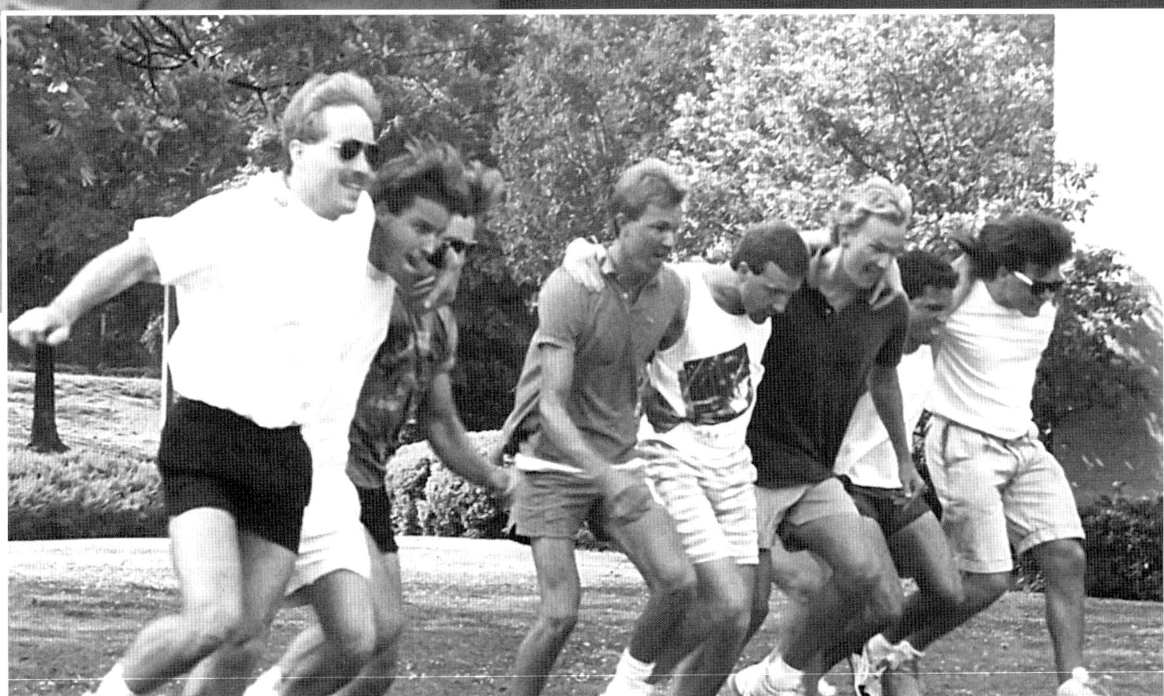

*Fitness Fights brought out the competitive spirit of MCG students at a 1989 Homecoming event.*

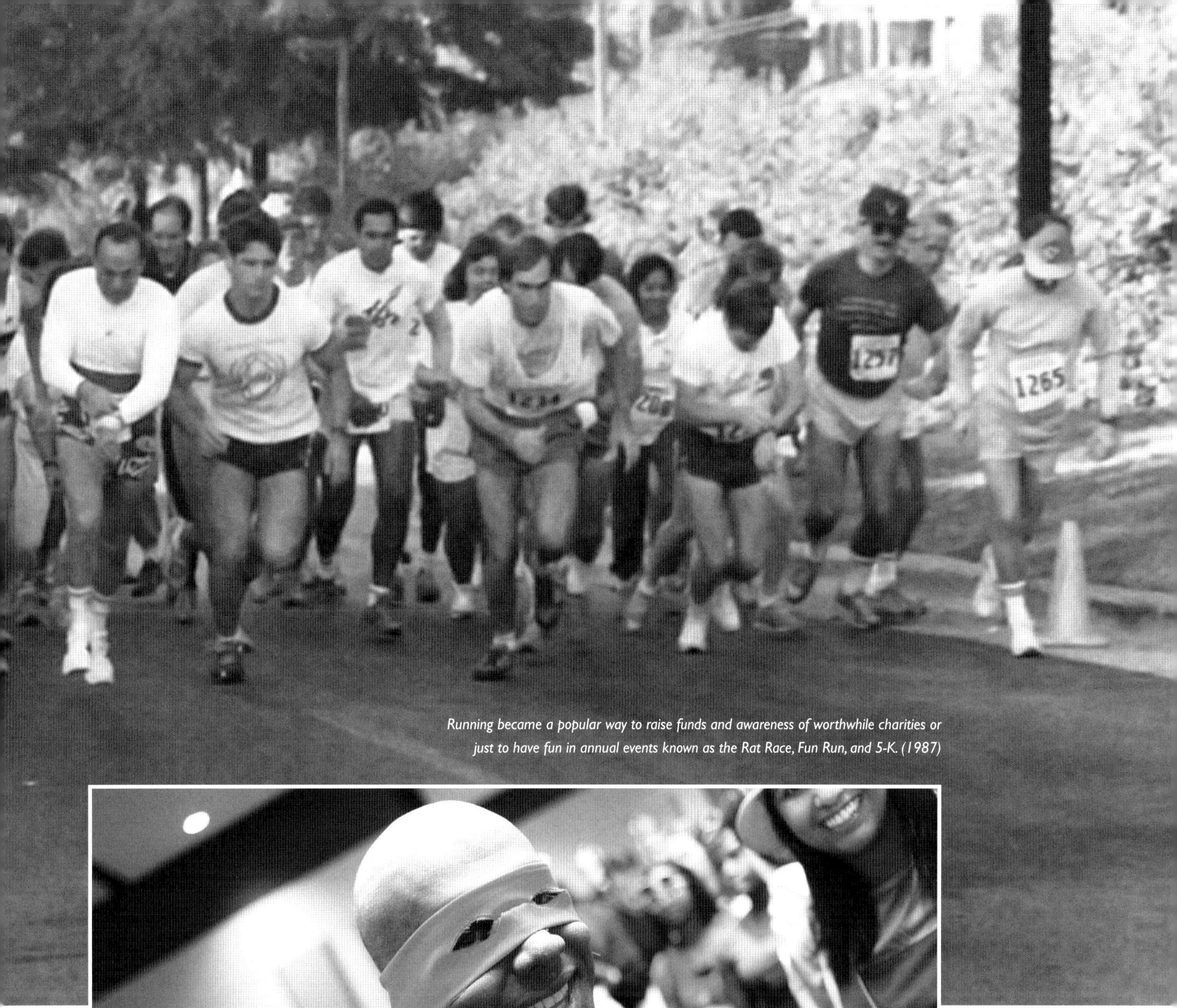


*Running became a popular way to raise funds and awareness of worthwhile charities or just to have fun in annual events known as the Rat Race, Fun Run, and 5-K. (1987)*

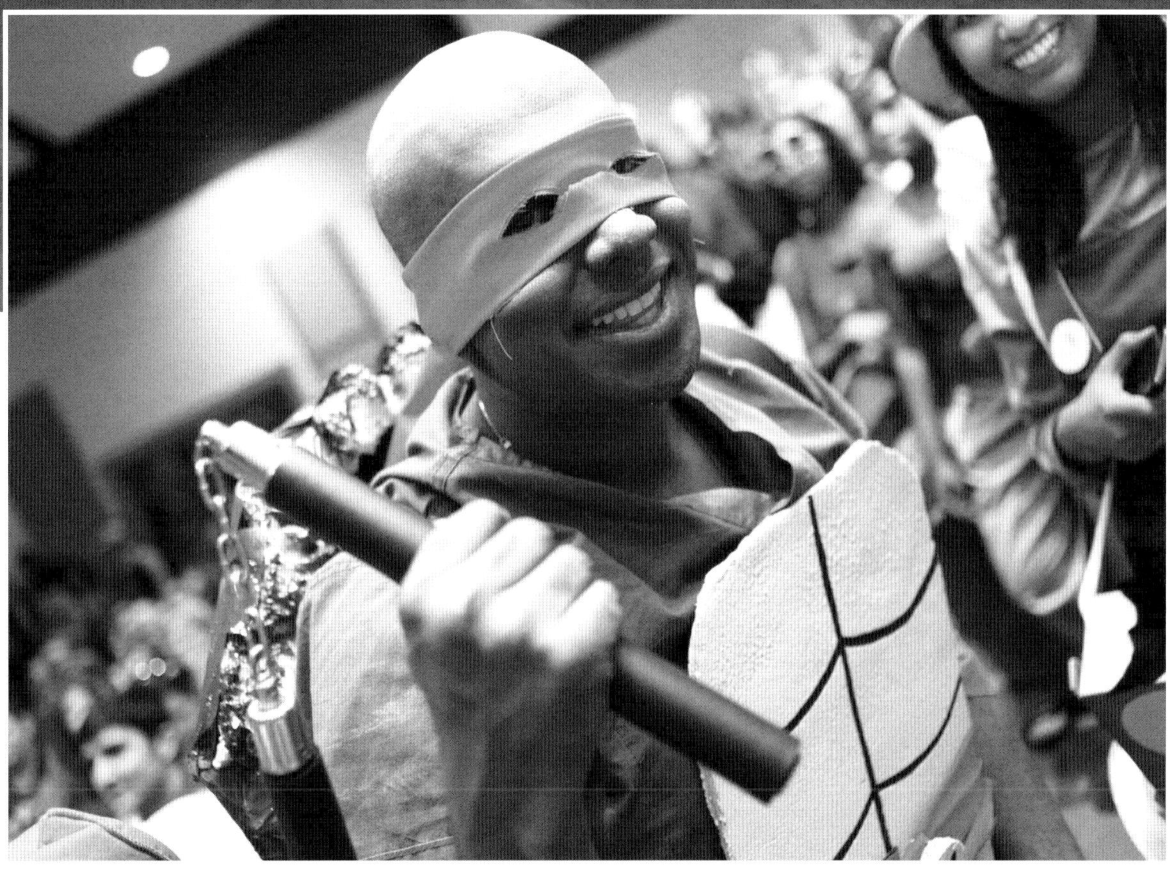

*Senior medical students dressed in costume at the annual "Match Day" activity to learn whether their top choices for continued medical training "matched" their placement by the National Resident Matching Program.*

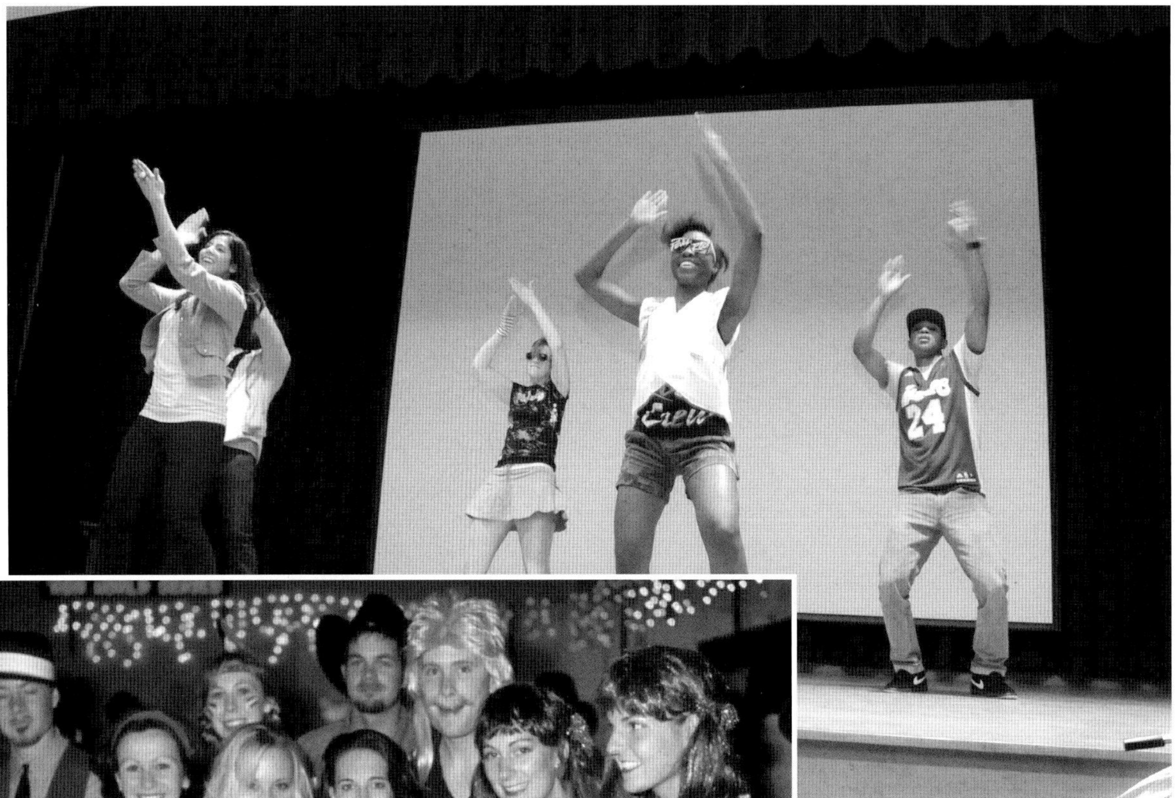


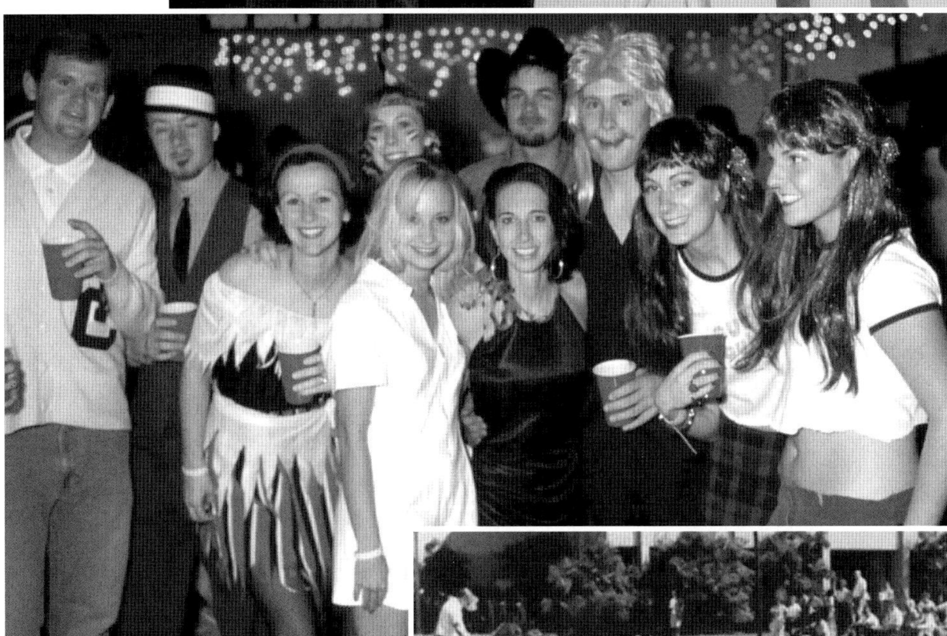

*Above: The annual talent show featured students competing in a variety of performances for MCG audiences.*

*Above: MCG's Student Government Association hosted TGIF parties, with the most popular being the Halloween party.*

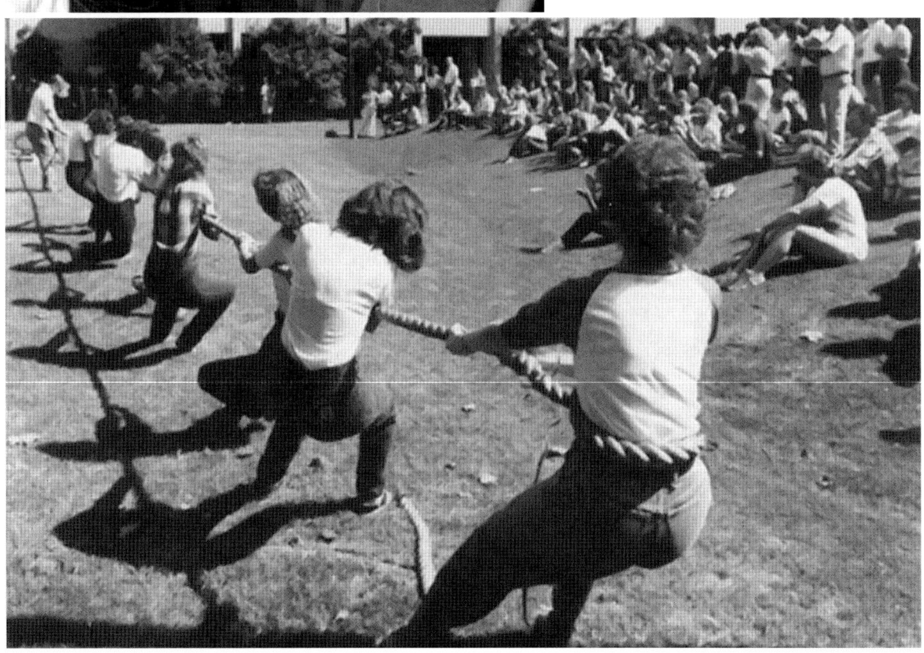

*Right: Students had fun in a 1986 tug-a-war contest to raise funds for the United Way.*

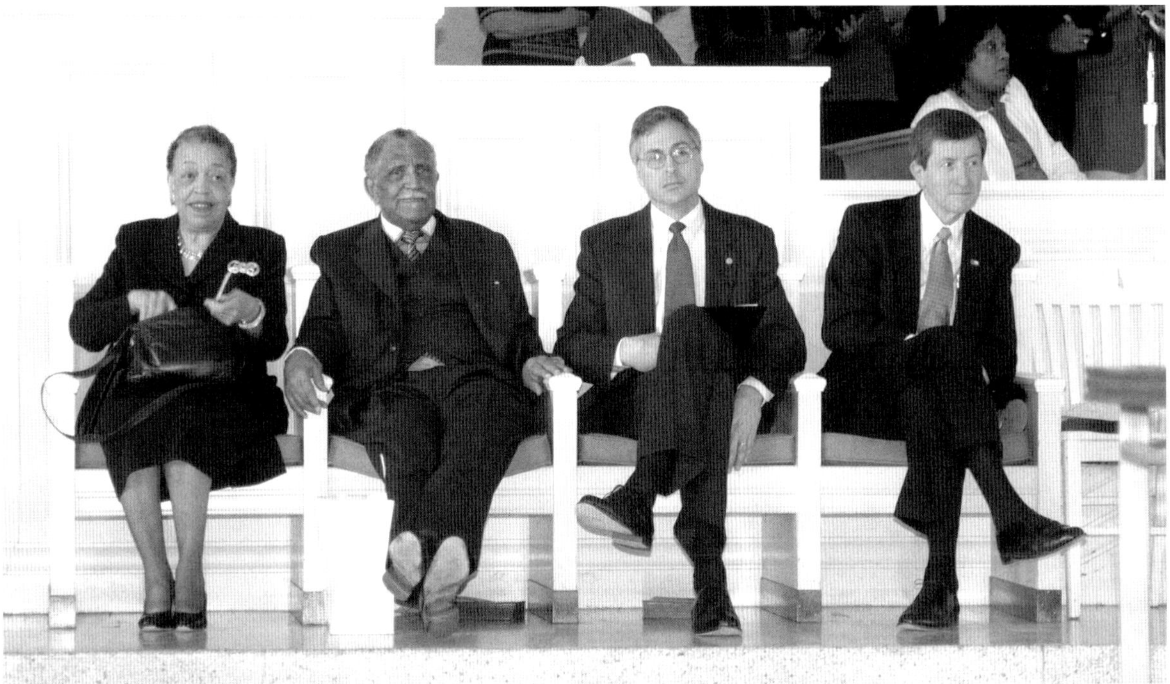

*The hosting of an annual observance of the birthday of Reverend Martin Luther King Jr. rotated among three, later four, Augusta colleges. Photo shows Paine College President Shirley Lewis, Speaker Joseph Lowery, MCG President Daniel Rahn, and ASU President William A. Bloodworth Jr.*

*In 2005, MCG held its first on-campus memorial service for cadaver donor families, students, and faculty. (Photo circa 2012)*

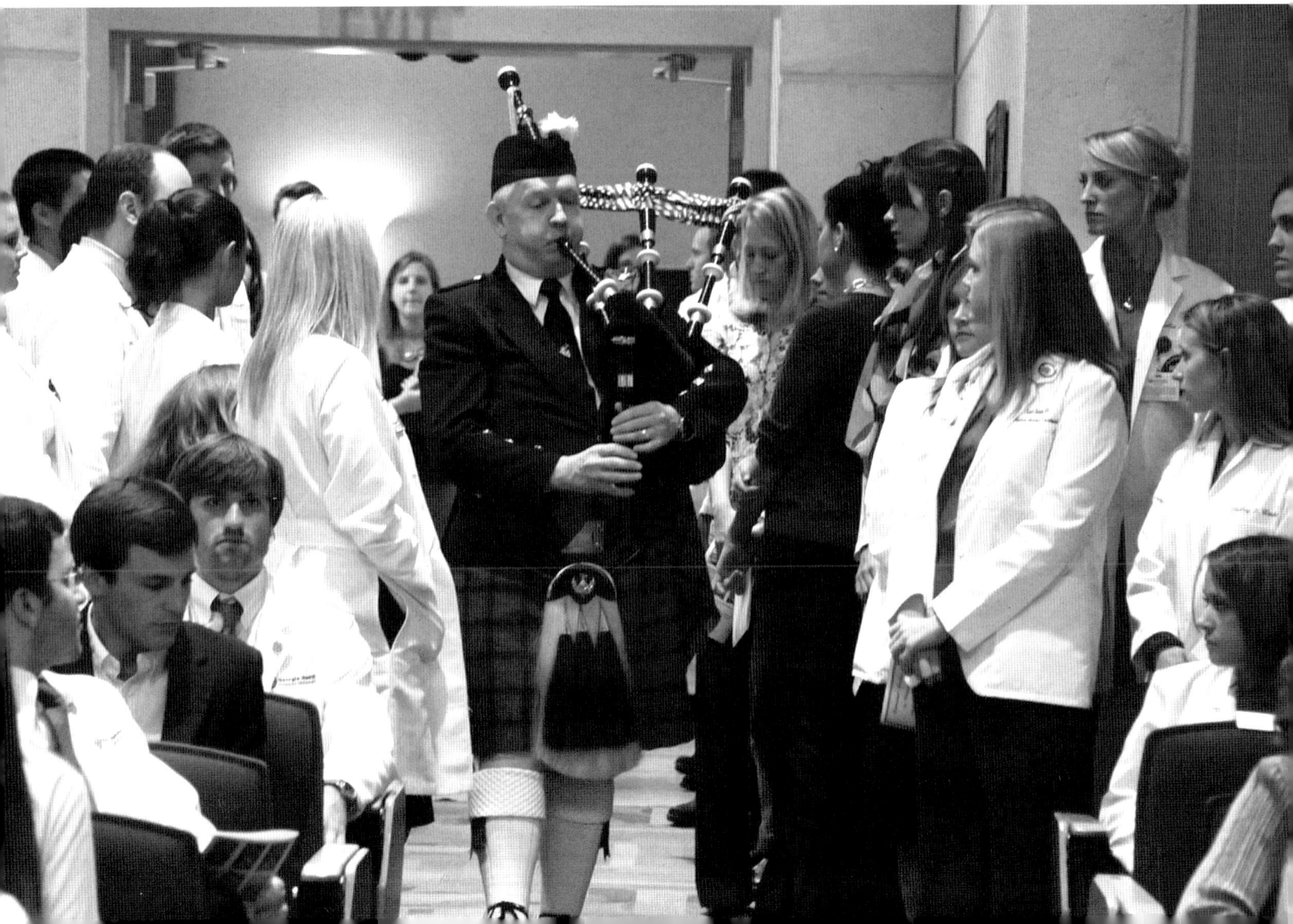

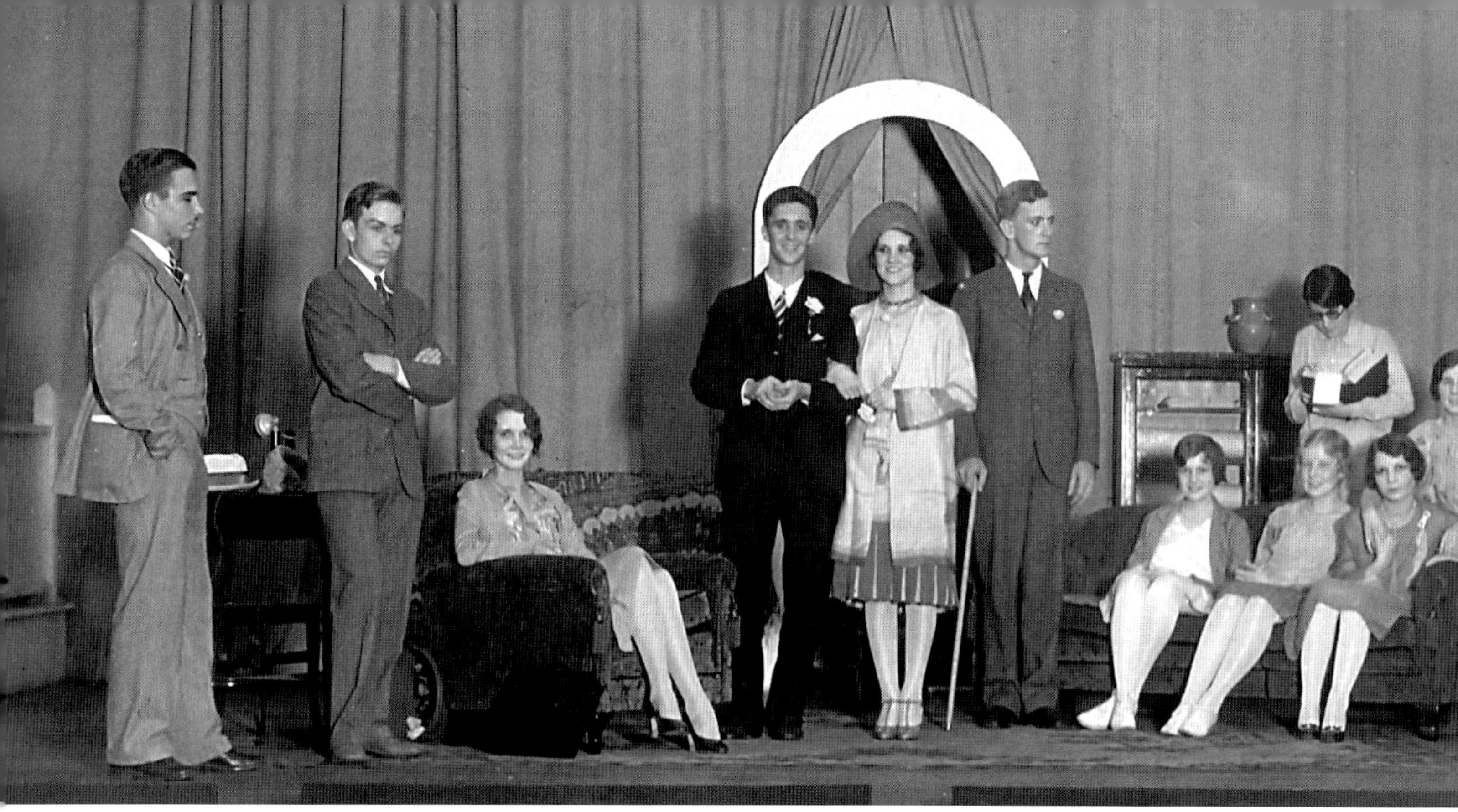

*The Dramatics Club produced a late 1928 production of* Charmed *at JCA, beginning a long tradition of theatrical performances by students.*

Outreach, activism, dances, and parties were also a part of an active student life that was launched almost immediately upon the creation of the Junior College of Augusta (JCA), which shared space with the Academy of Richmond County, its parent institution, and shared some activities as well. The first Student Council was formed, with the position of secretary designated a JCA student. The institution later established the Girls Council to address issues and concerns connected with the women's first co-ed educational opportunity since grade school.

By the mid-30s, a robust roster of activities was being offered that included a Dramatics Club, an orchestra, and the Sidney Lanier Literary Society. By 1938, a pre-law club was offered as well as a pre-med club, Rho Chi, where JCA students took trips to the hospital and interacted with medical students. A debate team, Hi-Y and Hi-Y-W, Phi Theta Kappa Honor Society, and more club options provided students a wide range of extracurricular activities.

The 1940s and '50s brought even more events and organizations. A Stunt Night presenting real talent, comedy, and "beauty;" a Sadie Hawkins Day; and a fashion show kicked off the 1940s. Women's activities took more of a role with the first campus sororities, Zeta Rho Sigma and Sigma Delta Chi, being formed. In the early 1950s, Hi-Y organizations had become so popular that more than one was offered to both sexes. The Psi Phalans social club for young men carried on charitable activities such as canned food drives and empty stocking funds, while they also hosted a rush party, a hop, and a Christmas party. Young women participated in Future Teachers, Future Nurses, and Future Homemakers, clubs reflecting the main options available to women of that era. When classes and activities were done for the day, collegians cruised down to Homefolks for the latest records or to the Dixie Pig on East Boundary for sandwiches and drinks.

When JCA severed its ties with the academy and moved to its new location on Walton Way in 1957, a new era in campus life began. Marking the school's first year as Augusta College (AC) in 1958, the *White Columns* yearbook and the *Bell Ringer* student newspaper both began publication, and new student organizations included the Drama Club, Student Association of Educators, and the Student Government Association (SGA). A bowling team and tennis club were outlets for the sports-minded, and by the following year, ten new organizations had formed.

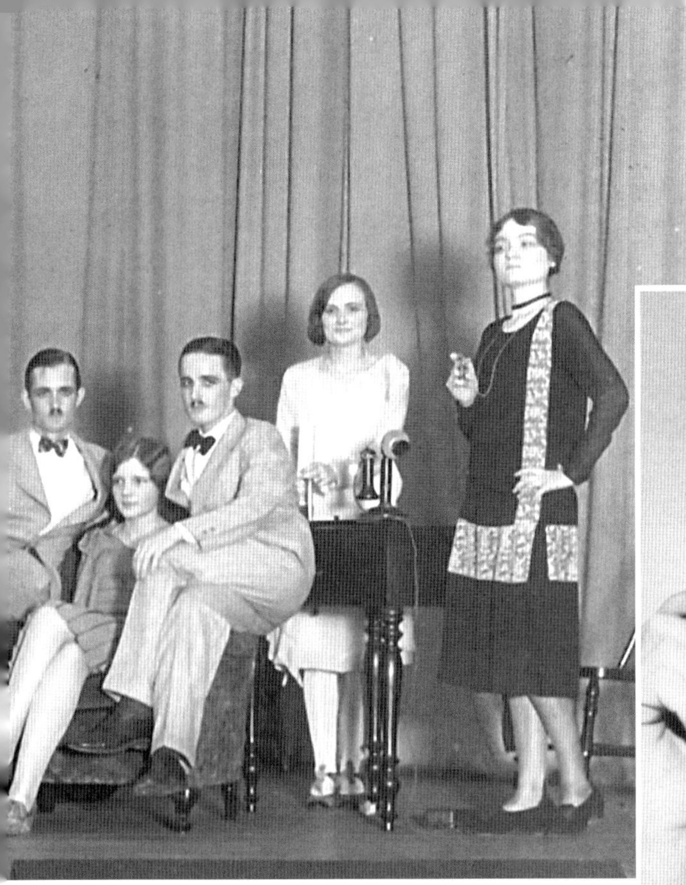

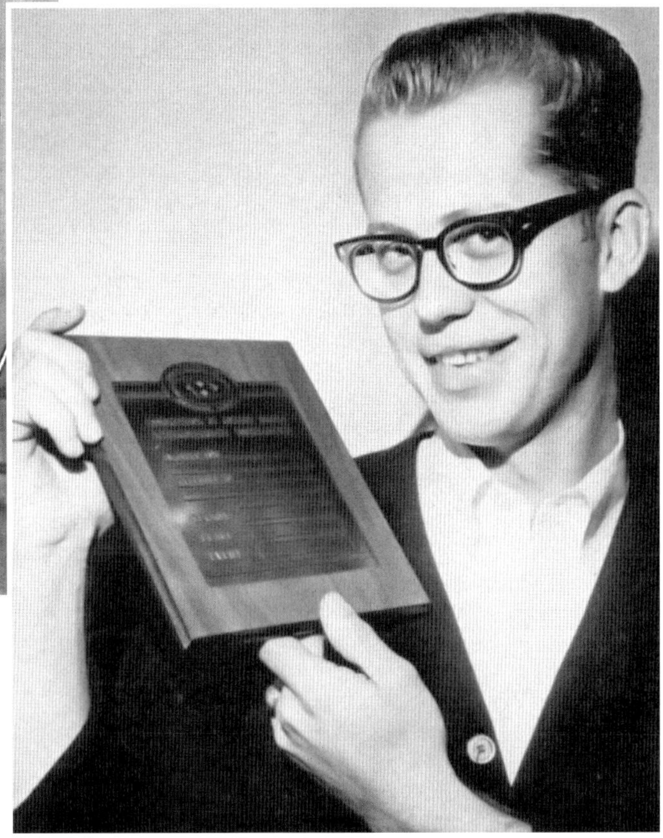

*Right: AC students organized a bowling league in 1960, and in 1965 pre-med major John Perry competed in the Association of College Unions national tournament after winning the regional singles championship.*

*Below: Playing cards was a favorite activity of students in the '60s at AC.*

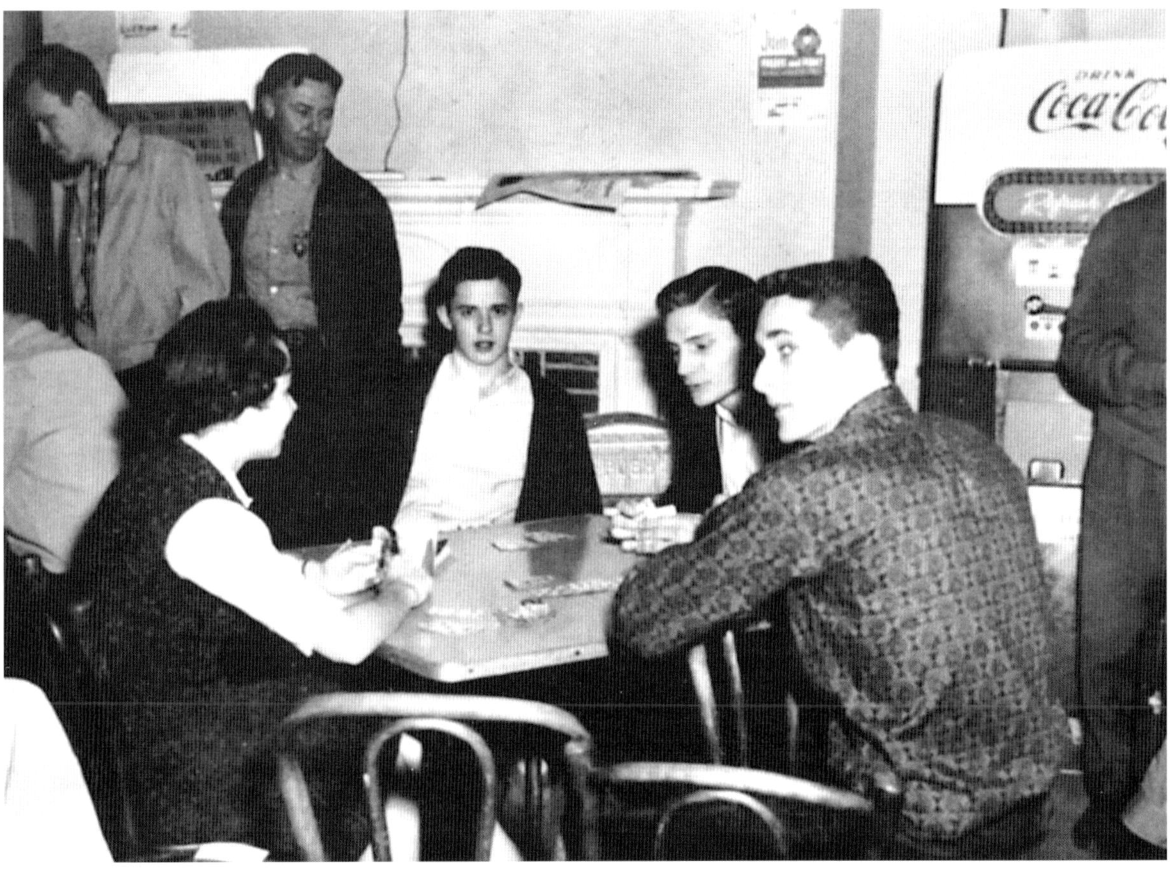

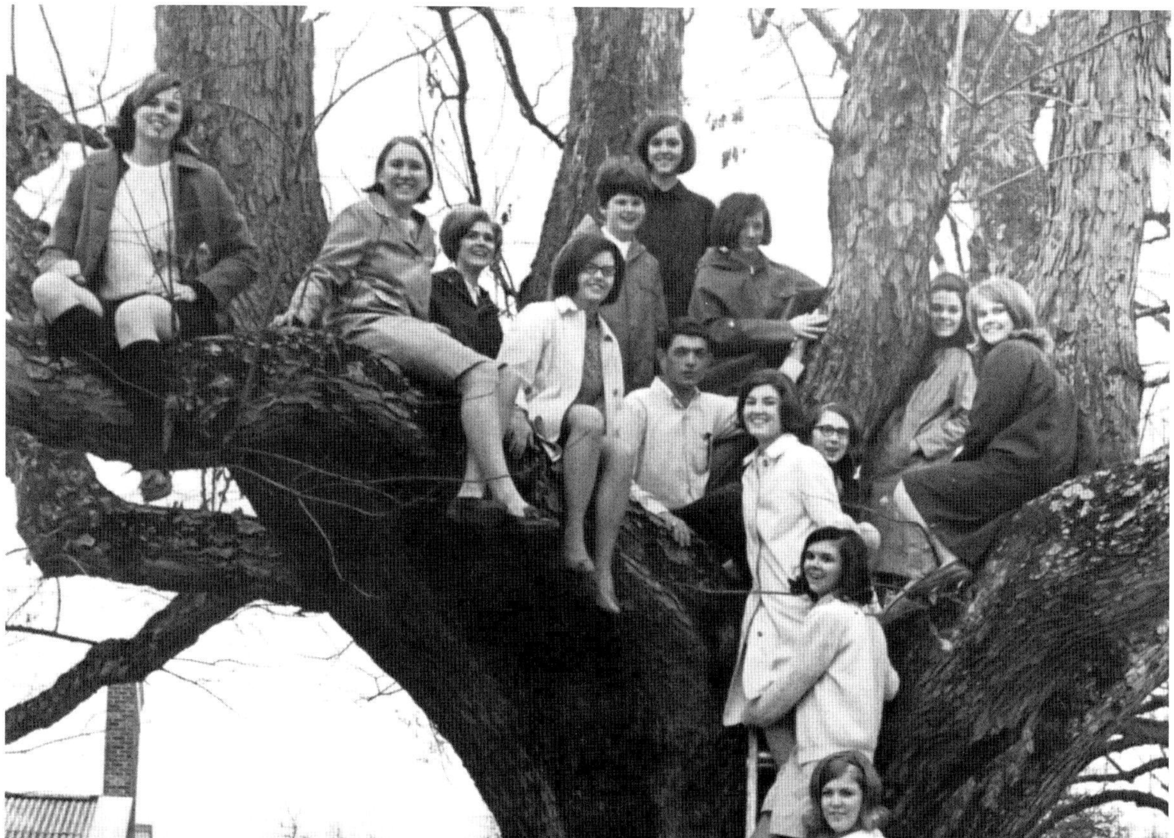

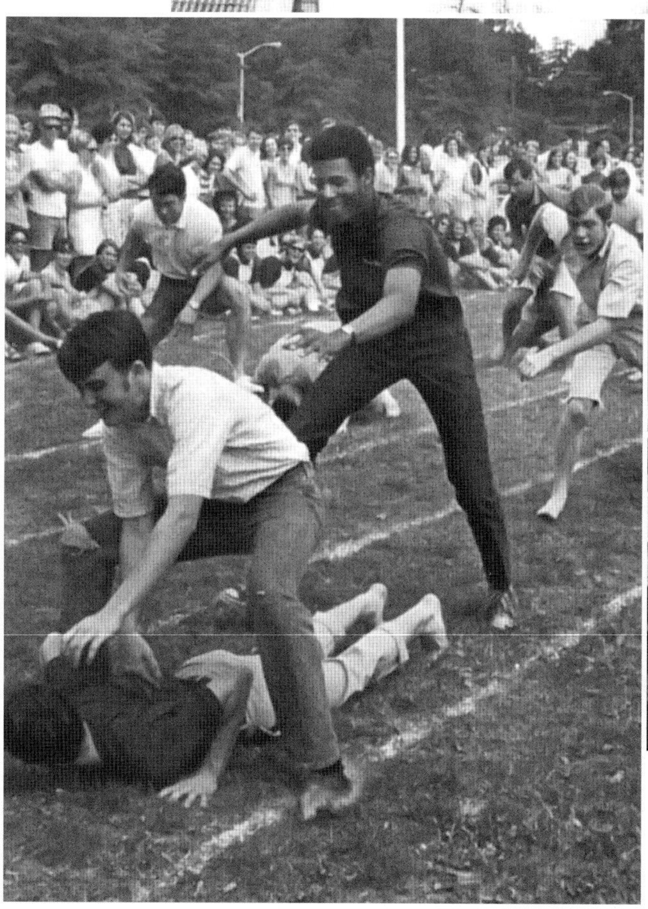

*The venerable Arsenal Oak provided a scenic backdrop for photos, and 1960s students found a creative pose to show its massive size.*

*Students joined in the fun during the '60s and '70s Field Day games.*

In the 1960s, students enjoyed dressing for Kids Day, "twisting" at a number of dances and hops, competing in Field Day events, playing powder puff football, and playing the faculty in basketball. New cultural opportunities included the AC Choir which toured in many states; the Cullum Lecture Series, which brought outstanding speakers to campus; and the still-active Lyceum Series, which provides outstanding artistic performances and speakers. The college went on the air with WACG-FM 90.7 in 1970, giving broadcasting experience to students and a strong outreach into the community.

Yet amid all the fun and cultural growth was the late '60s–early '70s undercurrent of social change that was also sweeping the

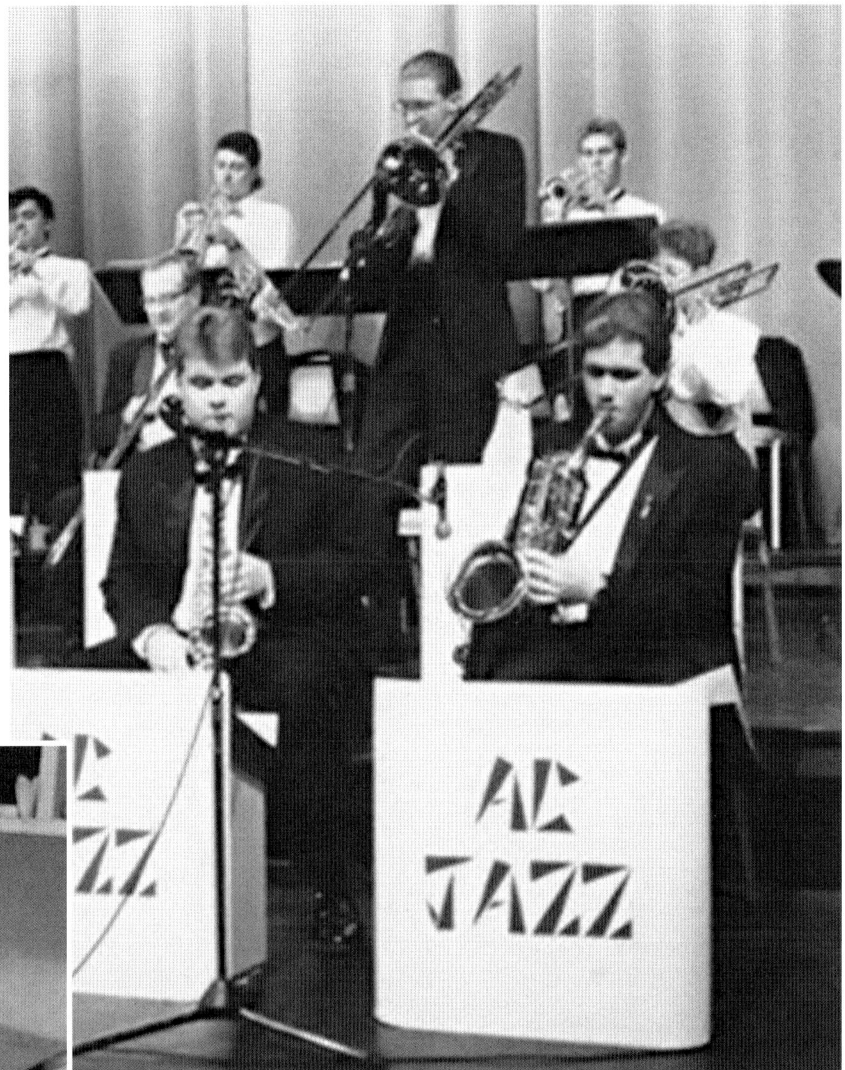


*Concerts gave student musicians the opportunity to perform before audiences.*

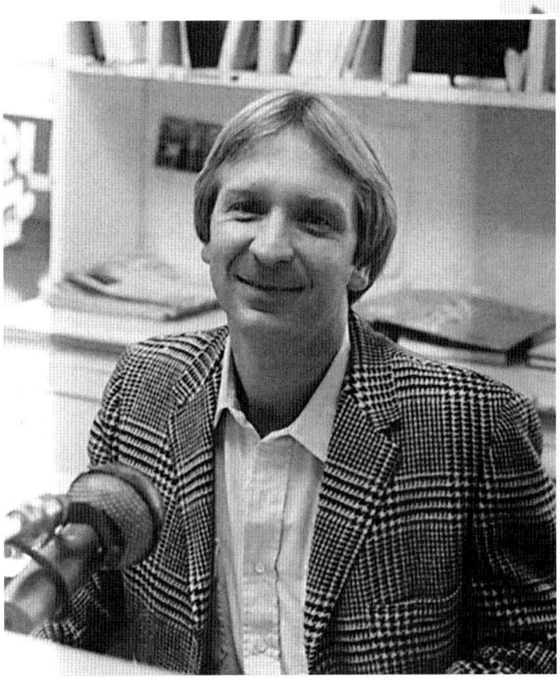

*Above: WACG began broadcasting in 1970, the university system's first non-commercial educational radio station. Alan Cooke (pictured) became station manager in 1979 and served in that role until his retirement in 2007.*

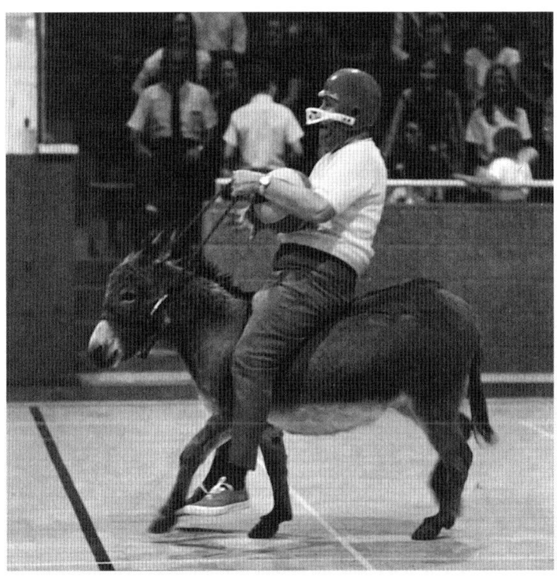

*Right: Halftime during the men's basketball game in the campus gym featured a then-popular donkey basketball game for faculty/staff. (Pictured is President George Christenberry)*

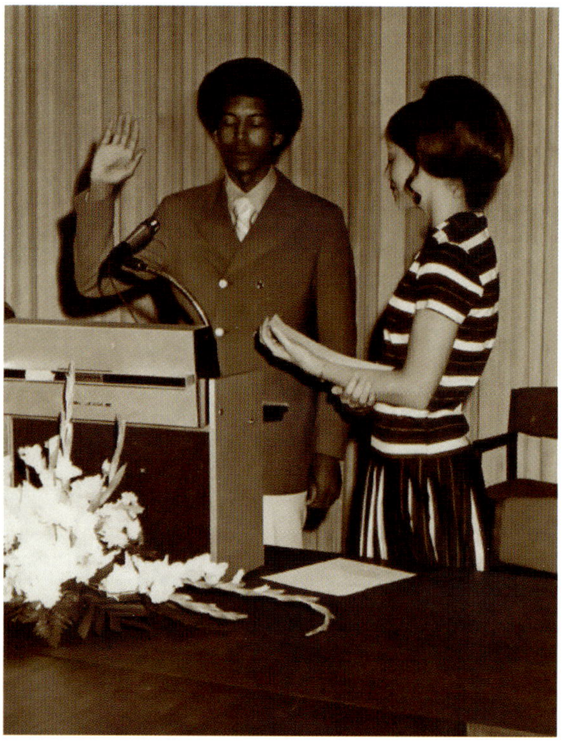

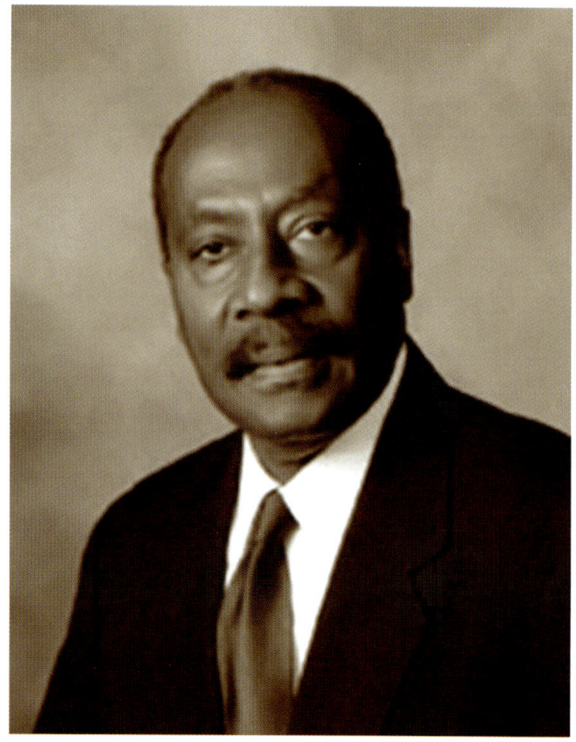

*Above: Allen Green took the oath of office in 1971, becoming the first African American elected president of the Student Government Association.*

*Above right: Dr. Joseph Greene was the first president of the Black Student Union, later becoming a member of the faculty and, ultimately, a member of the University System of Georgia Board of Regents.*

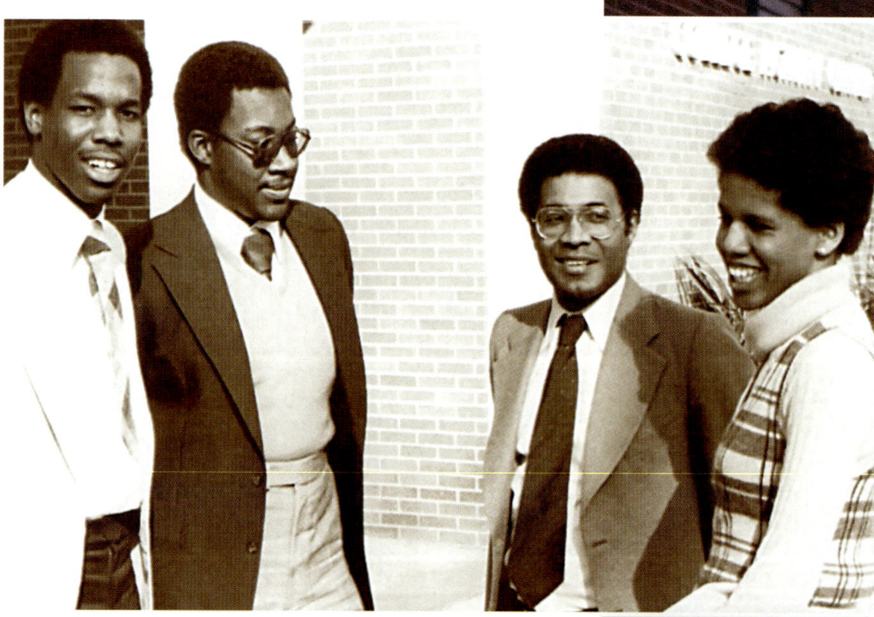

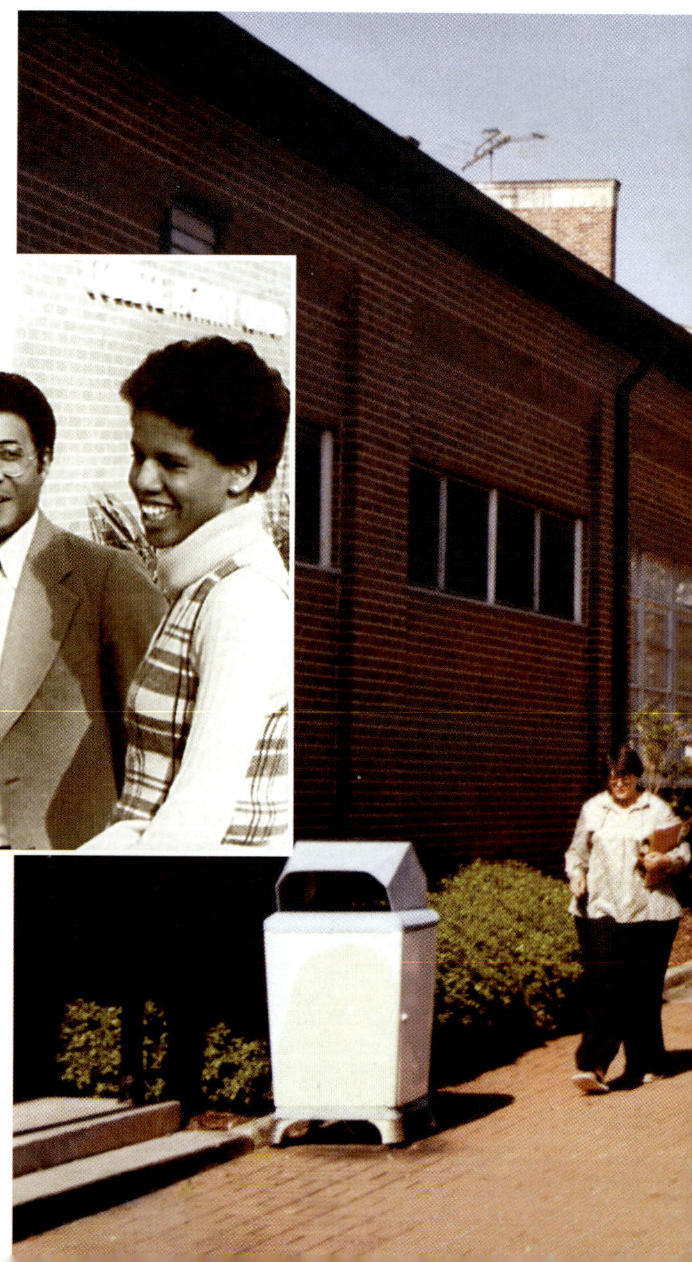

*The AC Student Union and Black Student Union co-sponsored a late 1970s campus visit from Dr. Alvin F. Poussaint. (Left to right: AC students Henry Kelly and Ed Tarver, Dr. Poussaint, and Beverly Myers)*

nation. In the late 1960s, the college became racially integrated and in 1968 African American student Sylvia Grant became the *Bell Ringer* beauty; two years later she was Miss Christmas Belle. In 1970, a group of African American students, prohibited from using the word "Black" in an organization it attempted to form, chartered the Progressive Student Alliance. Its first official act was to change its name to the Black Student Union. Joseph Greene, the first president of the Black Student Union, became the Cree-Walker Professor of Business Administration at AC as well as a member of the Board of Regents of the University System of Georgia. Also in 1970, African American Roscoe Williams began his twenty-plus years at AC, first as assistant dean of students and later as dean. The following year, students elected the first African American president of the Student Government Association, Allen Green. That year's valedictorian was Lillie Butler, who years later would come back to AC as Dr. Lillie Johnson, long-serving chair of the English program.

Amidst all the social change, there was still time for fun. Students enjoyed local watering holes such as Squeaky's Tip Top and Red Lion Pub, as well as swimming at the college's site on Clark's Hill Lake. Old AC traditions continued, including students gathering for those precious ten minutes between classes at the brick "Teardrop." Greek life gained footing after a Panhellenic Council, the Pi Kappa Phi fraternity, and the Zeta Tau Alpha and Alpha Delta Pi sororities were joined by other Greek organizations. A new fad on college campuses took AC by storm

*Students made their way to classes in the old "six-pack," finding places along the way to visit with friends.*

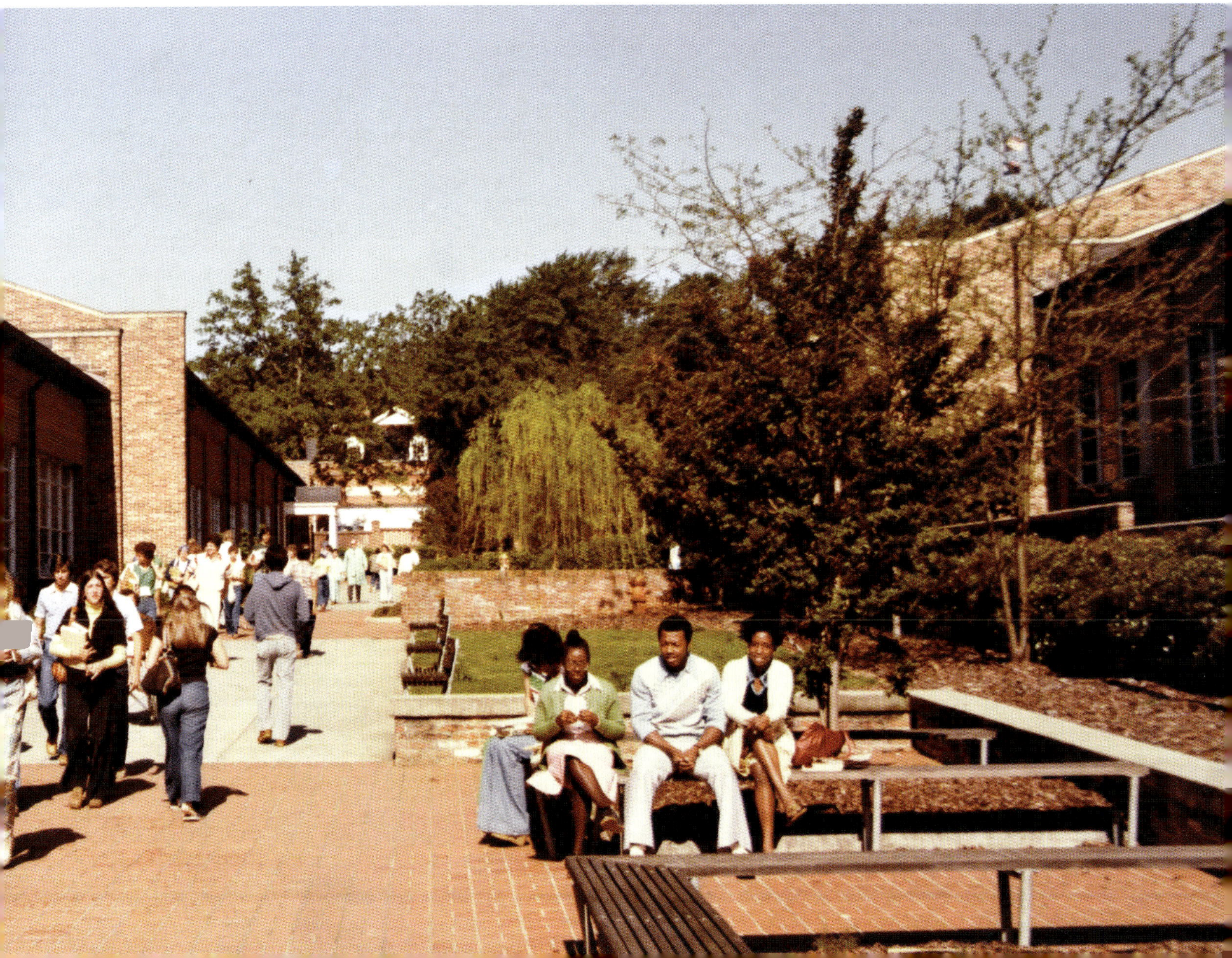

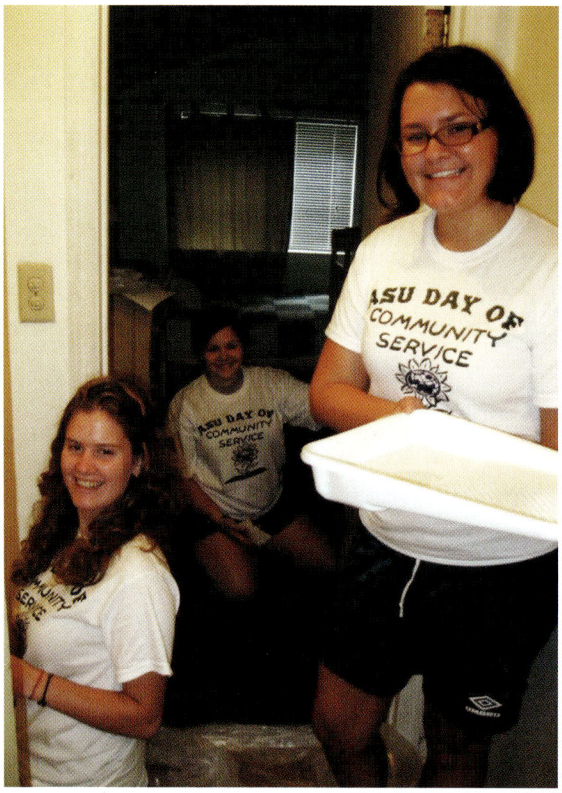


as a rash of "streaking" incidents disrupted classes, amused other students, and challenged administrators. After the 1973 incorporation of the AC Alumni Association, college alums had a voice in the institution and actively supported their alma mater.

Changes and additions continued in the 1980s with events such as Oktoberfest, Tug-a-War, Rocky Horror Picture Show, and dances in the College Activities Center. Patti Peabody became the first woman to be elected president of the SGA. The late 1980s/early 1990s drew international attention to AC when its table tennis team took the national Intercollegiate Table Tennis Team Championships from 1989 to 1992.

*Left: Students provided assistance to off-campus nonprofits in the annual day of community service.*

*Below: The ASU faculty and staff offer a welcome at fall convocation.*

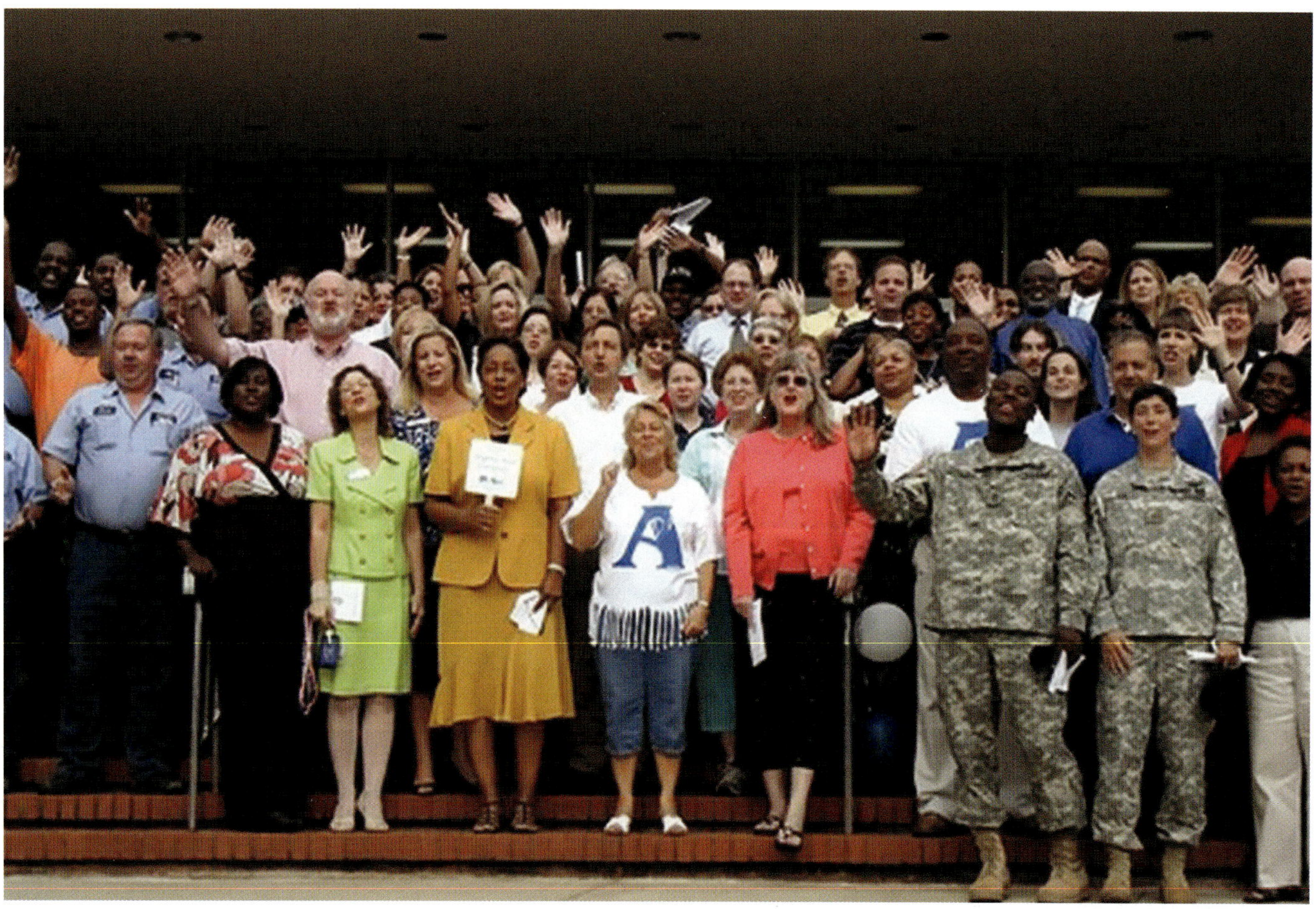

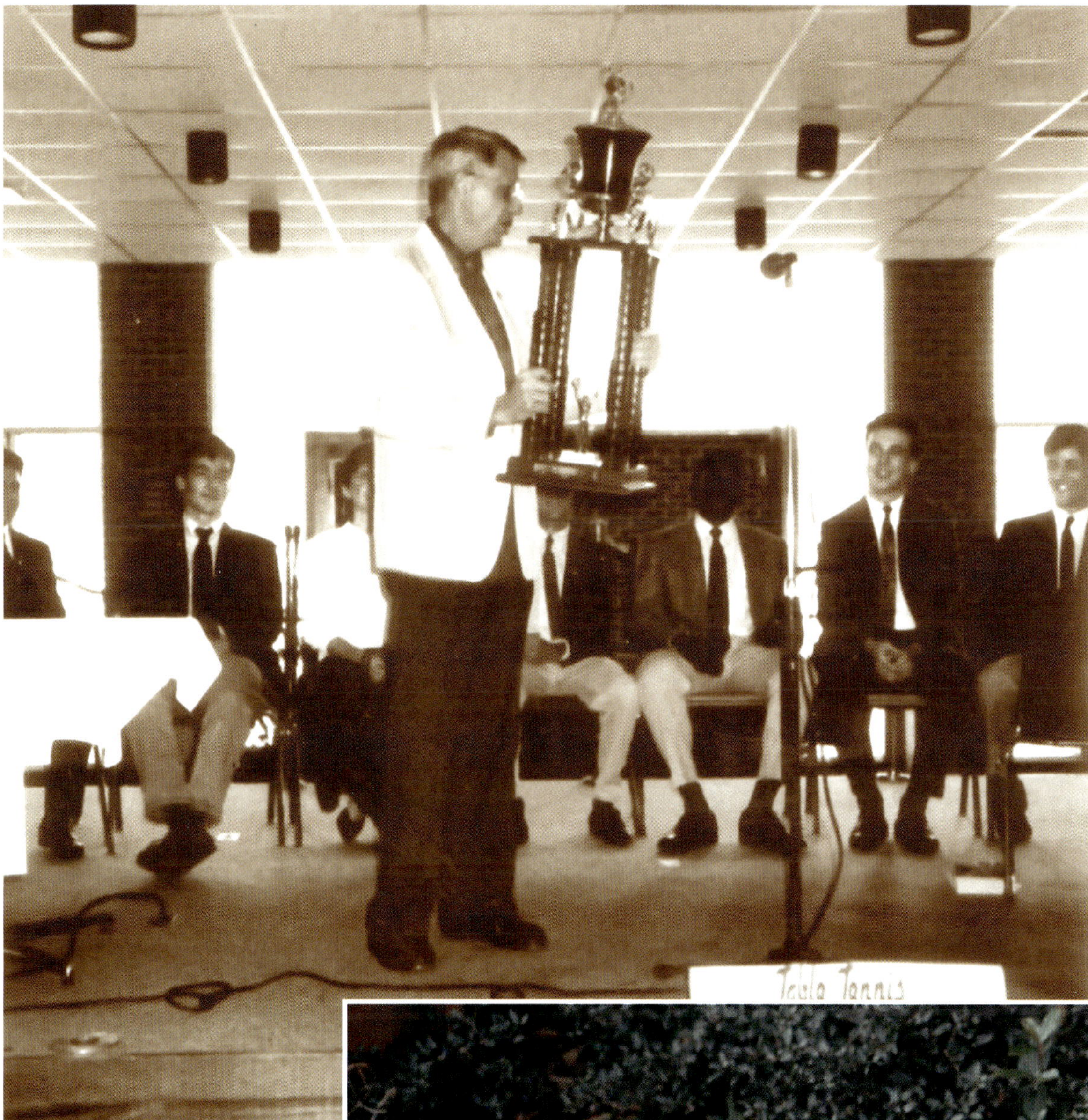

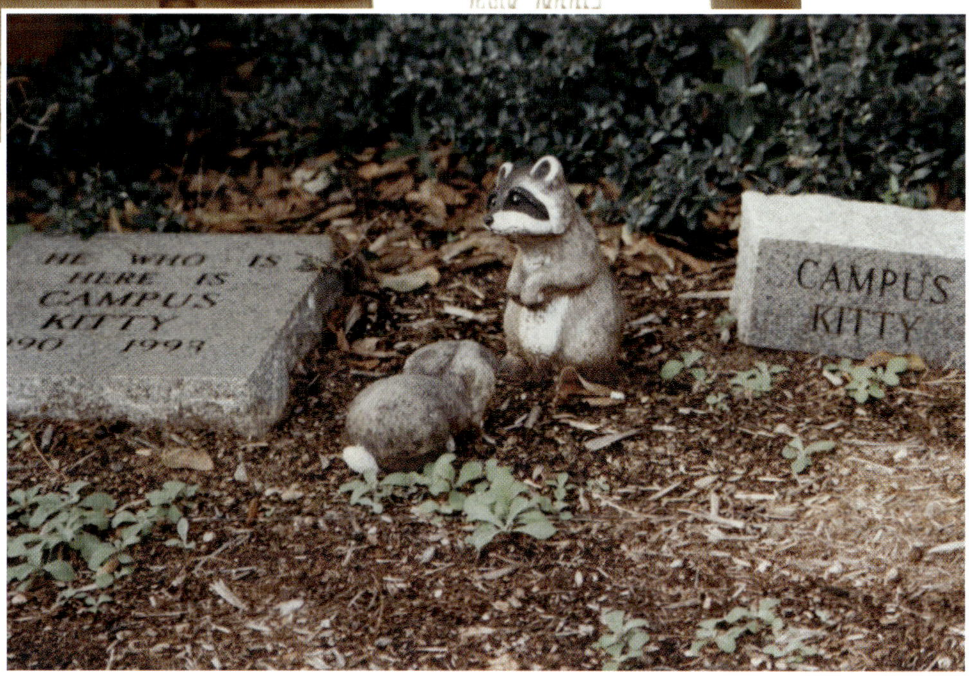


*Above: The table tennis team captured the national Intercollegiate Table Tennis Team Championships from 1989 to 1992, as well as the International Borrego Championship in 1990. Scott Butler, 1989 men's national singles champion, and Derek May, 1990 singles champion, won spots on the U.S. National Table Tennis Team and became contenders for the 1992 U.S. Olympic team. Magali Montes was the nation's women's singles champion in 1992.*

*Right: AC students memorialized the "campus kitties" with their own plot next to the "teardrop" in the early 1990s.*

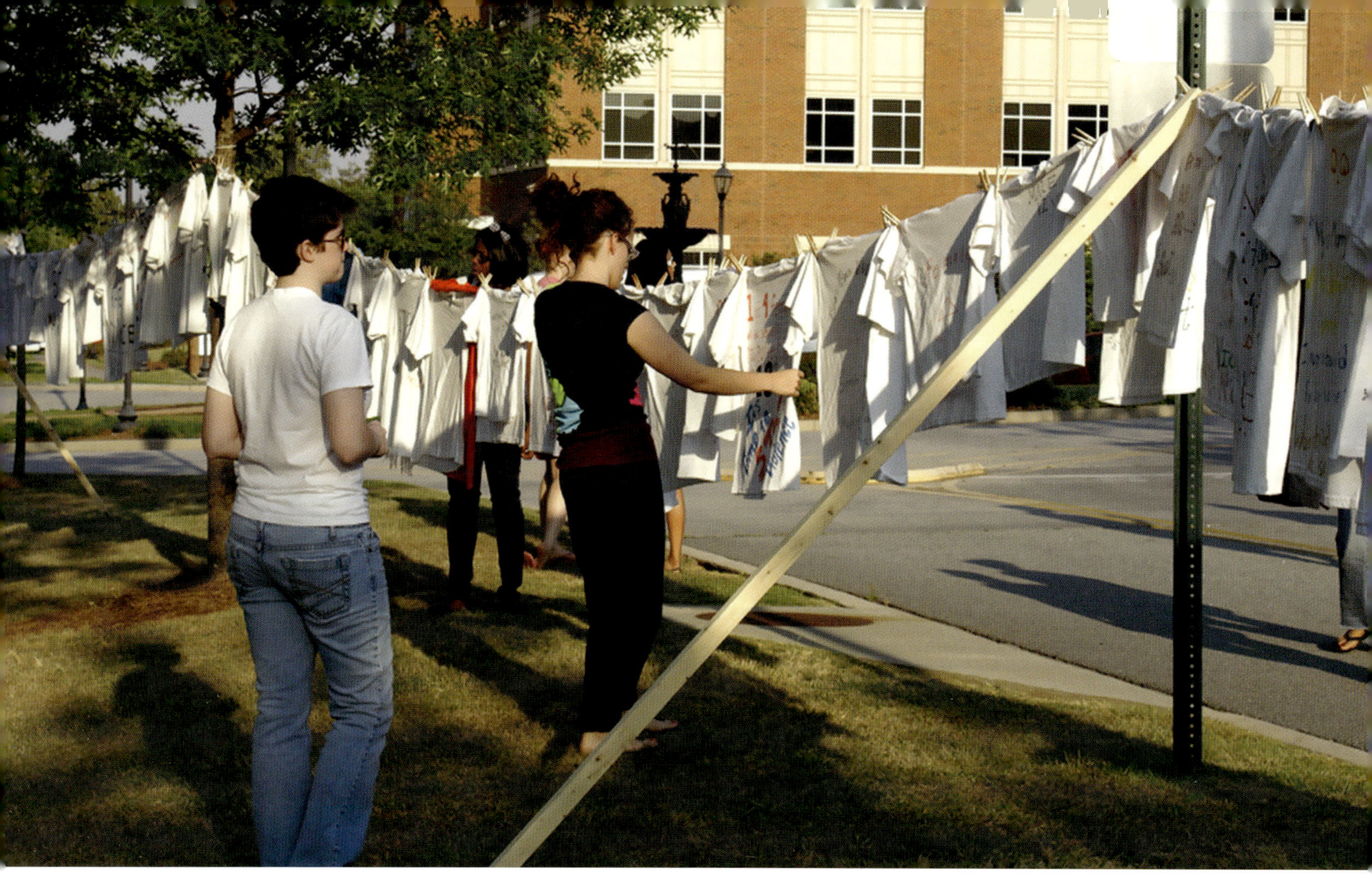

*Take Back the Night activities, held annually with Paine College and the Rape Crisis and Sexual Assault Services, focused attention on domestic and sexual violence.*

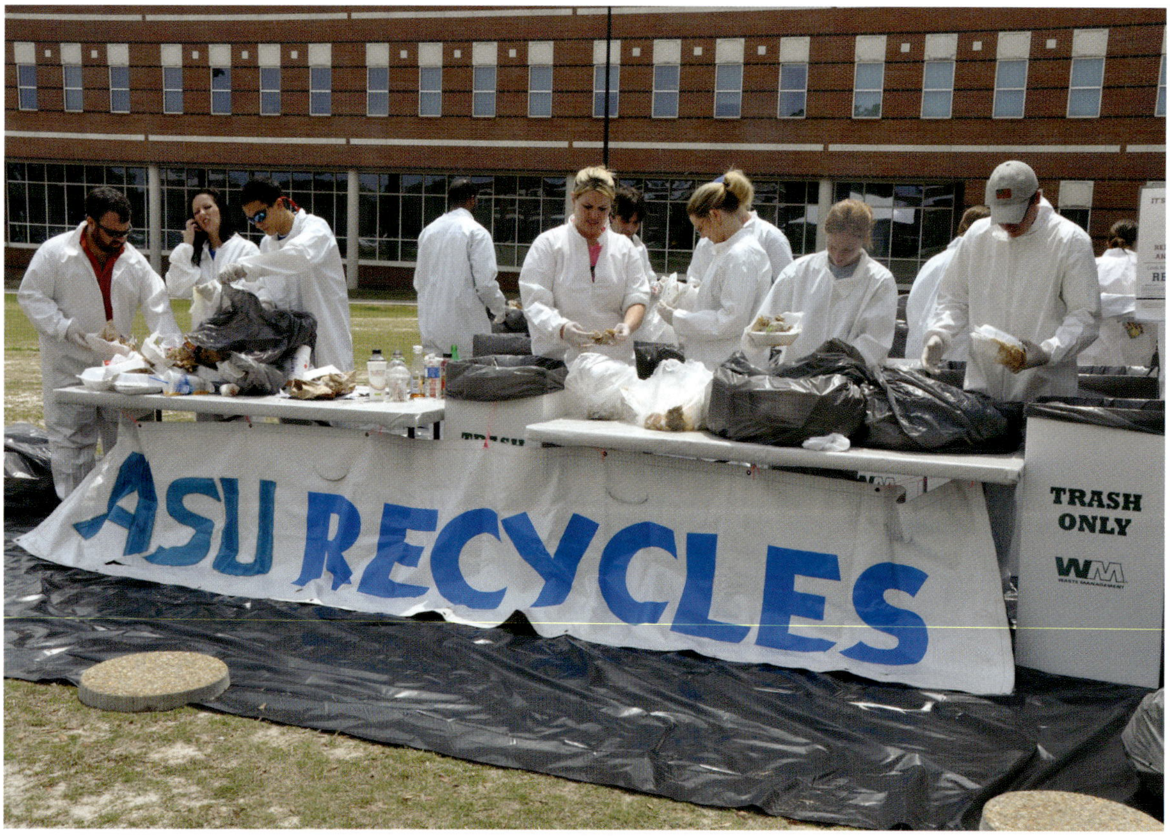


*Sorting recyclables from campus trash focused attention on the university's efforts to recycle.*

By this time, more nontraditional undergraduate students and older graduate students were entering AC's student population. An increased social awareness was also taking hold. "Students and faculty took interest in improving our campus by campaigning for recycling awareness, alcohol awareness, and safe-sex promotion," announced the 1992 yearbook. That same year, the campus continued to be alcohol free at all college functions and became smoke-free in all buildings other than the lower level of the CAC (College Activity Center).

The 1990s ushered in new traditions and activities—annual cookouts, fish fries, fall convocation, Pig-Out, SOS Day, and an international festival. A-Day for Augusta College became a friend-raising and fundraising campaign with its annual alumni barbecue.

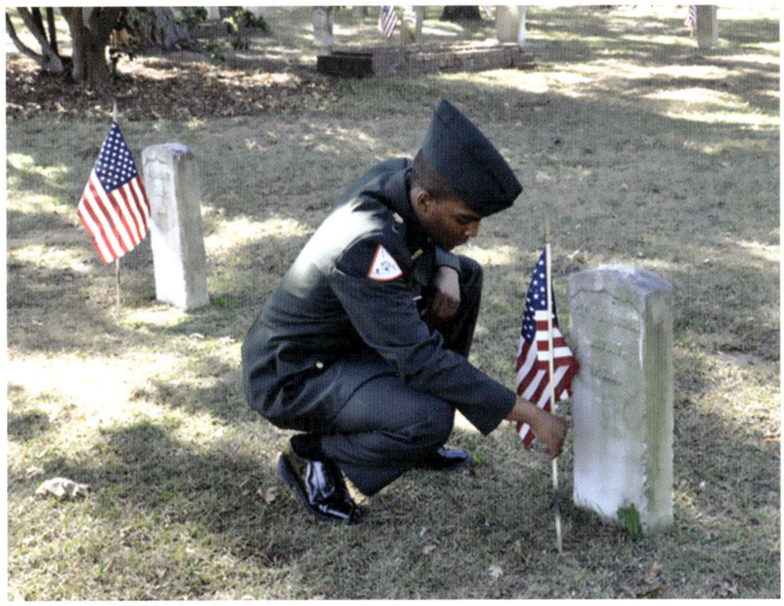

*Right: ROTC cadets honored veterans buried in the military cemetery on campus. ASU's cadre included students from other local colleges including MCG.*

*Below: Faculty and staff grilled and served food while students played games at Pig-Out, a tradition each semester.*

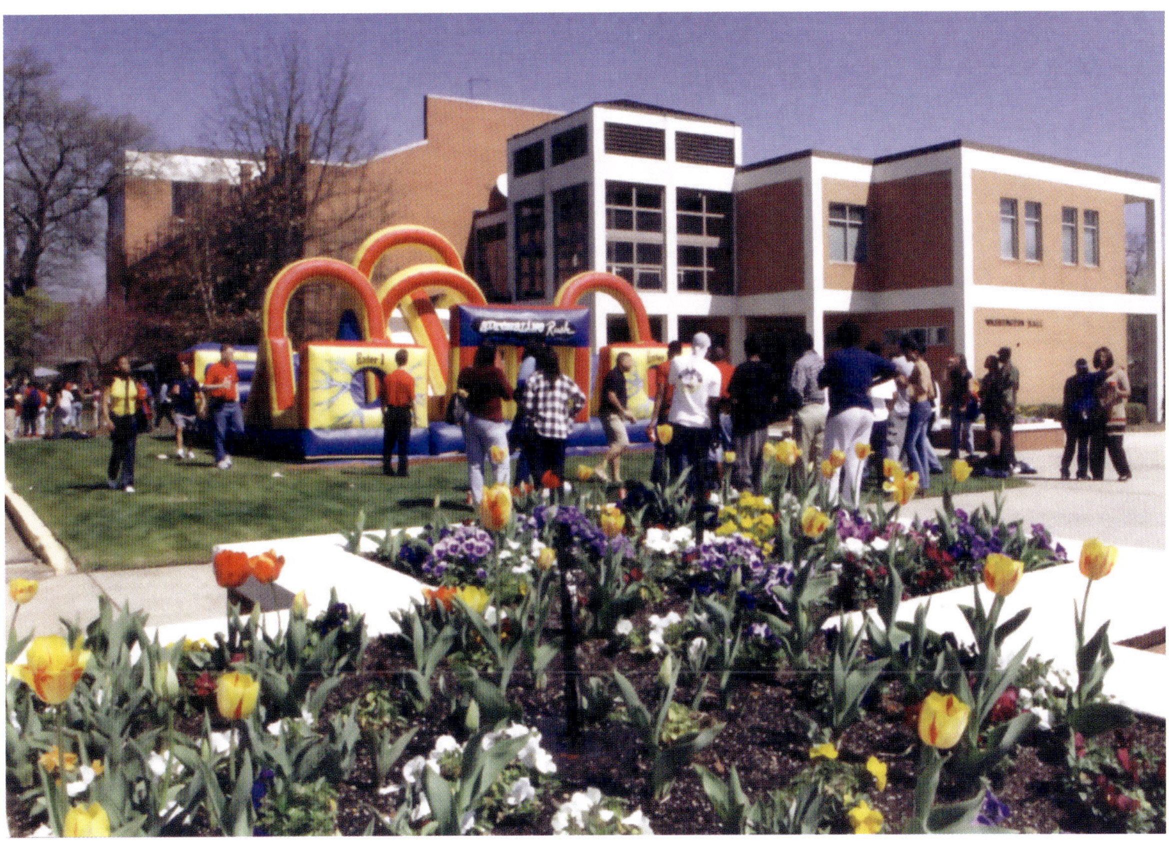

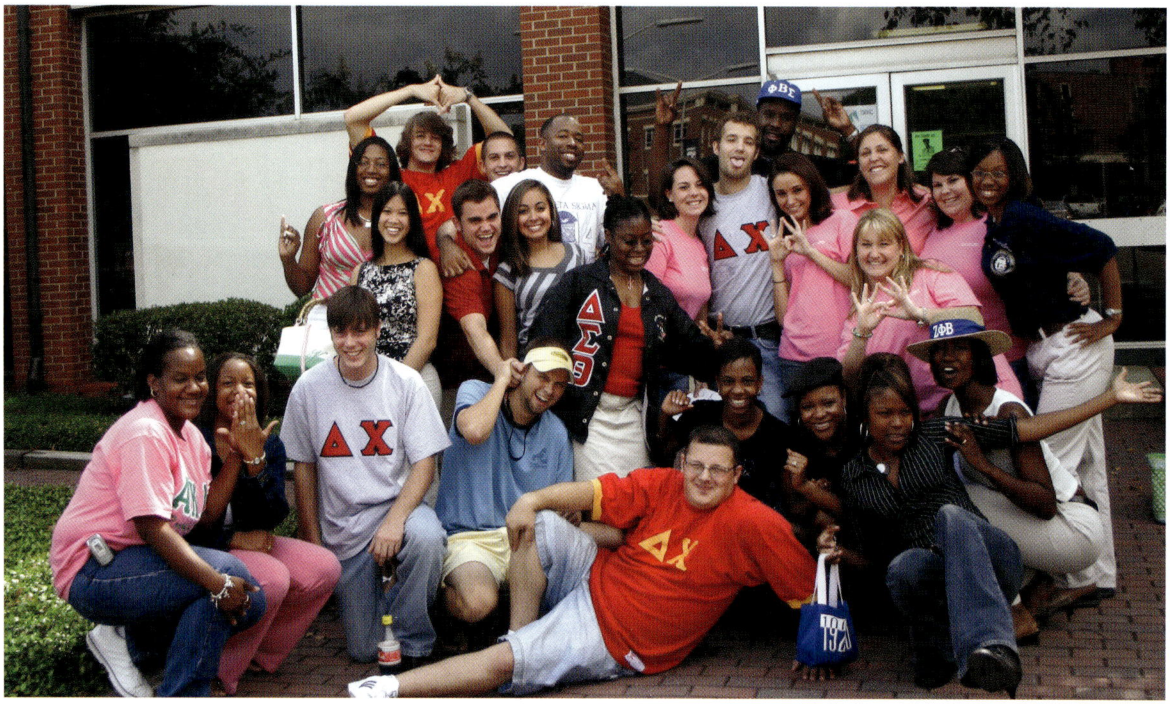


*Fraternities and sororities provided an added dimension to student life, rushing students in the first few weeks of classes. (late 1990s)*

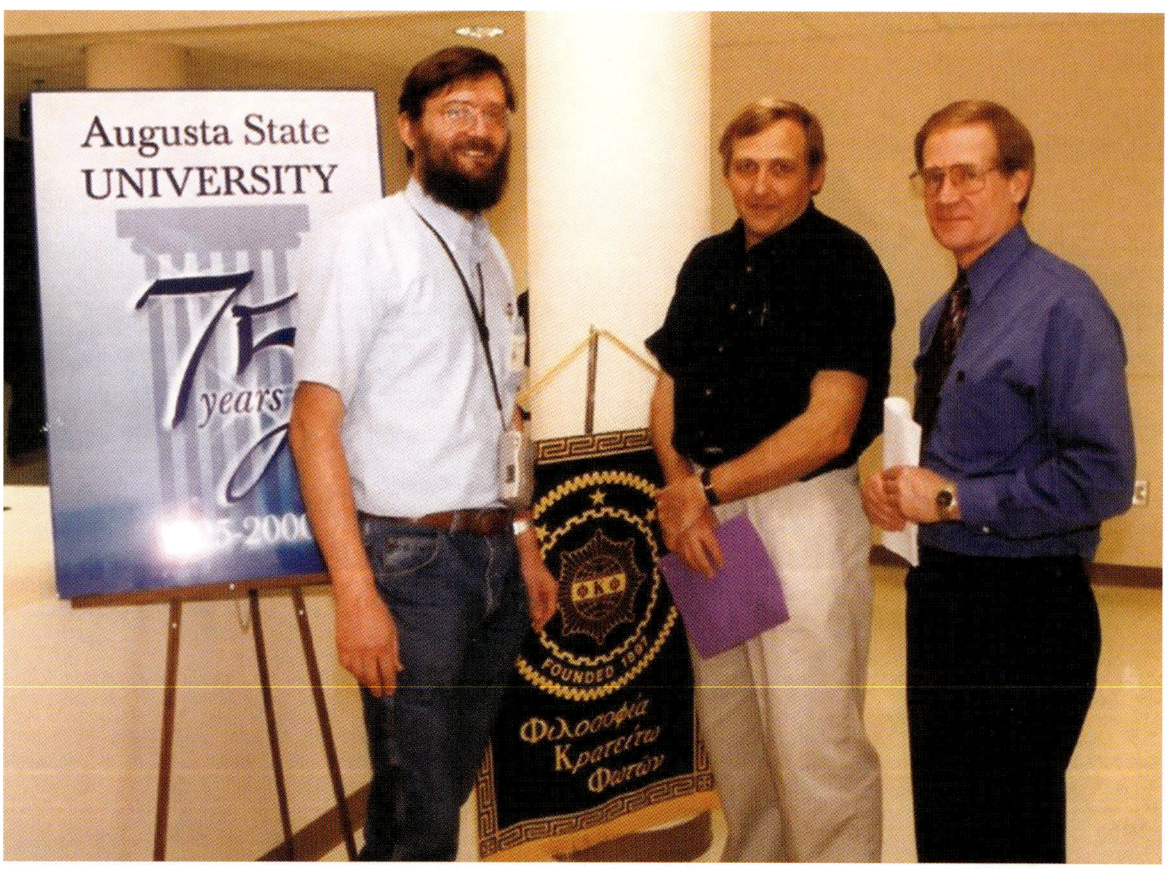


*The AC chapter of the interdisciplinary Honor Society of Phi Kappa Phi organized in 1974 and began holding a Student Research and Fine Arts Conference in 2000. A chapter began at GHSU in 2012 and the following year the chapters consolidated. Pictured left to right: Drs. Jurgen Brauer, Gary Stroebel, and Stephen Hobbs.*

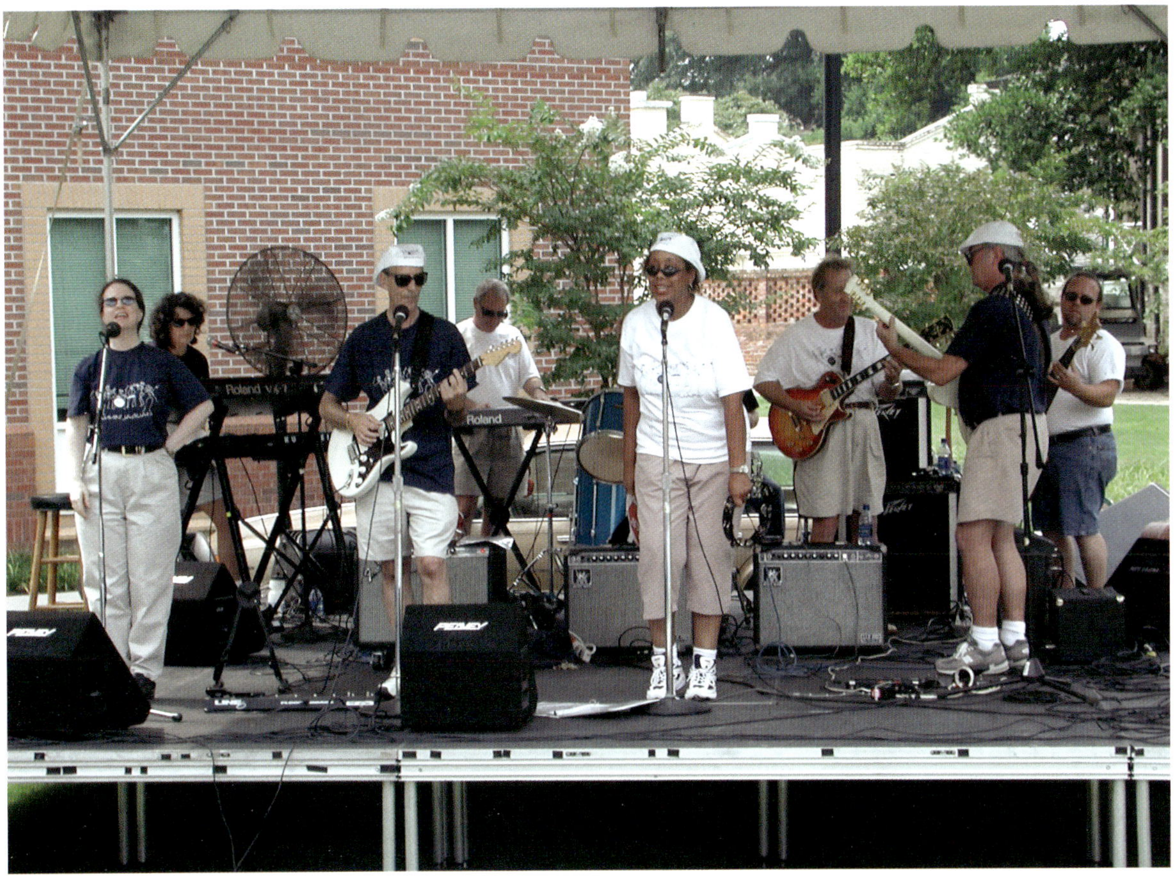


*The Jammin' Jags, an informal band led by math faculty members Jim and Michele Benedict, entertained at campus events in the 1990s and 2000s, recording a CD and donating the proceeds to the university.*

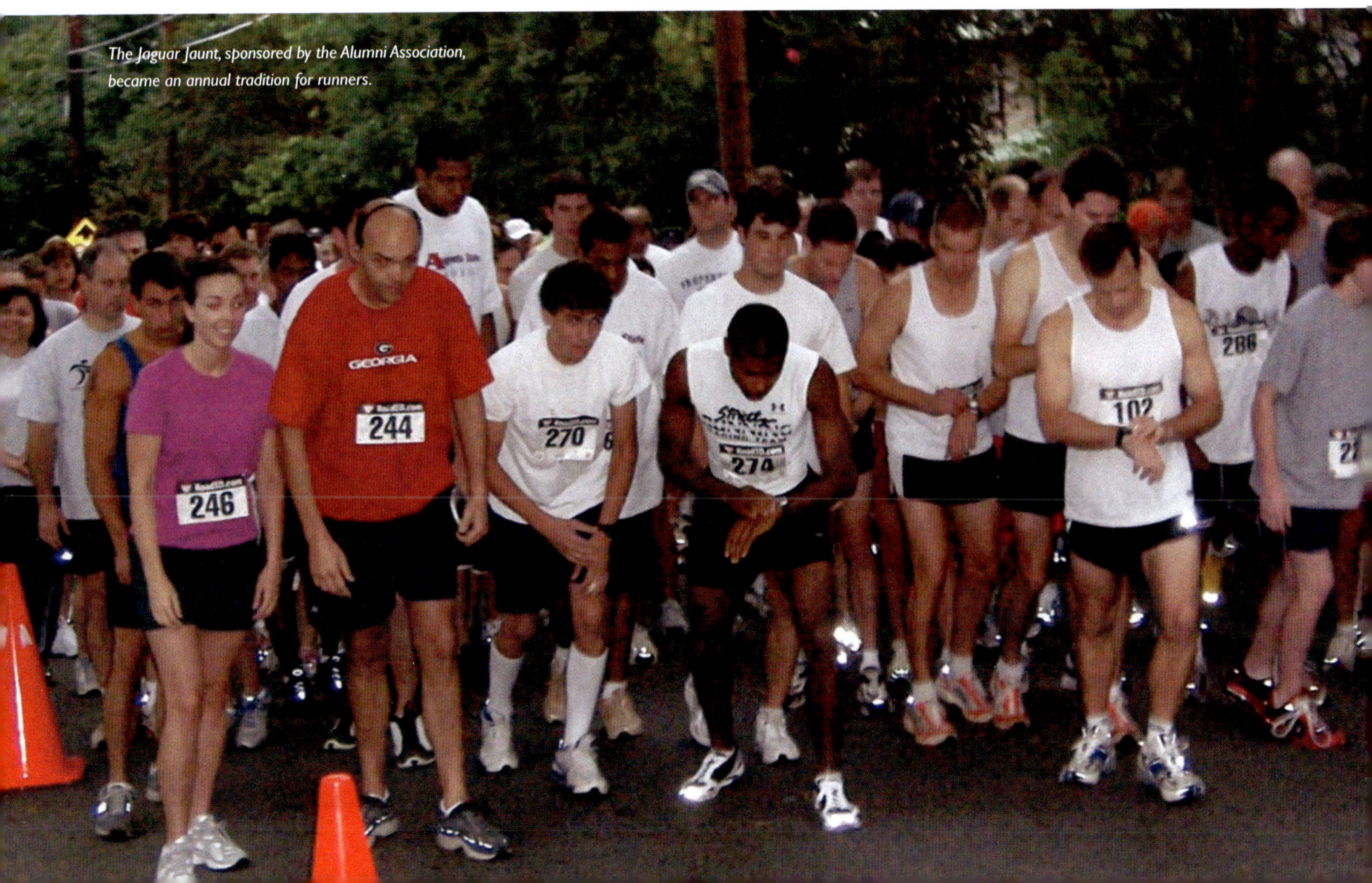


*The Jaguar Jaunt, sponsored by the Alumni Association, became an annual tradition for runners.*

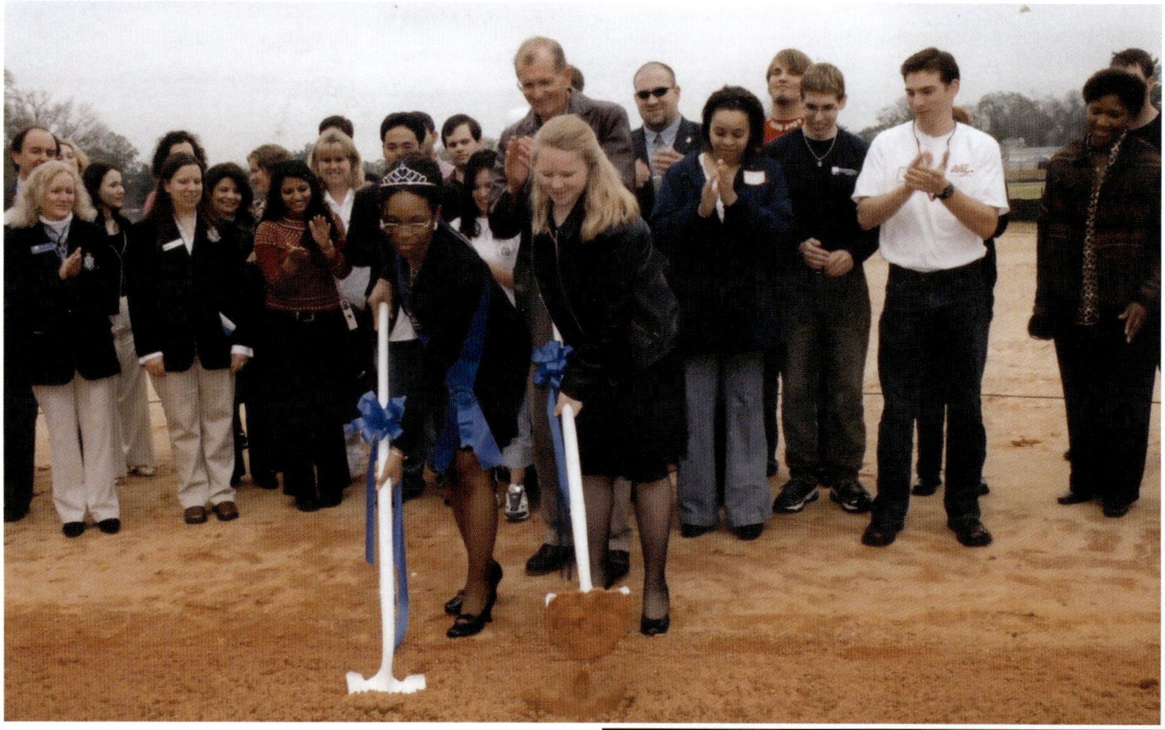

*Student leaders from 1928 to 2005 joined John Groves, thirty-five-year director of student activities, in breaking ground for the Jaguar Student Activities Center.*

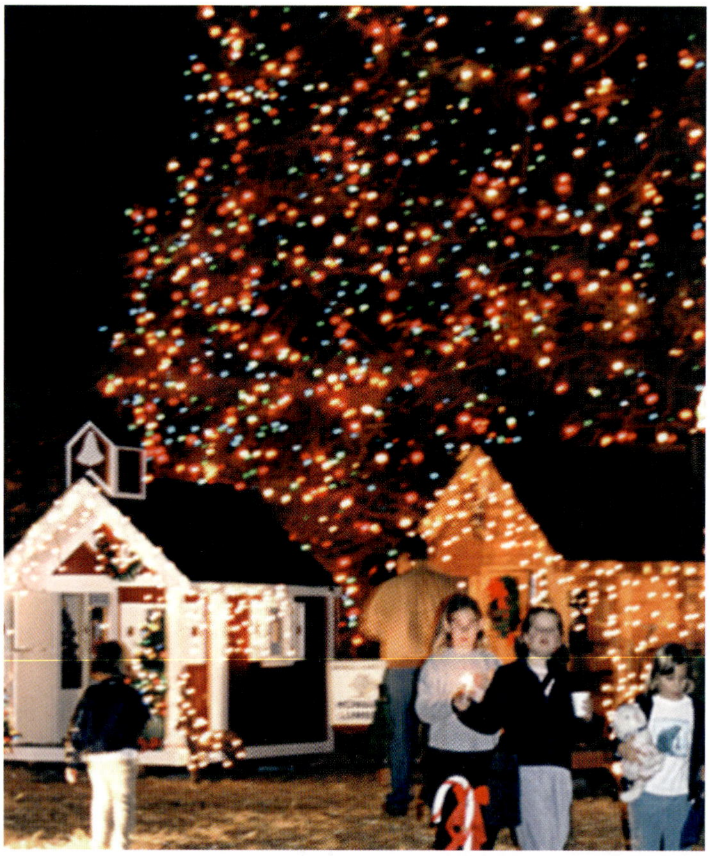

*The campus joined with the Summerville community for the annual tree lighting and to welcome Santa to the neighborhood.*

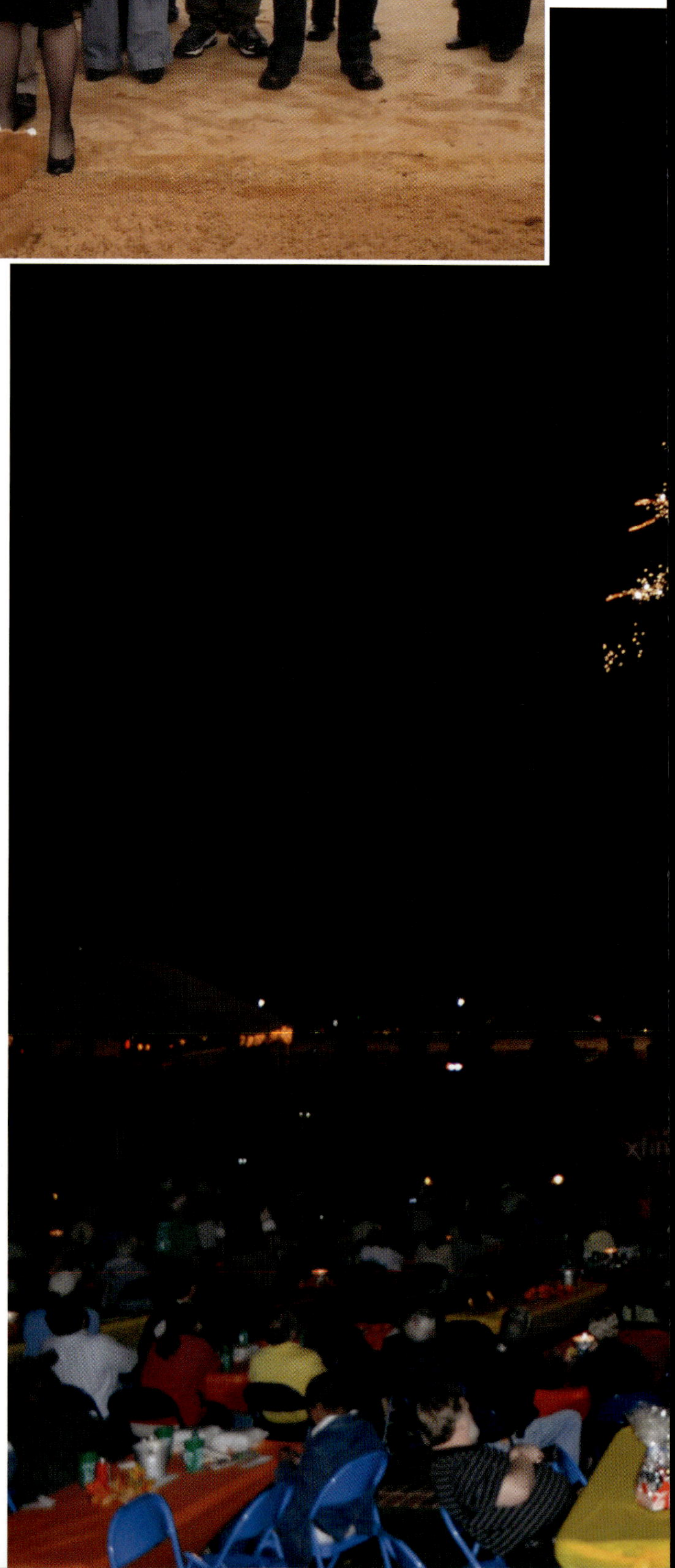

A new dimension to campus life was added in the mid-2000s with the openings of the first campus housing and the new Jaguar Student Activities Center. Students created YouTube videos, listened to touring bands in "Unplugged," danced as part of a flash mob, and competed in "Top Model" contests. Faculty shared their expertise with the community on a commercial radio station in *ASU Reports on Air*.

Upon consolidation in 2013, over 120 organizations, honor societies, fraternities, sororities, and activities created a sense of community on the campuses that became Georgia Regents University. They brought students together, nurtured a spirit of compassion and philanthropy, encouraged an enjoyment of leisure and fitness activities, and fostered an ability to focus on goals for success in academics and in life.

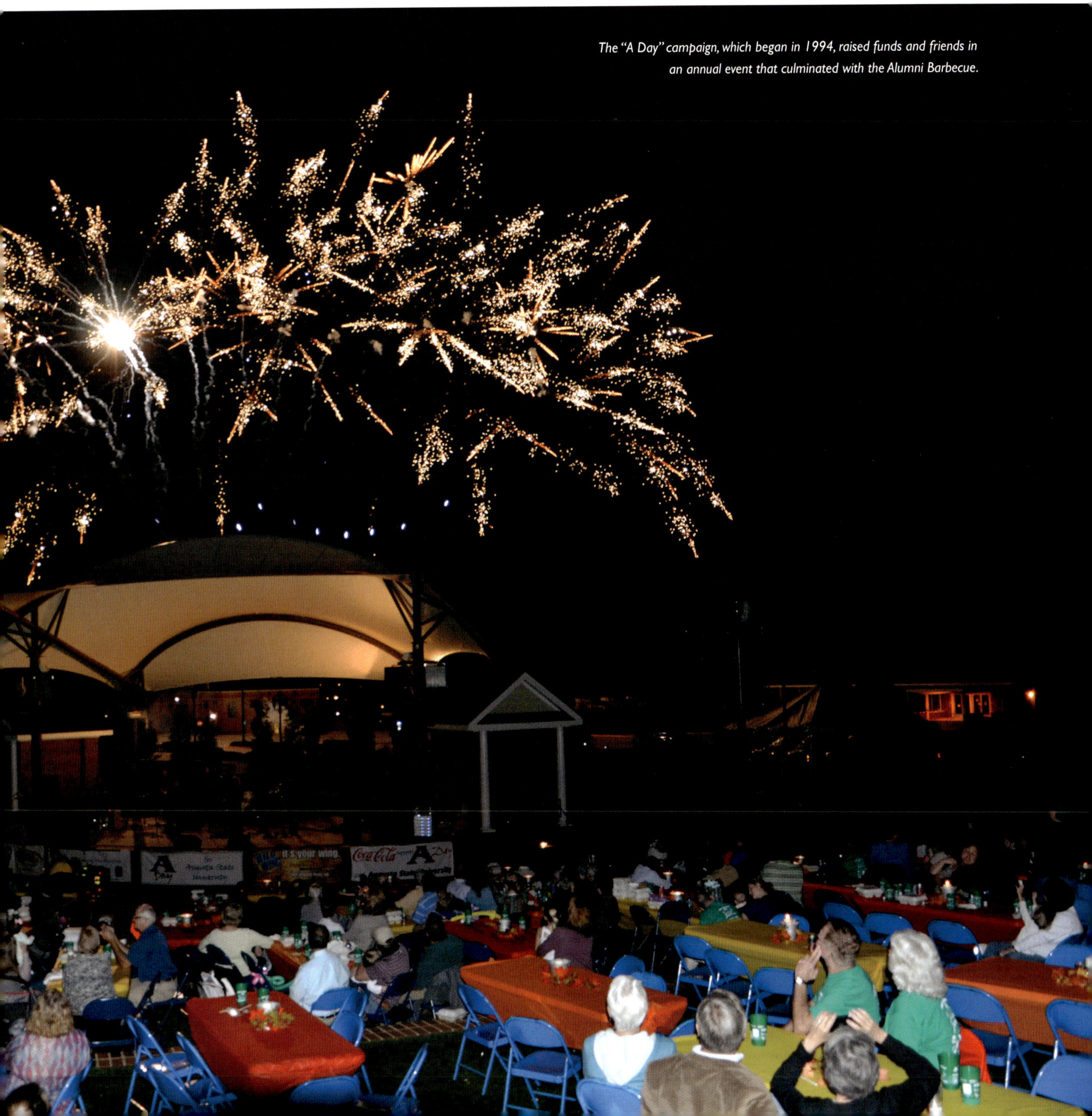

*The "A Day" campaign, which began in 1994, raised funds and friends in an annual event that culminated with the Alumni Barbecue.*

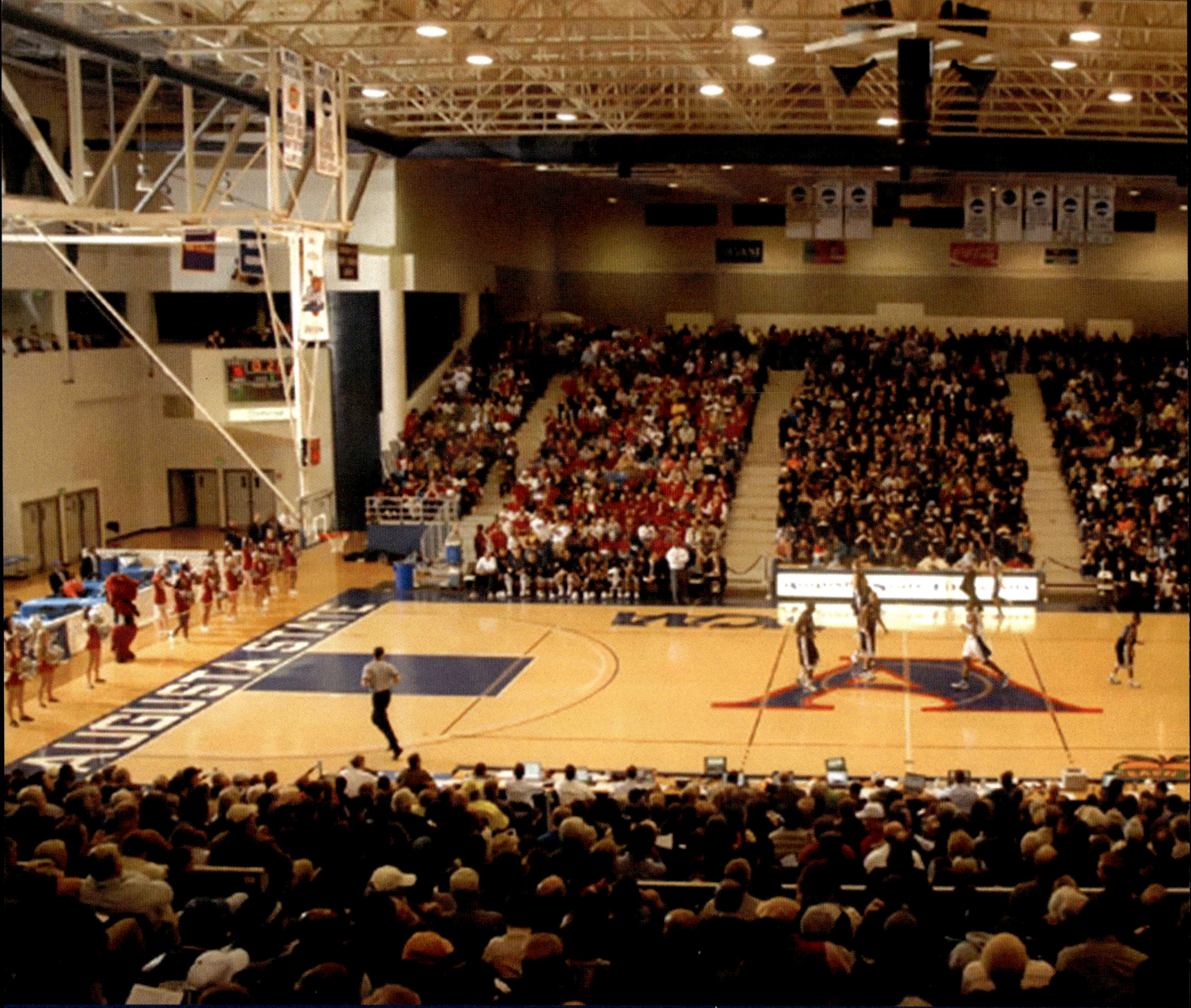


# ATHLETICS:

## *A Legacy of Performance and Competition in Sports*

**Before there were flights to Massachusetts and Oklahoma, there were train rides to Pennsylvania and Florida. Before there were national playoffs with the likes of the University of Georgia, Winona State, and Oklahoma State, there were matchups with Yale, Duke, and even Ireland's College of Surgeons.**

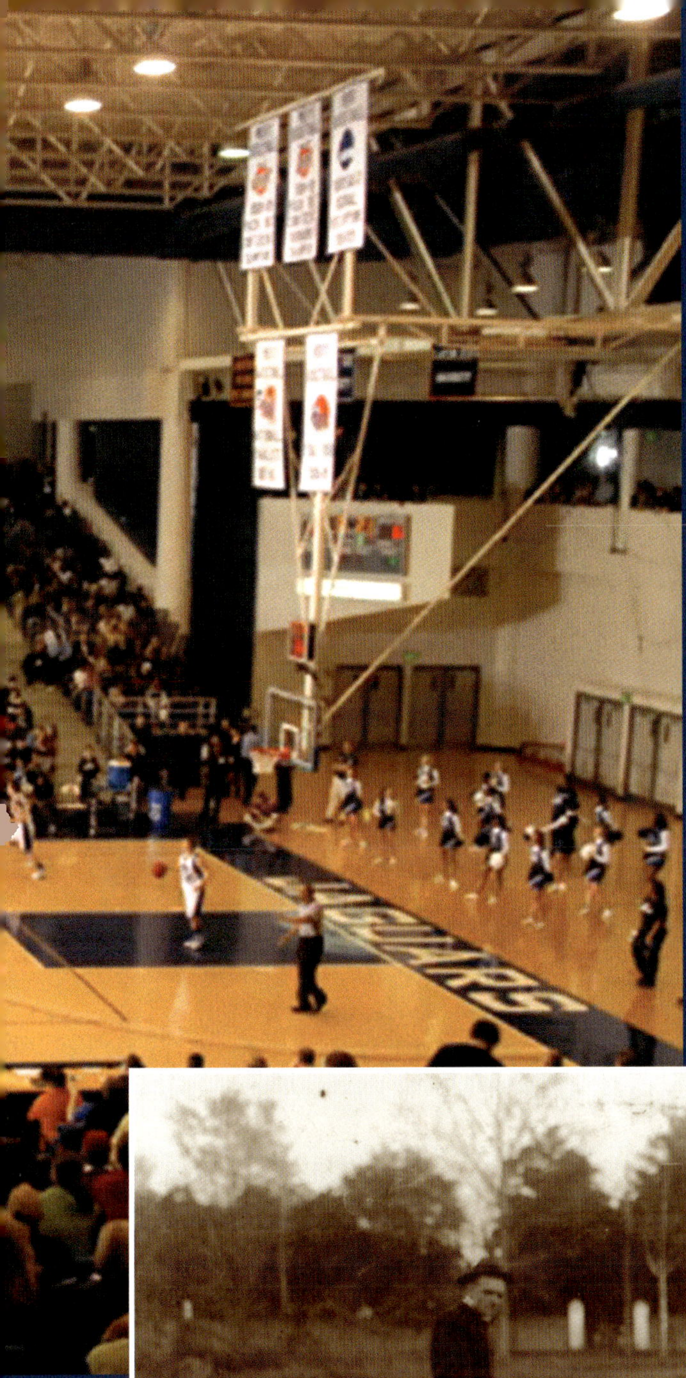

Athletics have been an integral part of Georgia Regents University, with teams from its legacy institutions of Augusta State University (ASU) and Georgia Health Sciences University (GHSU) competing in a number of sports. Before there were athletic conferences, teams competed against athletic clubs, military units, businesses, organizations, and other colleges and schools, including each other.

Sports teams of the Medical College of Georgia (MCG) were frequently called the "Medicos" or "Medics." As early as 1904, the Medicos were competing in a popular sport known as indoor baseball. The games drew large crowds, with nine hundred fans turning out in 1907 for a game played at the armory. MCG fielded a football team sporadically from 1907 to 1923, and students formed an athletic association in the fall of 1912 to raise funds to finance football and baseball.

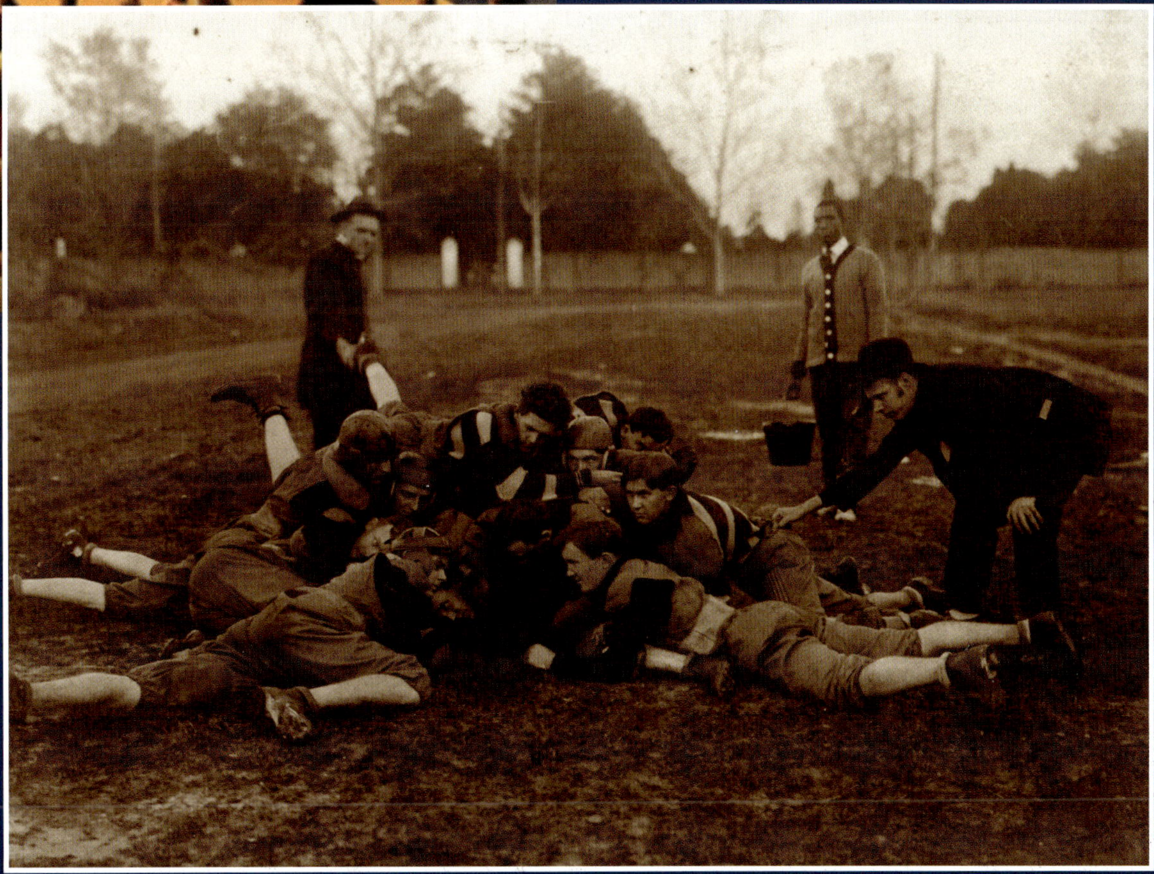

*MCG's first football game against South Carolina in Columbia ended prematurely in 1907 when the MCG team walked off the field after disagreeing with a referee's call. The following year, the Medicos defeated the University of South Carolina. (Photo of 1912 team)*

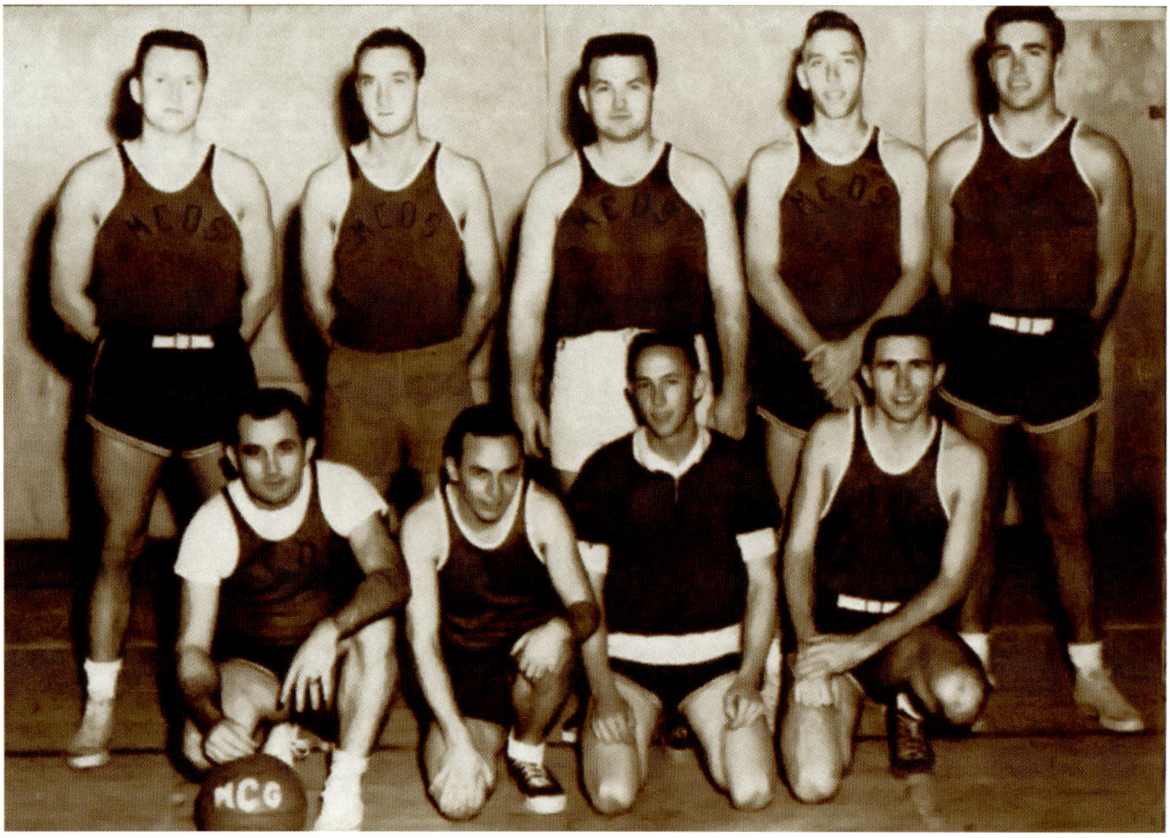


*MCG fielded teams in basketball as early as 1927, sometimes with both the "Doctors" and student "Medicos" competing. In 1955, Clyde Harrison (standing left) took the Most Valuable Player award in the city's recreation league.*

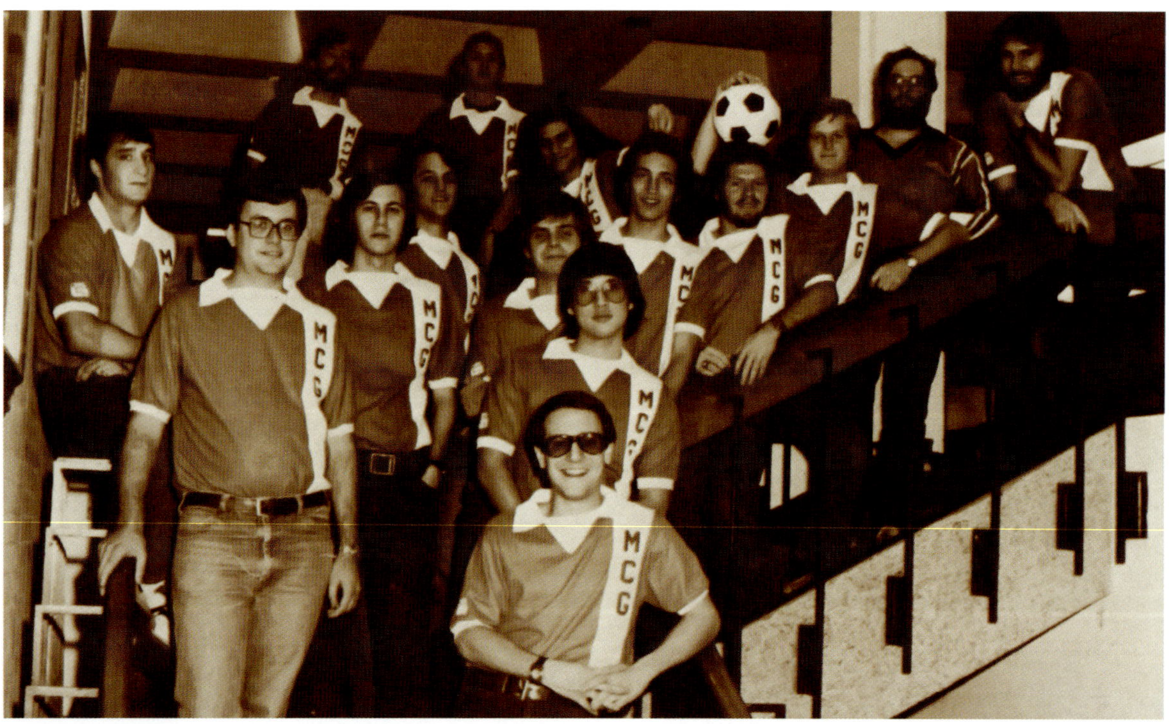


*MCG's soccer team won the Postseason Cup tournament in 1984, which the* Augusta Chronicle *reported was "its eighth postseason cup of the last 11 seasons." (1980)*

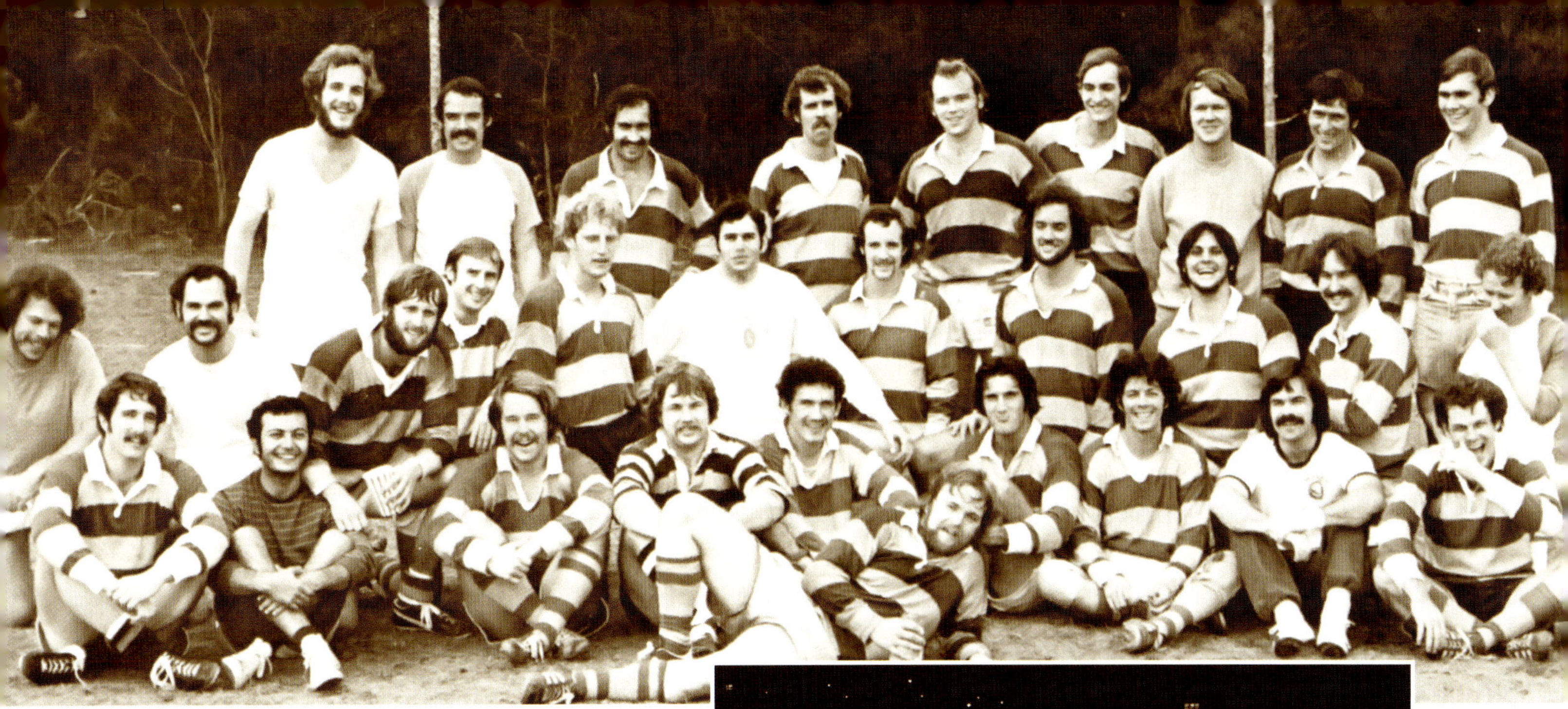

*Above: Jim McMillan (front row, third from right) and other students organized the MCG Rugby Football Club in 1973. Later led by player coach Edouard Servy, the team developed into one of the best programs in the Southeast and began playing internationally. Its name changed in 1985 to allow greater community participation. (Players cut down saplings to make goalposts for their first game.)*

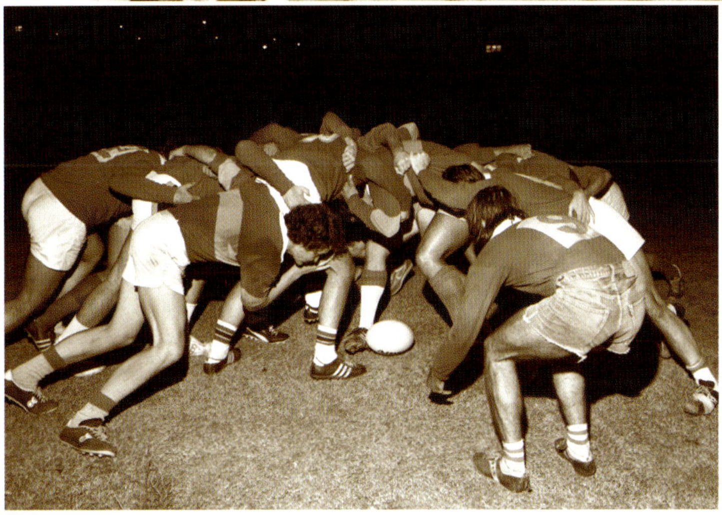

*Right: This 1974 photo showed the "Mad Dogs" facing off in a scrum. (Image@Lee Downing/The Augusta Chronicle/ZUMAPRESS.com)*

Men's basketball organized in 1927 and competitors included such teams as Parris Island Marines, Camp Gordon, Georgia Tech, College of Charleston, area businesses, and the Junior College of Augusta (JCA). The Medicos defeated a JCA team in 1947 comprised almost entirely of war veterans that was said to be the tallest in the state. Teams competed regularly until the late '60s when play continued less frequently in the city's recreation league.

MCG's women's basketball team took the city championship in 1971, the same year soccer was being played. Soccer enjoyed considerable success, with teams winning tournaments and postseason cups. A rugby program was added in 1973 and when celebrating its twentieth anniversary was said to have one of the most successful programs in the nation. The "Mad Dogs" rugby team competed internationally several times in the early 1980s. In the mid-1980s, an MCG rowing crew was organized and competed in the second annual Augusta Regatta, a year before the Augusta College (AC) sport was organized.

Many of the sports played at AC or ASU traced their roots to the junior college days. Sharing space, athletic facilities, and usually coaches, the Academy of Richmond County (ARC) and JCA teams frequently played a single schedule, with the opposing teams determining whether players competed as a combined

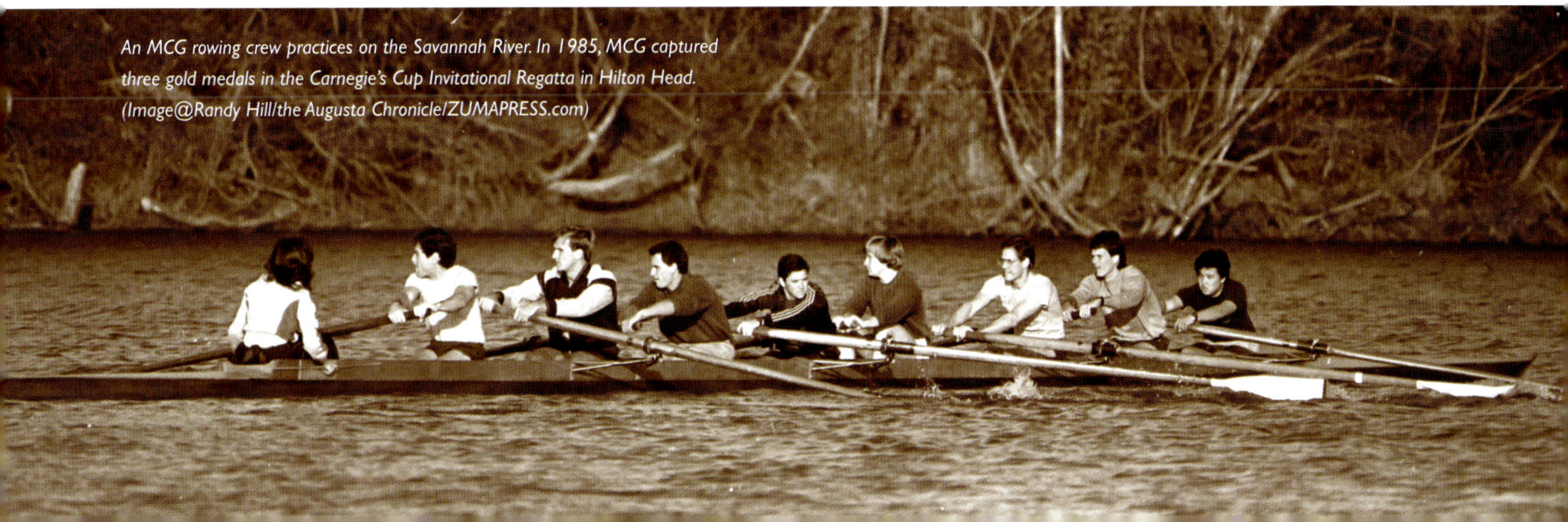

*An MCG rowing crew practices on the Savannah River. In 1985, MCG captured three gold medals in the Carnegie's Cup Invitational Regatta in Hilton Head. (Image@Randy Hill/the Augusta Chronicle/ZUMAPRESS.com)*

high school/college team. ARC-JCA teams competed in baseball, track, tennis, basketball, and football, with football's "wonder team" playing before thousands at a stadium in Pennsylvania in the early '30s. A short-lived JCA football program was formed in 1932 but discontinued due to financial reasons after a second unsuccessful season in 1933. The "minor sport of golf" was offered in 1932. College players took on Yale's Eli Squad in the early 1930s while the ARC players caddied or watched from the gallery. JCA formed its own golf team in 1934.

JCA fielded men's basketball teams consistently. A JCA women's basketball team was organized in 1934. When the junior college separated from ARC and moved to Walton Way in 1957, only men's basketball made the transition. The following year, golf was added. Teams began competing as Augusta College following the school's 1958 name change.

The year 1963 is considered the beginning of AC's intercollegiate athletics program, with Marvin Vanover being named athletic director and head men's basketball coach. Under his leadership, the Jaguars

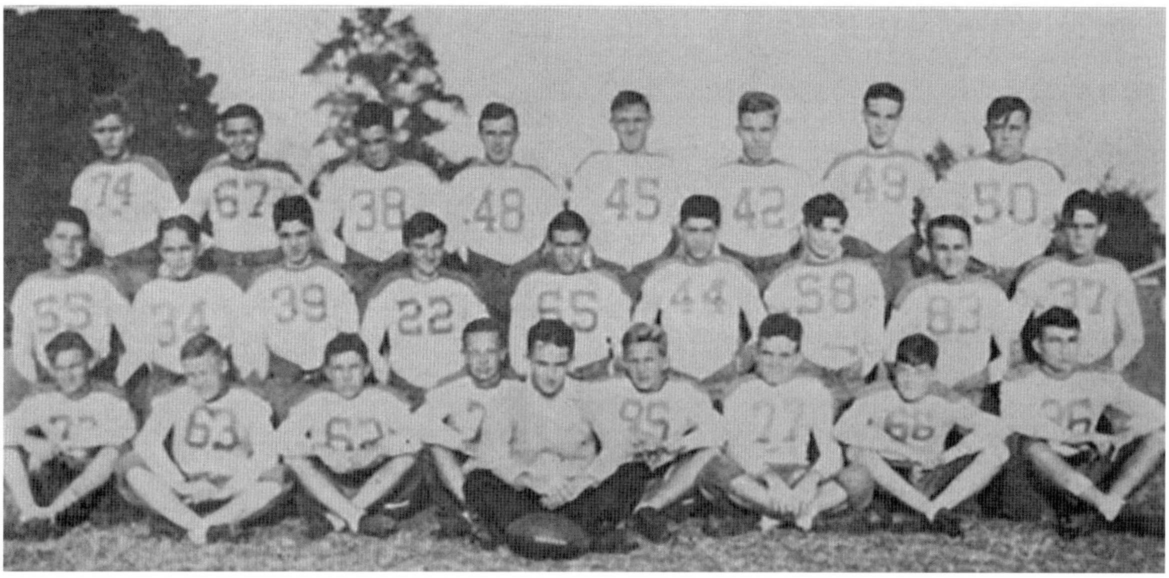

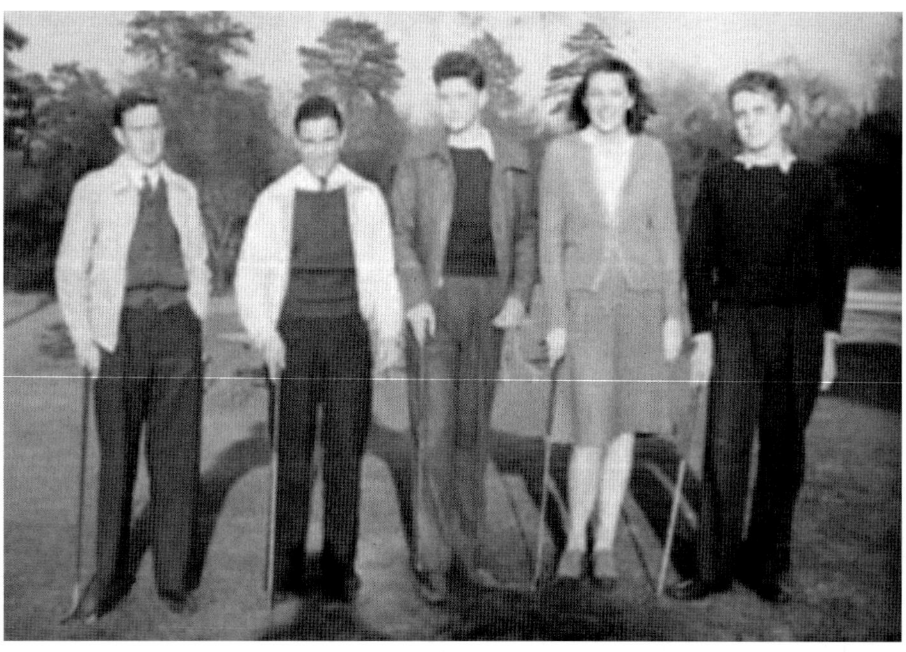

*Above: The JCA football team had no wins in its first season (1932) and scored only twelve points in its second and final season. The program was short lived due to the financial crisis of the early '30s.*

*Left: JCA's 1941 golf team included Eileen Stulb, who was inducted into the Georgia Golf Hall of Fame in 2004. College teams won state and regional championships in the 1950s and held conference titles in the '80s and '90s under coaches Ernie Langford, Jim Kelson, and Jay Seawell.*

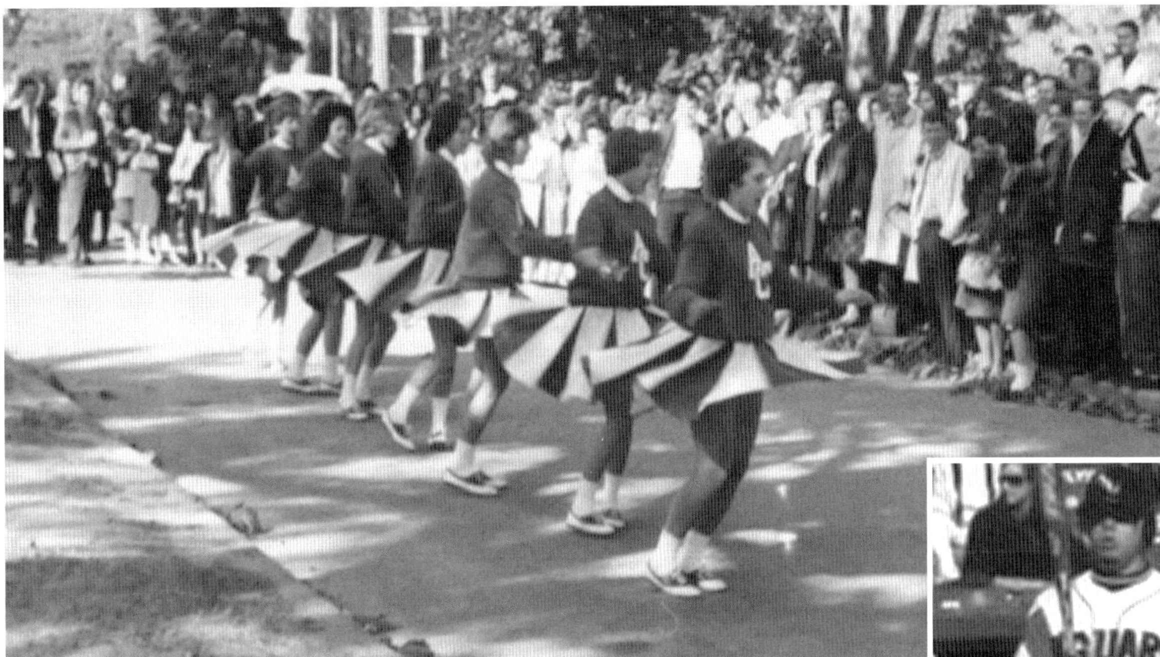

Cheerleaders have added spirit and enthusiasm to the sports program.

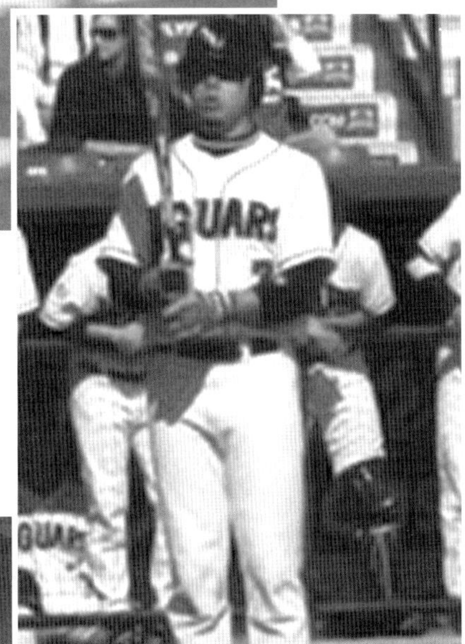


Baseball became a regular offering in 1966 with Head Coach Denny Bureau. In 2004, catcher Sam Barth set new Peach Belt Conference and NCAA records with hits in forty-seven consecutive games, the third-longest streak in history among all divisions. In 2009, Shannon Wilkerson (pictured) was named Division II Player of the Year and was drafted by the Boston Red Sox.

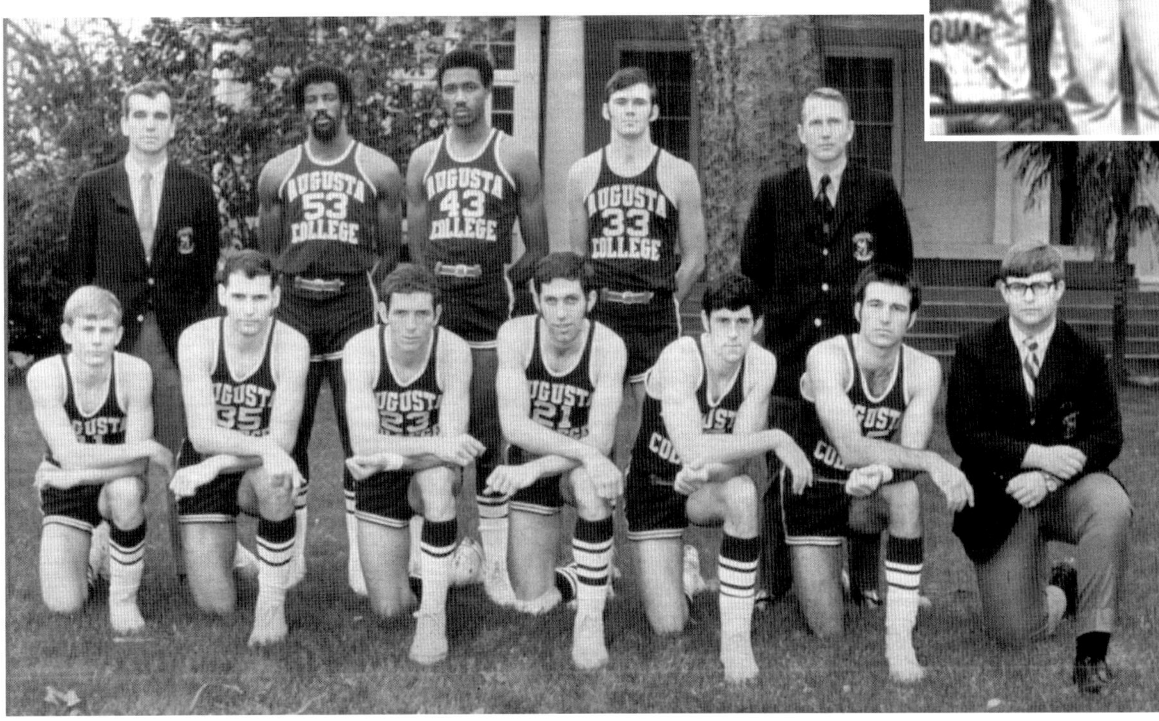


Under Coach Vanover, the Jags made the NAIA national tournament three of four years, 1968–1971. Bill Domen became the college's first All-State player, followed by Steve Brown. Jumpin' Joe McBride earned the first All-America honors, followed by Chip Johnson and Henry "Chicken Man" Davis. (1969–1970 Jaguars)

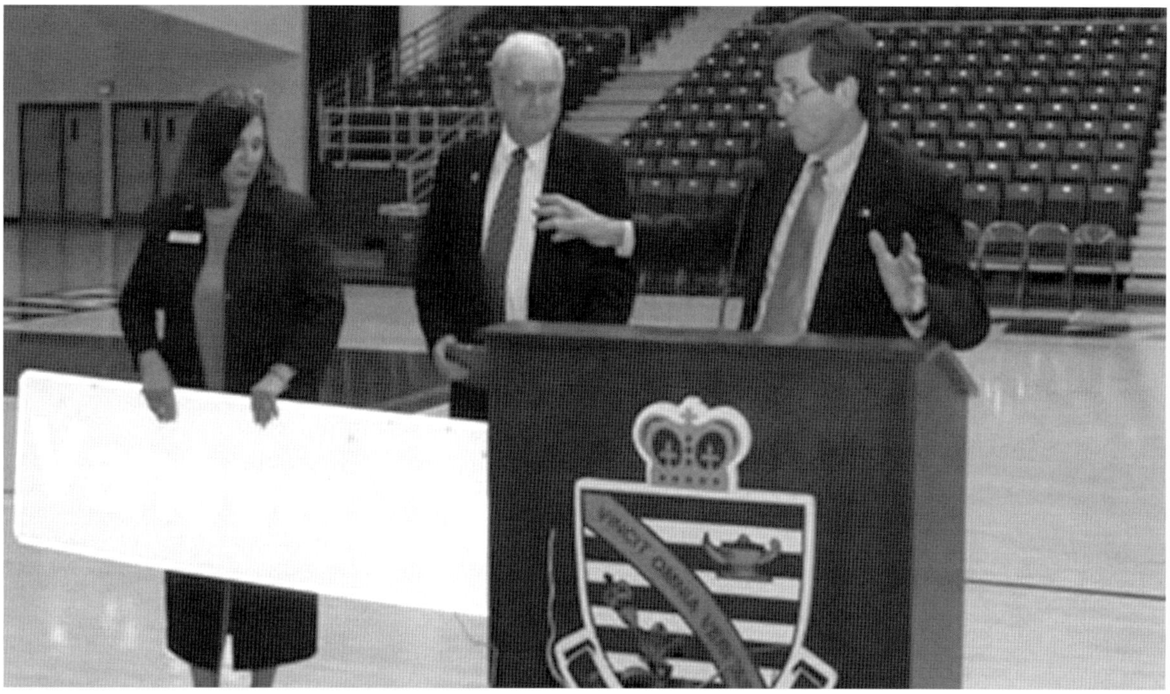

*Athletics Director Marvin Vanover (center) coached basketball, golf, tennis, and cross country and taught physical education classes. He is credited with being the first in the conference to integrate sports and to recruit international students. Before retiring in 1988, he had received five Coach of the Year awards and two Marvin Vanover Days in Augusta. In 2003, the road leading up to the fieldhouse was named in his honor.*

joined the NAIA (National Association of Intercollegiate Athletics), then the NCAA (National Collegiate Athletic Association) Division II, and later Division I Big South Conference. Vanover led the basketball team to three national tournament appearances, oversaw construction of a gym on the Walton Way campus, and added additional sports to the line-up: volleyball, baseball, men's and women's tennis, and cross country.

After a twenty-five-year stellar career, Vanover retired and Clint Bryant was named athletic director and head men's basketball coach. Bryant oversaw a move back to Division II as well as construction of a new physical education/athletic complex (now known as Christenberry Fieldhouse). Men's golf remained in Division I and a women's team was added in 2000. Bryant gave up his coaching role in 1997 to focus on his responsibilities as athletics director.

*Clint Bryant oversaw the growth of a thirteen-sport department that competitively battled for conference, regional, and national honors. He received a Coach of the Year award in 1991 as well as Division II Athletics Director of the Year honors for the Southeast Region in 2007. In the 2000s, forty-three teams qualified for NCAA regionals while twenty-eight earned national rankings in their respective sports.*

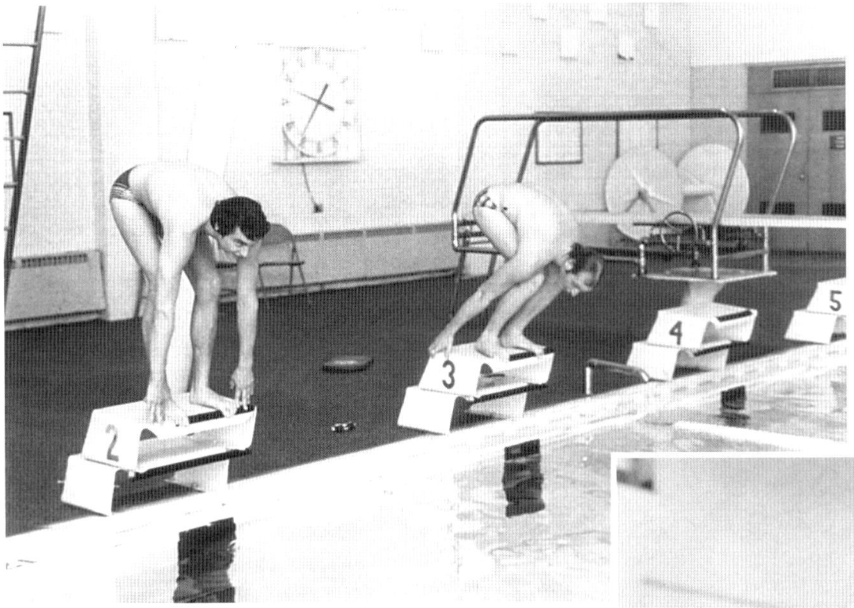

*Left: The Aqua Jags debuted in 1971 and ended in 1992–1993, the same year the three-year Lady Jaguar program ended. Richard Harrison coached both teams.*

*Below: Scott Stamper performs a push-up on the arms of his fellow "AC Crazies," a group of AC soccer and tennis team members who supported basketball in 1993.*

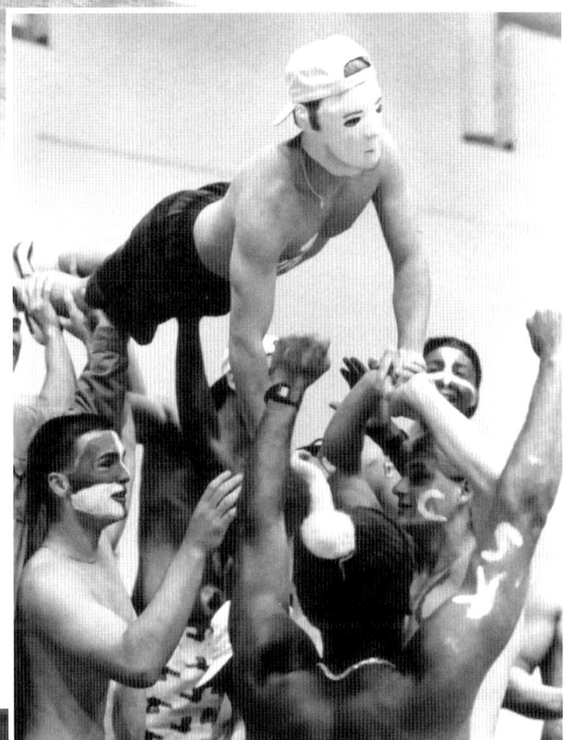

During the 2000s, the basketball teams again found a national arena as the women earned a berth in the 2004 Elite Eight tournament. The men's team competed in three Elite Eight tournaments, making it to the final four once. Eight players went on to play professionally in several countries, including the United States.

National attention also continued to follow the men's golf program. Ranked by *Golf Digest* magazine as the eleventh best collegiate program in history, the Jags frequently made it to the national championship. In

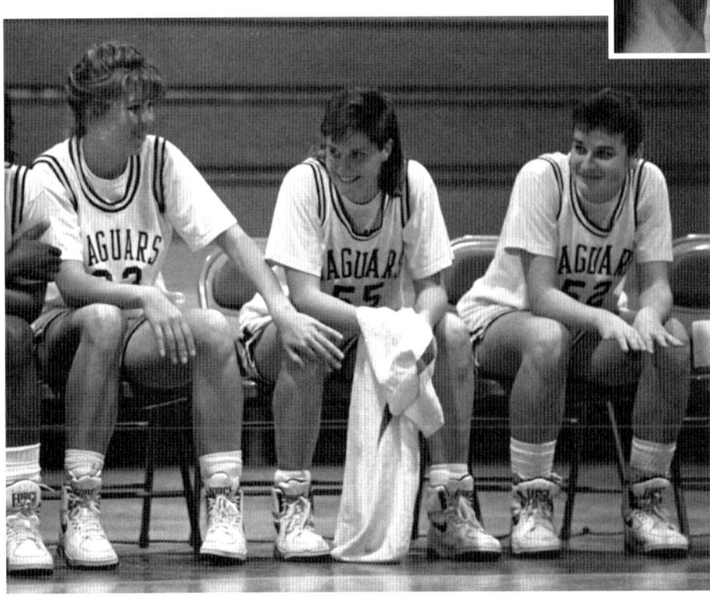


*En route to the 1988–1989 Big South Conference National Tournament, the bus carrying the women's basketball team crashed, injuring Coach Lowell Barnhart and several players. The following year was the last for star player Debbie Born, the first AC athlete to earn All Conference in two sports (basketball and softball). She set six school records, two of which still stand. In 2013, she was named to the Big South's first-ever All Decade Team, 1990–1999. (1990 photo shows Born with teammates Krysti Boeck (left) and Terese Smith. Image@Walt Unks/the Augusta Chronicle/ZUMAPRESS.com)*

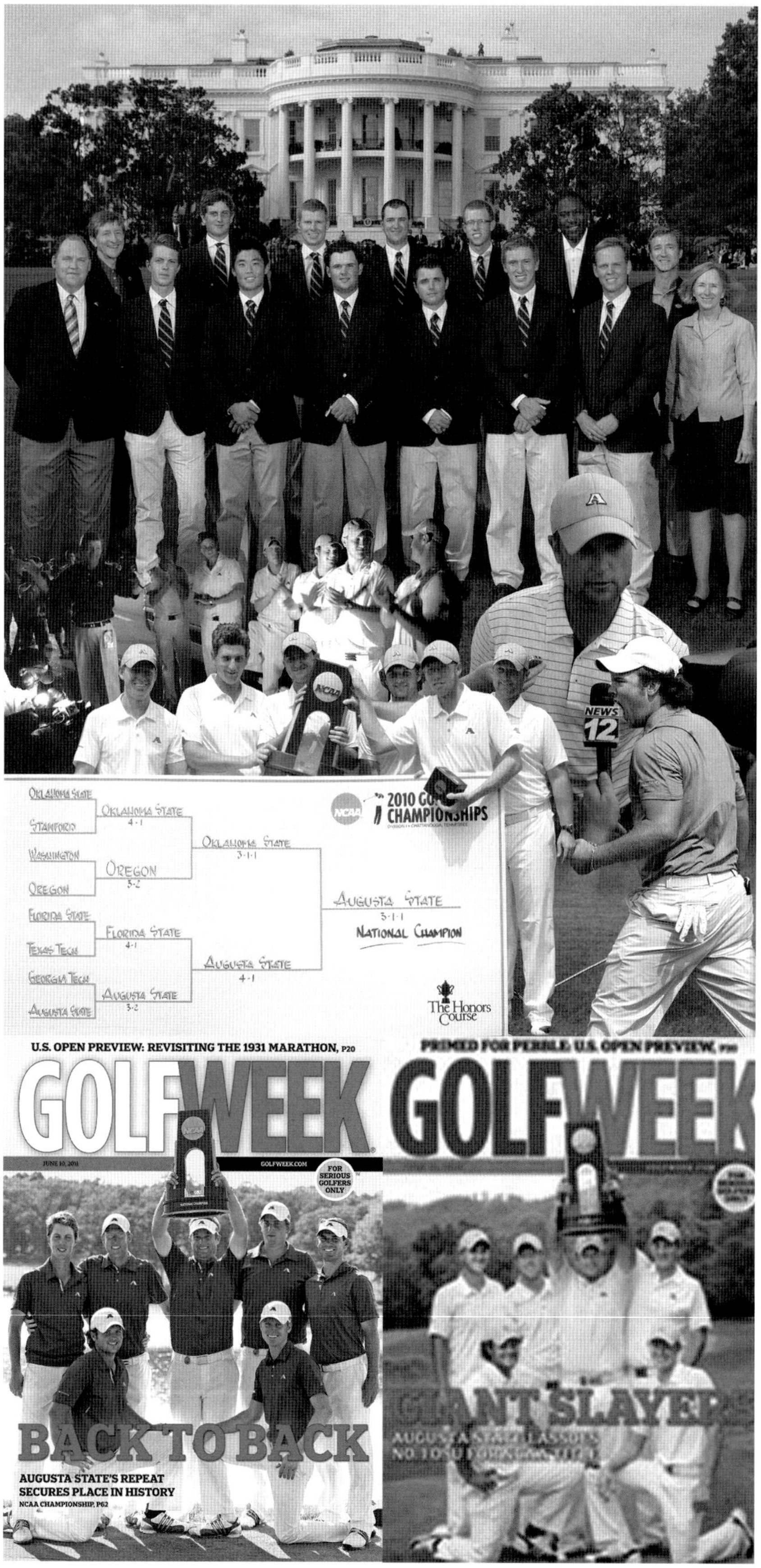


2005, the men finished the season ranked fifth in the nation and made their ninth appearance in thirteen years in the NCAA Division I Championships. In 2010, the Jags captured the national title by defeating golf powerhouse Oklahoma State University. The following year, the team took the title again by defeating the University of Georgia, becoming the only team to repeat as national champions since 1984. Private support for the golf teams provided a state-of-the-art practice facility and collegiate golf house adjacent to the university's eighteen-hole golf course.

Teams have been known as the Jaguars since 1933 (Junior College of Augusta), but the name wasn't used consistently until the institution became Augusta College. In 2013, the Jaguars were competing in thirteen sports: baseball, softball, and volleyball, and men's and women's basketball, cross country, golf, tennis, and outdoor track and field. As Georgia Regents University teams, the Jaguars will continue to be the moniker and athletics will continue to be an important part of the university's life and culture.

*Under Head Coach Josh Gregory, the Jags won the NCAA Division I golf championship in 2010. Henrik Norlander and Patrick Reed earned multiple All-America honors. The team received an invitation to the White House, was given a city parade and reception, and treated to a banquet with over one thousand supporters. The following year, the Jags captured their second consecutive national championship, a feat that hadn't been accomplished since 1984.*

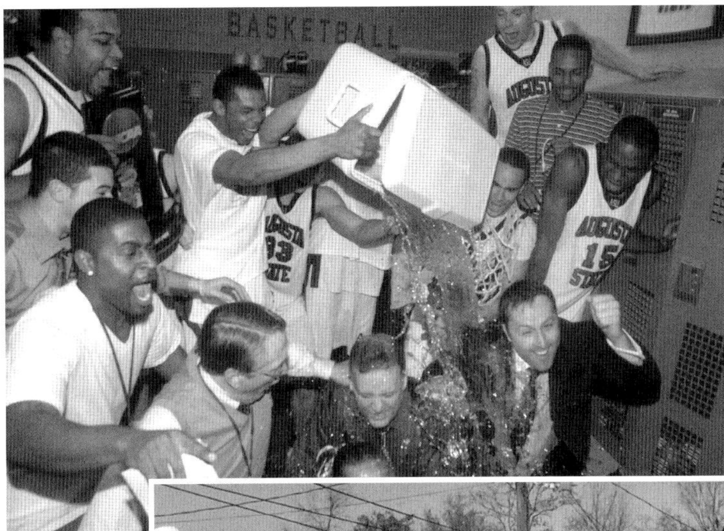


Coach "Dip" Metress led the Jags to a number one national ranking and three consecutive trips to the NCAA's Elite Eight. Playing on the championship teams were A. J. Bowman, who competed in ESPN's televised Slam Dunk contest and was twice named best college player in the state (joining Gary Boodnikoff who took the honor in 2002); Garret Siler, who holds the NCAA record among all divisions for career field goal percentages; and Ben Madgen, holder of the conference's scoring record and only the second ASU player ever named All Conference four years.

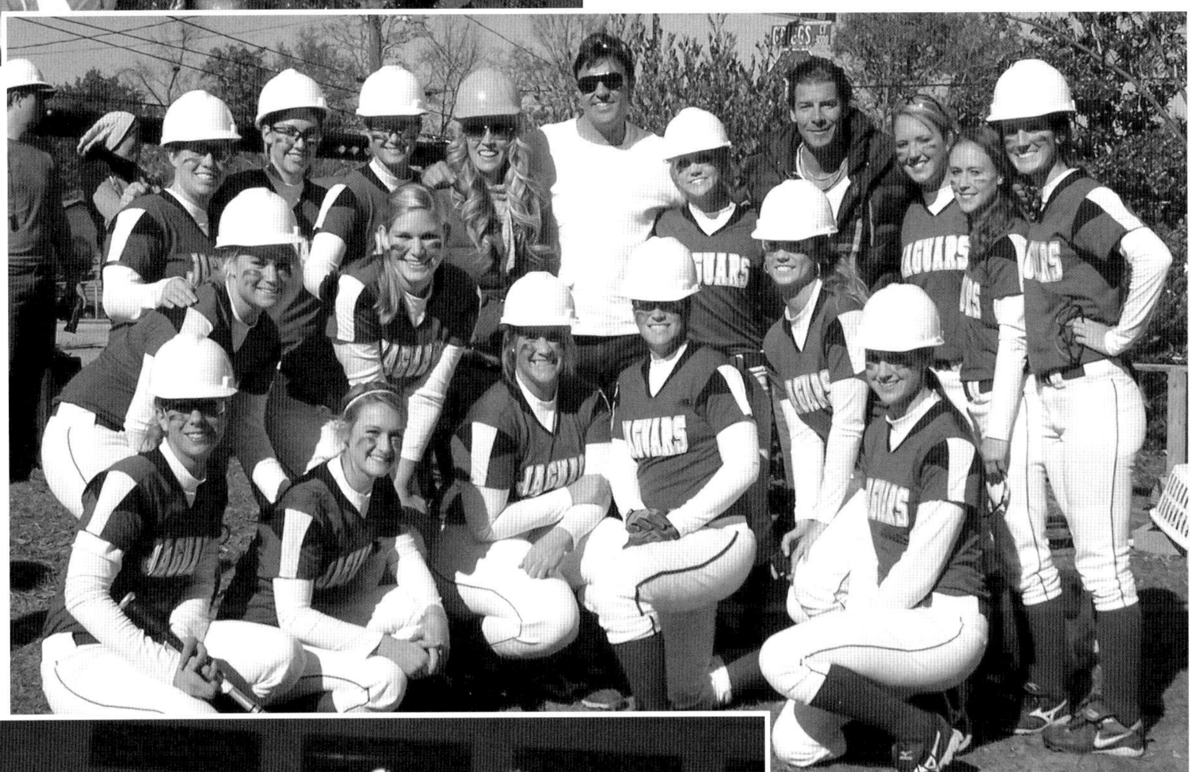


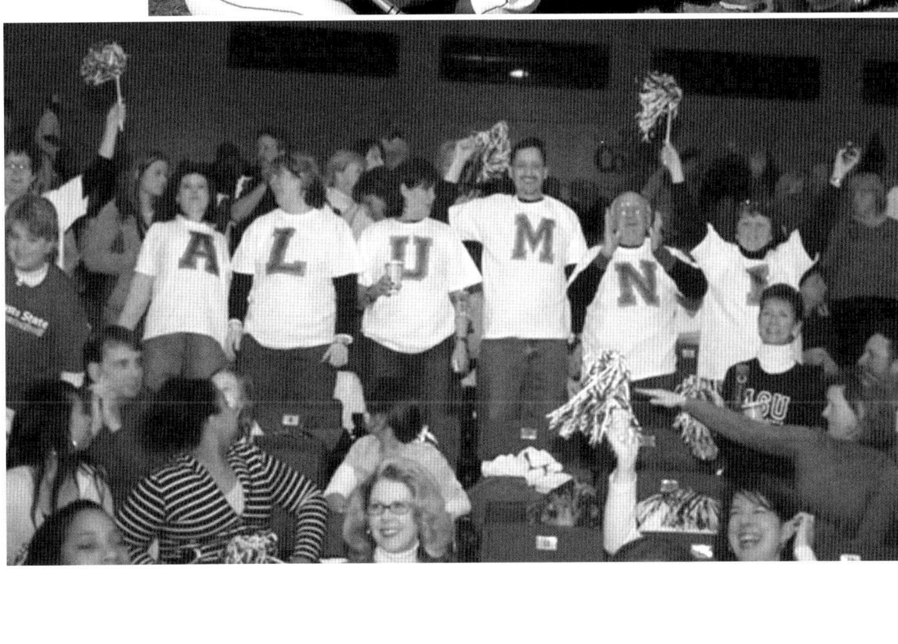

Above: The 2005 women's softball team joined celebrities in demolishing an Augusta home for rebuilding in the nationally broadcast television show Extreme Makeover.

Left: Helen Hendee (far right), alumna and long-time administrator, led alumni in supporting ASU sports and activities.

# EPILOGUE

In 2012, the Board of Regents of the University System of Georgia voted to consolidate Augusta State University with Georgia Health Sciences University to create the system's fourth broad-based research university, naming the new institution Georgia Regents University. With its nine colleges and schools, four on the Summerville Campus (the former ASU) and five on the Health Sciences Campus (the former GHSU), the university began its own history on January 8, 2013, with almost ten thousand students, one thousand faculty, and five thousand staff members. While merging two entities with different backgrounds, cultures, and missions had its challenges, dedicated faculty and staff worked diligently to create the consolidated institution. New governance was formulated, new programs created, new collaborations established, and physical improvements started. In this volume the long history of these parent schools is honored, even as a future as one distinctive university is being built on that legacy.

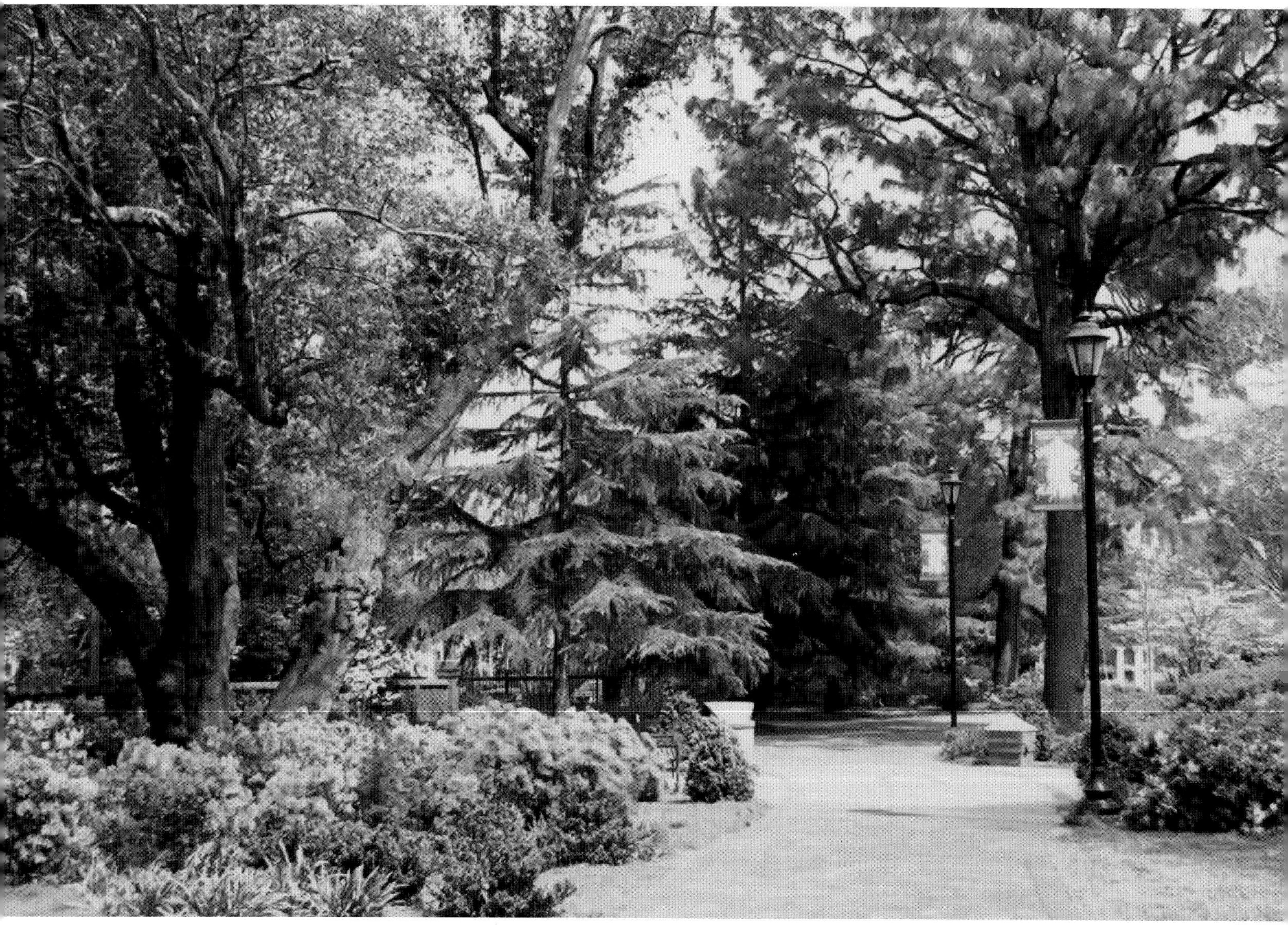

*The first phase of the History Walk opened in 2003, offering an attractive and informative walk around and through campus. Pediments, markers, the Guardhouse Museum, a military cemetery, and other historical features may be found along the walk, which was completed in 2011.*

# Appendices: A Look at Our Heritage

## Appendix I: Timelines: Moments in History

### Georgia Health Sciences University

1826 Dr. Milton Antony started informally teaching a handful of aspiring students at Augusta's City Hospital.

1828 The legislature chartered the Medical Academy of Georgia to award a bachelor of medicine degree.

1829 The academy's name changed to the Medical Institute of Georgia, authorized by the legislature to award the doctorate of medicine.

1833 The state legislature changed the institution's name to the Medical College of Georgia (MCG) to better depict the school's status and mission.

1835 The college opened in a new, unfinished building on Telfair Street.

1836 Dr. Antony and Dr. Joseph Eve began publishing the *Southern Medical and Surgical Journal* to report medical advances and practices.

1861 Classes were suspended during the Civil War while the building served Confederate surgeons as headquarters and at times as a hospital.

1865 The college reopened with forty-four southern students and three northern soldiers.

1873 The name changed to the Medical Department of the University of Georgia, a loose affiliation with local board of trustees retaining actual control.

1888 The first formal residency training began at City Hospital.

1896 The State Board of Medical Examiners required graduates of Georgia's medical colleges to pass an examination.

1911 The state legislature assigned control of the school to the University of Georgia trustees.

1912 Classes ended in December at the Old Medical College building on Telfair Street and began in January in a building on the present campus that was later called the Newton Building.

1922 The college admitted its first female.

1933 The regents closed the medical department but reinstated it due to public outcry, renaming it the University of Georgia School of Medicine.

1937 Basic science classrooms and labs found a home with construction of the Dugas Building, named for Dr. Louis A. Dugas.

1939 Funding by the Public Works Administration provided for construction of the Murphey Building, named for Dr. Eugene E. Murphey.

1941 MCG joined other medical schools in starting a twelve-month, three-year accelerated program to aid the World War II effort.

1945 The addition of the Jennings Wing, named for Dr. William D. Jennings, an MCG graduate and former mayor, provided forty-two private patient rooms.

1946 Students began publishing *The Cadaver* newspaper, and the following year, the school's yearbook, the *Aesculapian*.

1950 The regents made the medical school an independent unit of the university system, restoring the name of Medical College of Georgia and changing the title from dean to president.

1951 The Board of Regents authorized MCG to grant master's degrees in anatomy, microbiology, biochemistry, physiology, pharmacology, endocrinology, and medical arts.

The legislature authorized a state teaching hospital and named it for the late Governor Eugene Talmadge.

1954 The Kelly Administration Building, named for Dr. G. Lombard Kelly, opened.

Five physicians contributed private funds to help form the MCG Foundation.

1956 Talmadge Hospital opened as a teaching hospital.

Regents authorized the transfer of UGA Nursing program to MCG, renaming it the School of Nursing.

1957 The first male enrolled in the School of Nursing.

1960s Regents approved three schools: Graduate Studies ('65), Allied Health Sciences ('68), and Dentistry ('65), as well as degrees in medical records science, dental hygiene, medical technology, and radiologic technology.

1961 Talmadge Hospital gained a research wing.

1962 The college purchased twenty-five acres of land on Gwinnett Street to build the Student Center and a Research and Education Building.

1963 The first freestanding library opened, later named for Dr. Robert B. Greenblatt.

1968 The first African Americans entered the School of Medicine.

1970s Advanced degree programs started in oral surgery, periodontics, oral biology, and prosthodontics as well as joint MS/MD and PhD/MD degrees; doctoral degrees in dental medicine were awarded.

1971 Regents authorized the master of health education, encompassing the disciplines of medical technology and dental hygiene.

Two new buildings opened: the School of Dentistry Building and the Research and Education Building, named in honor of the father of Governor Carl E. Sanders.

1972 A Sickle Cell Center was established.

1973 MCG bought "Old" University Hospital, remodeling the Jennings Wing and the Milton Antony Wing, which was renamed the Walter L. Shepeard Building.

1976 The Virgil P. Sydenstricker Wing of Talmadge Memorial Hospital opened.

1979 The addition of the Hamilton Wing to the R&E Building relieved overcrowded classrooms.

1980 Basic and clinical research saw encouragement through the establishment of the Research Institute.

1981 Student Health Services and the Georgia Radiation Therapy Center opened.

Talmadge Hospital received the first triple organ donation in Georgia.

The college gained new bachelor's and certificate programs in diagnostic sonography.

1983 Talmadge added a Pediatric Intensive Care Unit.

1984 MCG offered an associate degree of science in occupational therapy.

1984–1985 Patients saw enhanced care through the first magnetic resonance imaging (MRI) scan; the addition of extracorporeal membrane oxygenation (ECMO) to aid in treating newborns; the addition of children to the kidney transplant program; and the offer of embryo freezing, allowing childless couples a higher success rate for in vitro fertilization.

1990s MCG established the Pediatric Care Transport Program ('90), Vascular Biology, Telemedicine ('92), Institute of Molecular Medicine and Genetics ('93), Senior Health, and the Heart and Cardiovascular Health Center ('95), and Center for Sports Medicine ('99).

1992–1993 The Specialized Care Center adds an emergency room, trauma center, outpatient clinics, and four intensive care units.

1993 Regents authorized MCG's first external degree program, a bachelor's degree in medical technology.

1996 The Interdisciplinary Research Building opened, followed two years later by the Children's Medical Center.

1999 Regents authorized an early retirement plan, resulting in 89 percent of eligible employees participating.

2000 MCG Health Inc. formed to manage clinical facilities the following year.

2003 The new affiliation agreement provided an automatic pathway for Augusta State University (ASU) students with associate degrees to get a bachelor's degree from MCG in five programs.

A Student Wellness Center opened, providing space for fitness and recreation.

2004 Construction ended on the second phase of the Interdisciplinary Research Center.

2006 MCG opened the Cancer Research Center.

Private funding enabled the addition of the Betty Browning Tollison Reflection Garden.

2007 The Health Sciences Building opened.

2008 Regents authorized purchase of the Gilbert Manor housing property, enabling campus expansion. The Augusta Commission provided $10 million to purchase the property.

2010 A new governance structure integrated MCG clinical, education, and research activities.

MCG Health Cancer Center opened in January, featuring a café, library, meditation retreat, and gardens on both floors.

2011 The university, hospital, and Physicians Practice Group became one enterprise. The institution's name changed to Georgia Health Sciences University (GHSU); the schools were renamed colleges while maintaining Medical College of Georgia for the School of Medicine; and dentistry changed to Dental Medicine.

The new College of Dental Medicine building opened.

2013 Consolidation of GHSU and ASU created Georgia Regents University.

## Augusta State University

1783 Legislation called for the establishment of a "seminary of learning." Two years later, the Academy of Richmond County (ARC) opened.

1802 ARC moved from its Bay Street location to a newly constructed building on Telfair Street.

1863–1865 The building became a hospital treating Confederate soldiers during the Civil War.

1865–1867 Federal troops used the building as headquarters following the end of the war.

1868 The academy reopened with CSA Colonel George Washington Rains as regent.

1910 ARC began offering a formal course of study for the first year of college.

1925 The Junior College of Augusta (JCA) chartered, becoming the first in the state.

1926 JCA held registration at the building on Telfair Street.

1927 JCA and ARC moved into a new building on Baker Avenue, which they would share for the next thirty-one years.

1955 Efforts began to acquire the recently decommissioned Augusta Arsenal on Walton Way for the JCA.

1957 The army conveyed a portion of the Augusta Arsenal to the Richmond County Board of Education for use by JCA.

1958 JCA joined the University System of Georgia (USG) and its name changed to Augusta College (AC).

1959 AC acquired fifteen additional acres of the arsenal, which included six warehouses that became the principal academic units for over forty years.

1963 The Board of Regents authorized senior (four-year) status for AC, approving programs leading to the bachelor of arts, bachelor of science, and bachelor of business administration degrees.

The Augusta College Foundation chartered on May 24.

1965 The college admitted its first African American students.

1967 AC conferred its first baccalaureate degrees (181).

1968 The Board of Regents authorized the bachelor of science in education degree.

The newly completed Fine Arts Center and Performing Arts Theatre opened.

Students elected the first African American president of the Student Government Association (SGA).

The regents authorized the MBA and master's degrees in elementary and special education.

1974 The Board of Regents authorized master's degrees in psychology and reading education.

1977 The college expanded with the acquisition of the last parcel of arsenal property and the opening of Reese Library.

1978 The college acquired the Armed Forces Golf Course, which would be managed by the Augusta Golf Association.

1980 The college offered a computer science major, the first at a senior college in the USG.

1981 Regents approved a specialist in education degree.

1986 Students elected the first female president of SGA.

1988 AC became the first senior institution in the USG to have an eminent scholar chair.

The regents' new border tuition policy offered students from the South Carolina counties of Aiken and Edgefield in-state tuition.

1991 The new Physical Education/Athletic Complex opened.

The college became a member of the Peach Belt Athletic Conference.

1994 The college held its first A Day campaign.

1996 Regents changed the names of many USG institutions; AC became Augusta State University (ASU).

The university assumed the master of public administration degree program, after offering a joint program with Georgia Southern University.

1997 U.S. President William J. Clinton visited Augusta State University to discuss his new national education program.

The College Activity Center became known as Washington Hall in honor of local educators, Drs. I. E. and Justine Washington.

Alumna Katherine Reese Pamplin's major gift led to the university naming the College of Arts and Sciences in her honor.

1998 The academic semester system replaced the quarter system at all USG institutions.

2000 The new Science Building opened, ushering in a decade-long $104 million building program.

2002 The first classroom replacement building opened, named in honor of Thomas F. Allgood and his wife "T."

2003 The physical education/athletic complex was renamed Christenberry Fieldhouse in honor of former president George Christenberry. The road to the fieldhouse was named Vanover Drive in honor of long-time athletics director Marvin Vanover.

2004 University Hall, the second classroom replacement building, opened along with a new, gated entrance to campus. The six old academic buildings were demolished.

2005 University Village opened, providing housing for about five hundred students.

2006 The Jaguar Student Activities Center and privately funded-Golf Pavilion at Forest Hills opened.

The College of Business Administration became the James M. Hull College of Business, marking the benefactor's philanthropy.

2007 The J. Fleming Norvell Collegiate Golf House opened.

2008 The D. Douglas Barnard Jr. Amphitheatre opened.

The College of Business Administration proposed a management information systems (MIS) major; regents authorized a bachelor of social work degree.

2009 A major gift from the Knox Foundation established the Knox School of Accountancy and the Peter S. Knox Distinguished Chair.

Regents approved a bachelor of science in nursing degree program to begin 2010.

ASU and Ga Tech-Savannah signed a pre-engineering articulation agreement.

2010 Men's golf team won the National NCAA Division I championship.

2011 ASU began offering a master of education in teacher leadership degree.

The art gallery is named in honor of Mary S. Byrd.

Men's golf took its second consecutive National NCAA Division I championship.

Construction ended on the fourth and final stage of the History Walk.

2012 USG Regents vote to consolidate ASU and GHSU—one of four consolidations.

2013 ASU and GHSU consolidate, creating Georgia Regents University.

# Appendix II: The Changing Face of Our Campuses

The founding fathers of the two legacy institutions could not have envisioned the expansive campuses that grew from their two adjoining buildings on Telfair Street. With help from the city, state, and federal governments as well as generous donors, the two consolidated institutions have grown into one research university with 650 acres and over 150 buildings. Aerial shots of the three campuses show the amazing growth of Georgia Health Sciences University and Augusta State University.

## Georgia Health Sciences University

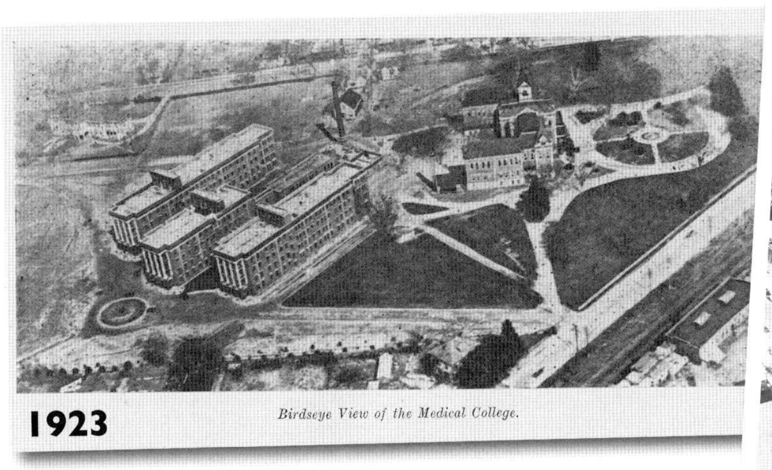


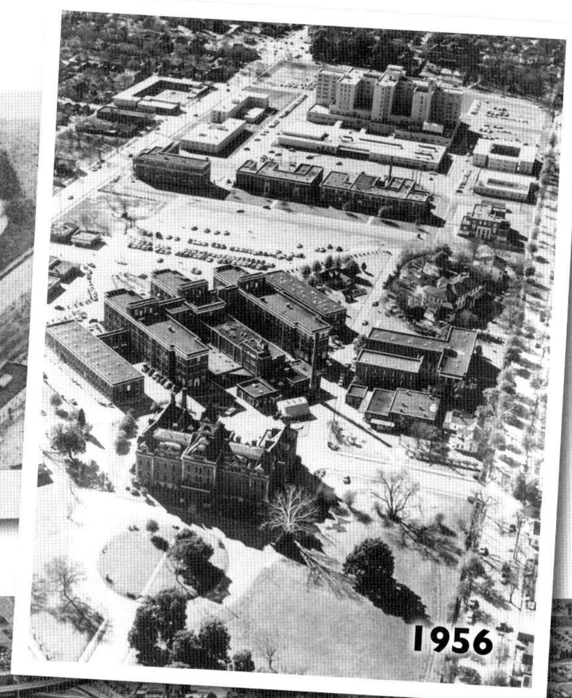


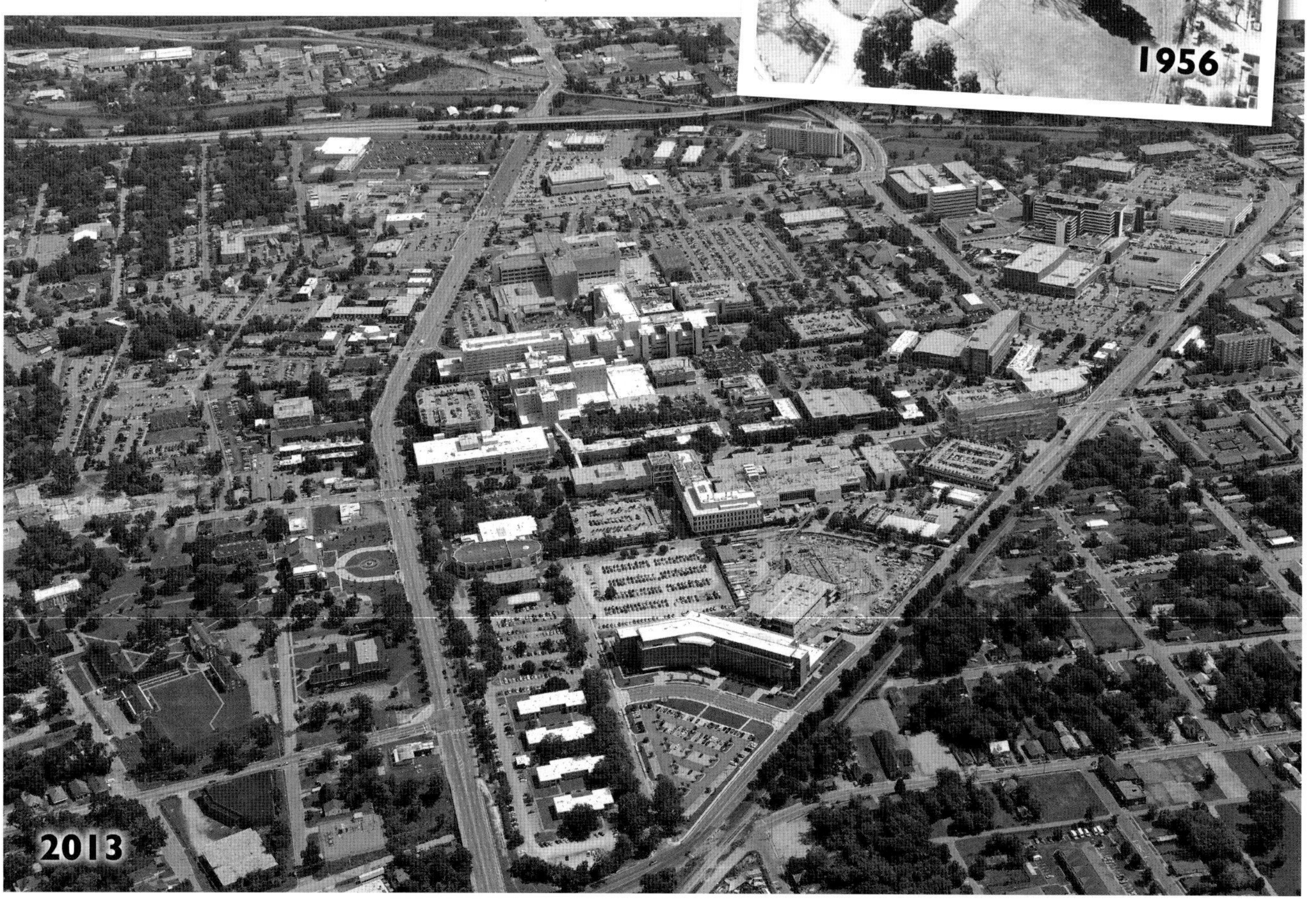

## Augusta State University: Summerville Campus

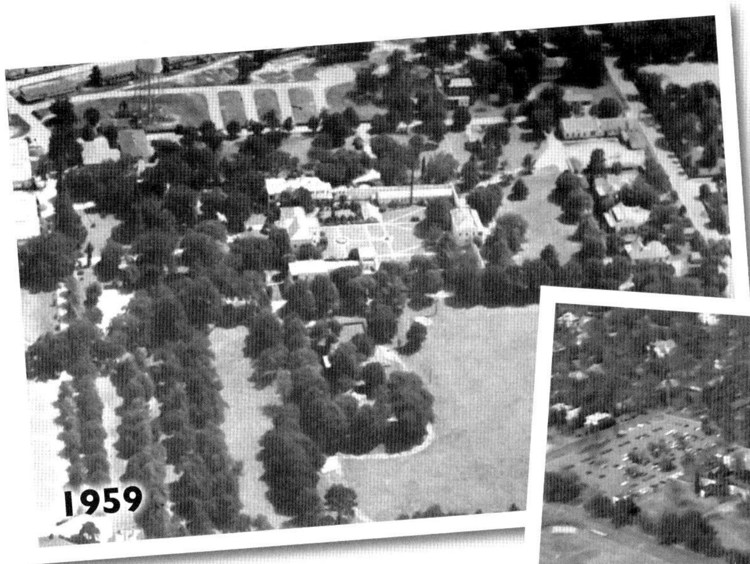


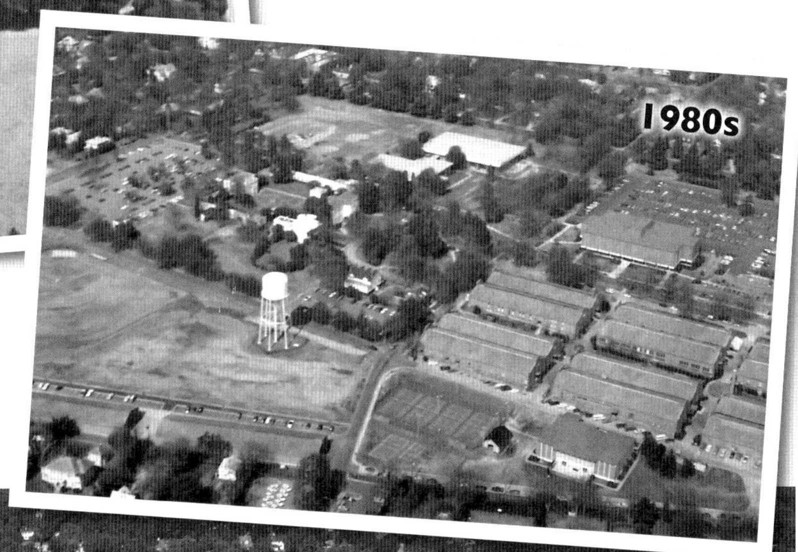


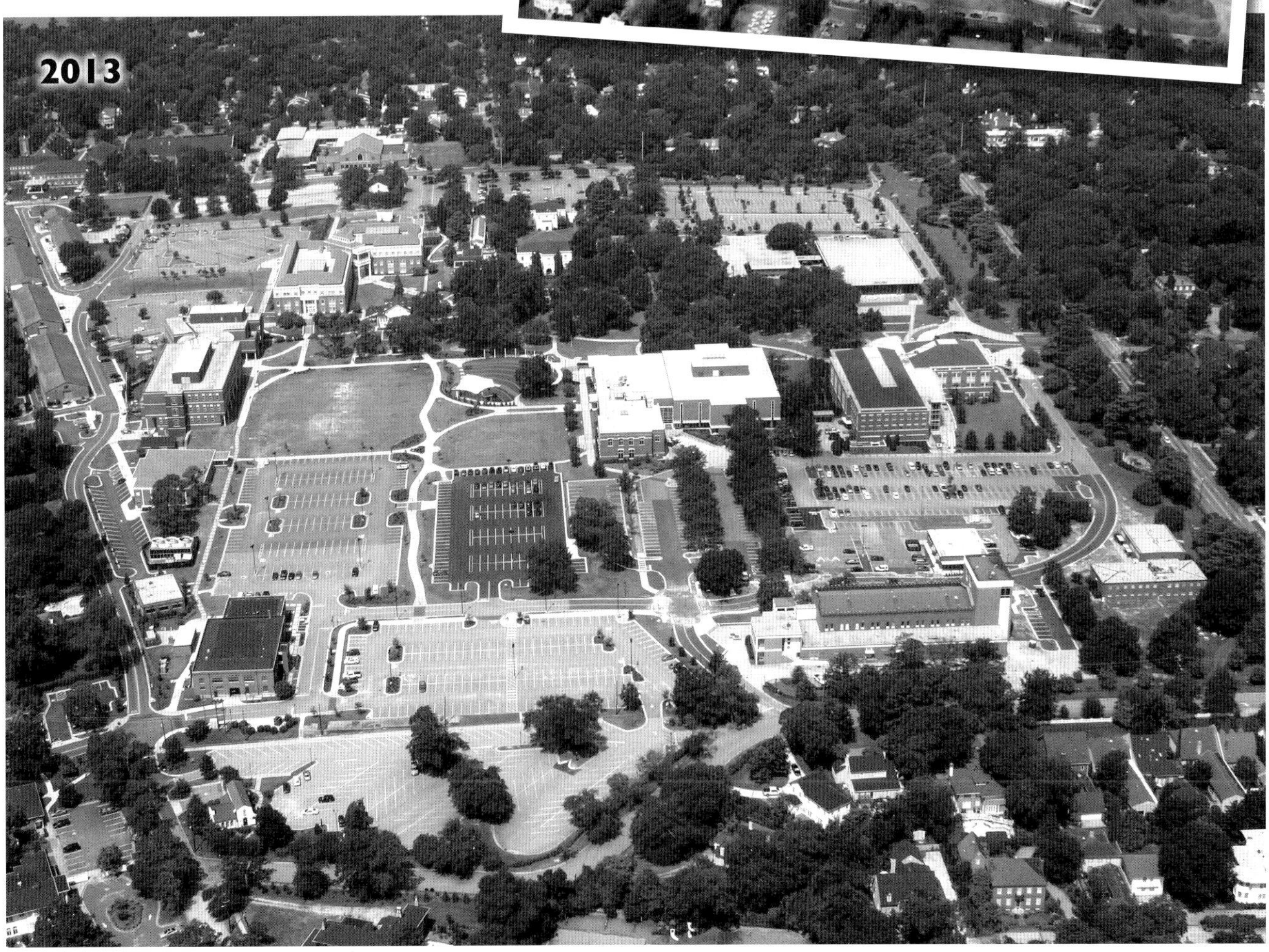

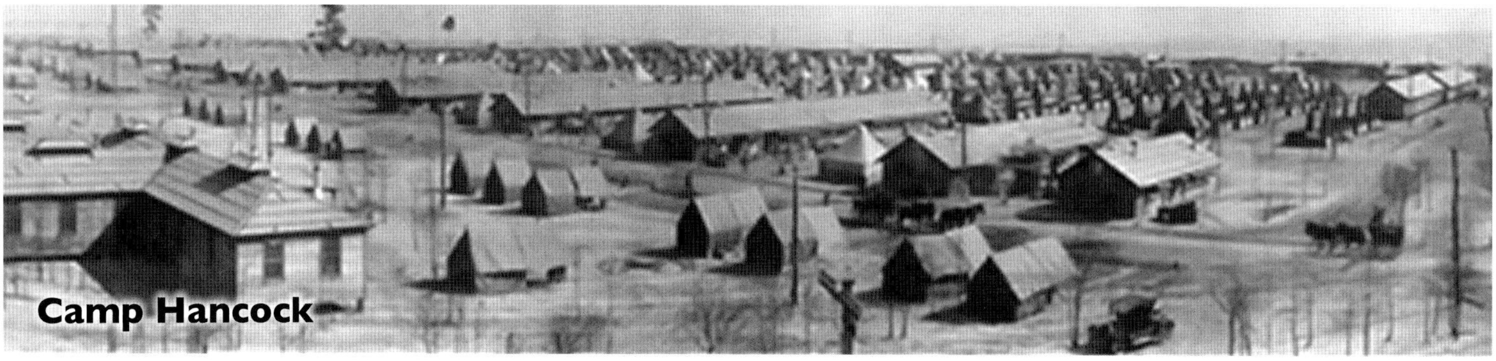


**Augusta State University:**
**Forest Hills Campus**

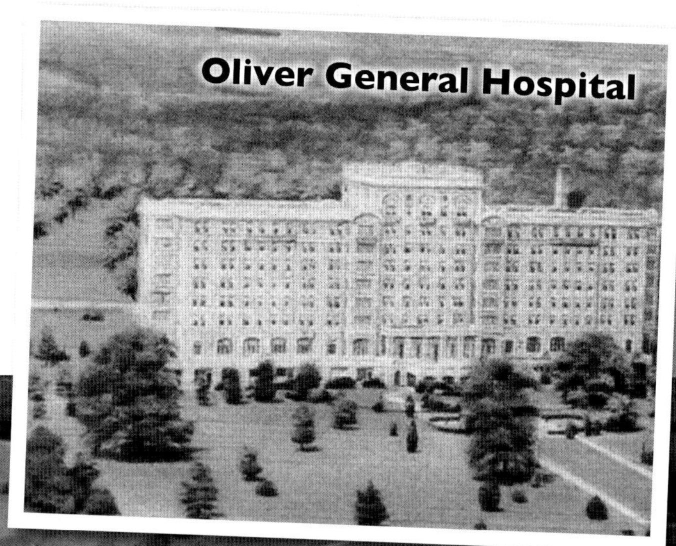


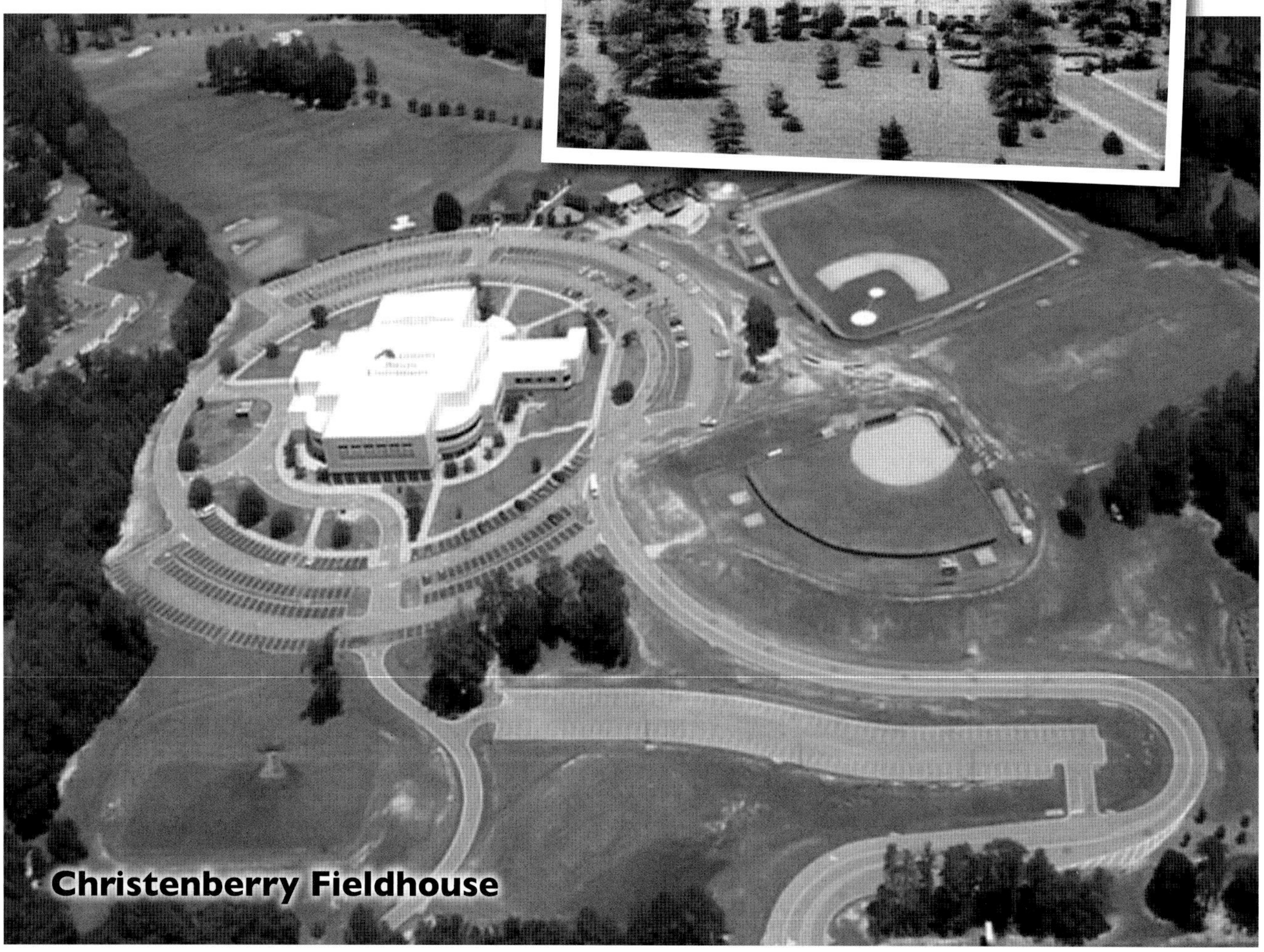

# Index

# Acknowledgments

Compiling a pictorial history of Georgia Regents University (GRU) that incorporates the historic development of two legacy institutions, which spans almost four hundred combined years, was a massive undertaking requiring extensive help from writers, researchers, photographers, editors, and others. We found many talented and informed individuals who provided this assistance. To all of them, we offer our deepest appreciation and thanks, beginning with President Ricardo Azziz whose desire to preserve and share the unique histories of Augusta State University and Georgia Health Sciences University—GRU's legacy institutions—led to the production of this volume.

We also thank the contributing writers whose preliminary work laid the foundation for this book: Jim Garvey, Paula Hinely, Danielle Moores, Caleb Rule, and Joey Warren. GRU Archivists Carol Waggoner-Angleton and Renee Sharrock located photographs, documented facts, and assisted with other research questions, as did Sarah Braswell, Office of the Medical Historian in Residence; Patricia Johnson and Toni Baker, GRU Communications; and Rhonda Banks, GRU Office of Advancement.

Marvin Vanover, Augusta College athletics director and coach, made his scrapbooks and himself available, and both he and current Athletics Director Clint Bryant provided much needed assistance with athletics documentation. Rule, Warren, and Taylor Lamb tracked down athletics photographs and provided other editorial assistance.

We relied heavily on three books, *The History of the Medical College of Georgia* by Phinizy Spalding, *The Medical College of Georgia from 1829-1963* by S. Joseph Lewis Jr. with contributions from Lois Taylor Ellison, and *The History of Augusta College* by Edward Cashin. Dr. Cashin's notes on news articles found in the archives of the *Augusta Chronicle* were invaluable in developing hard-to-find details as were the archives themselves.

Unless otherwise noted, images came from university files, archives, or special collections taken by contract for hire or staff photographers. Phil Jones, senior photographer with the Office of Communications and Marketing (OCM), supplied images and expert advice that saved countless hours in formatting. Other individuals in OCM—Kim Ratliffe and, in particular, Robin Medlock—provided research, editorial, or technical assistance. We also thank other individuals in GRU's Offices of Student Affairs, Alumni Relations, Research, Facilities, and Auxiliary Services for their contributions to this book.

The Editorial Committee of Lois Ellison, MD, Medical Historian in Residence; Lee Ann Caldwell, PhD, Historian in Residence; Sarah Braswell, Historical Research Coordinator, and myself read and re-read the content to ensure historical accuracy. Dr. Caldwell spent many hours rewriting the narrative and strengthening the content, and I am particularly grateful she was able to give life to this history. If there are errors, I must take ultimate responsibility but beg your understanding and forgiveness.

And finally, the committee charged with producing this volume is grateful to the many other individuals associated with our legacy institutions who expressed their support and appreciation for this project. Without all of you, this volume would not have been possible.

Kathy Schofe
Director of Community Relations and Museums (retired)

*The Editorial Committee wishes to express gratitude to Deb Barshafsky, GRU Heritage Project, and Dr. Karla Leeper, executive vice president for University Relations and chief of staff, for their advocacy and work in crafting the Leadership chapter of this pictorial history. We thank them for partnering with us to get this wonderful volume about GRU's history across the finish line.*

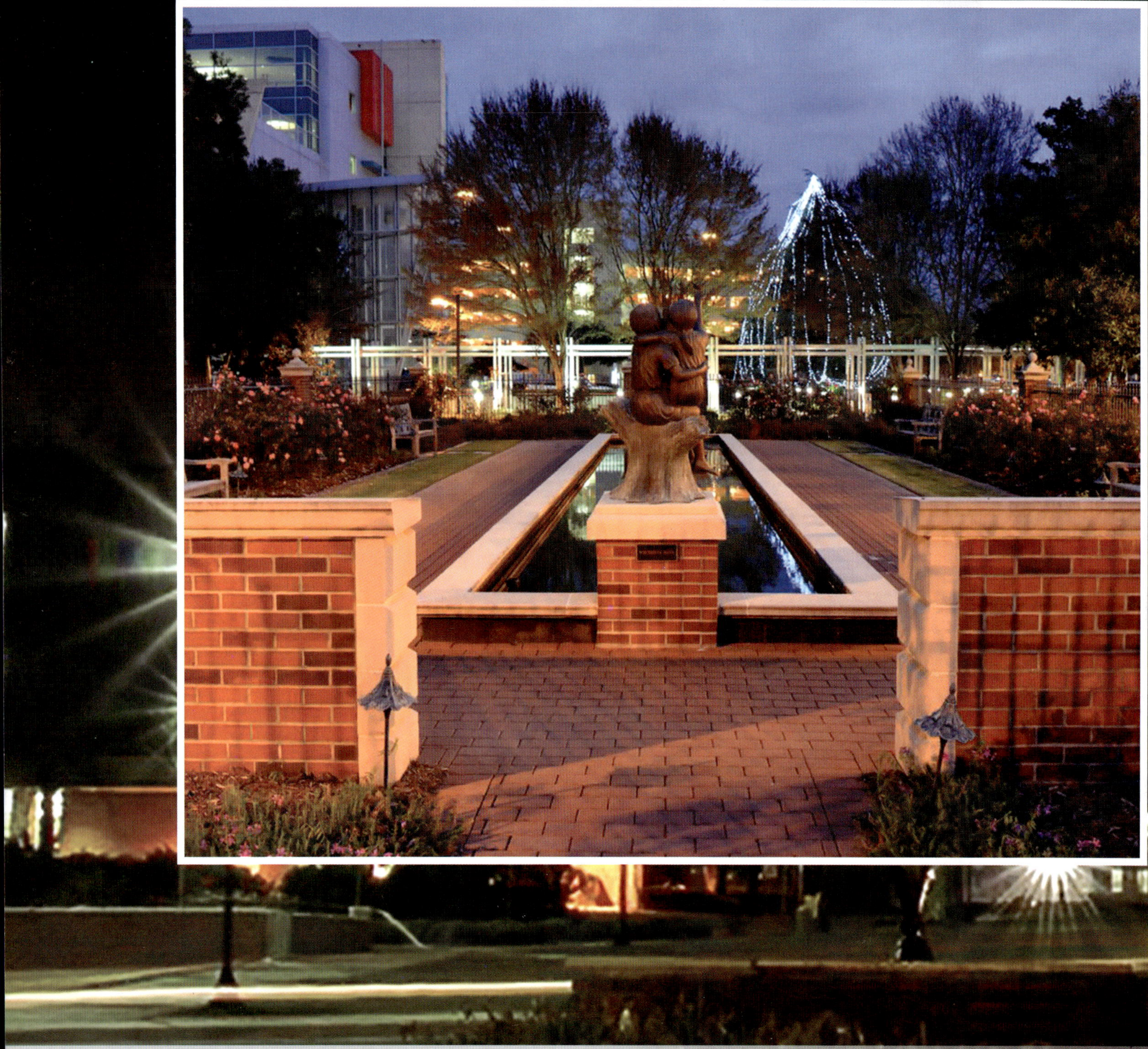

GRU GEORGIA REGENTS UNIVERSITY
AUGUSTA